THE BOTANICAL WELLNESS GUIDE

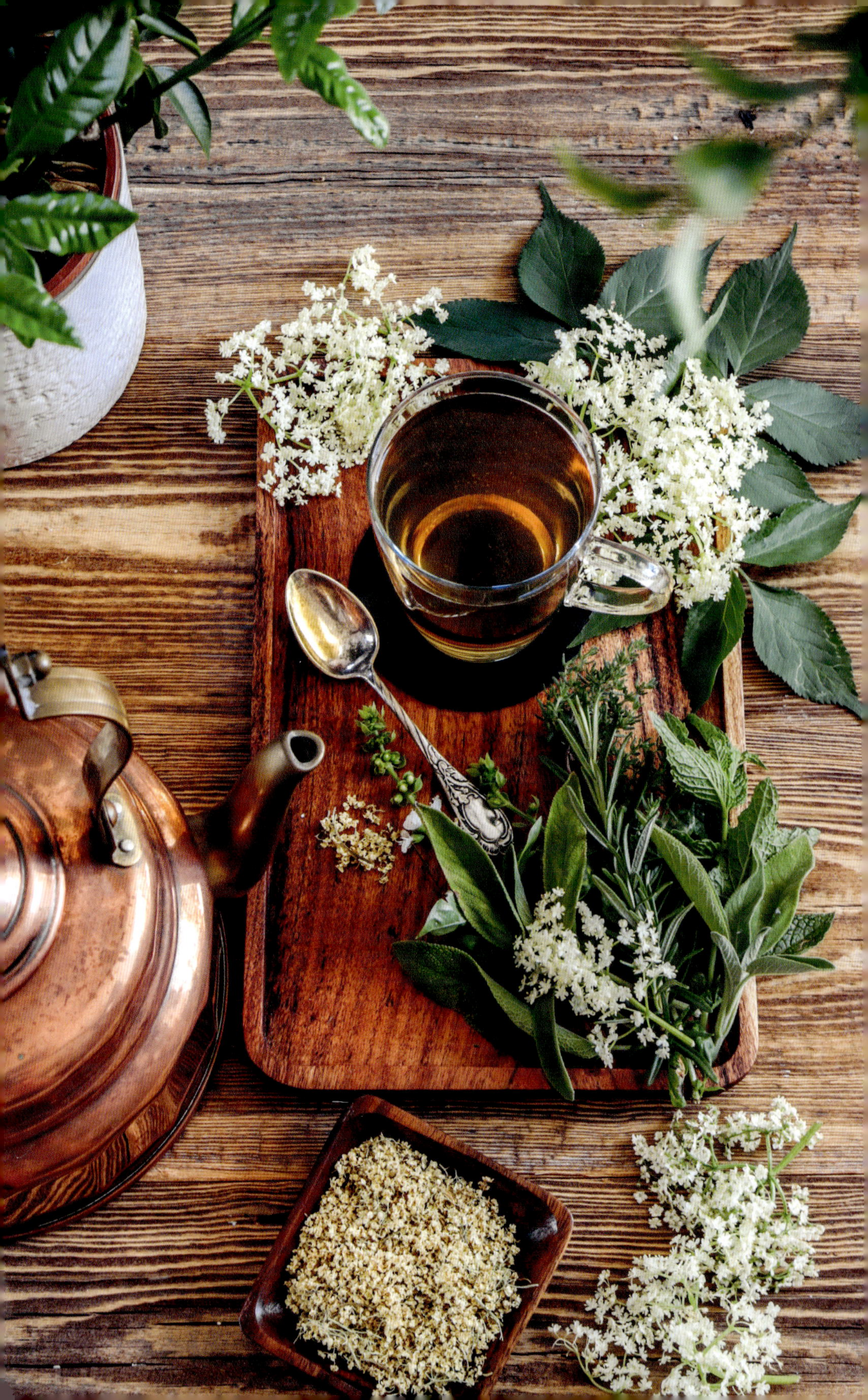

THE BOTANICAL WELLNESS GUIDE

Natural Herbal Treatments for Common Ailments

Anna Newton

GREEN BOOKS

LONDON • OXFORD • NEW YORK • NEW DELHI • SYDNEY

To Rosie and Heather

GREEN BOOKS
Bloomsbury Publishing Plc
50 Bedford Square, London, WC1B 3DP, UK
Bloomsbury Publishing Ireland Limited,
29 Earlsfort Terrace, Dublin 2, D02 AY28,
Ireland

BLOOMSBURY, GREEN BOOKS and the Green Books logo are trademarks of Bloomsbury Publishing Plc
First edition published in 2010 as *Herbs for Home Treatment* by Green Books Ltd
This edition published 2026 by Bloomsbury Publishing Plc

A catalogue record for this book is available from the British Library

ISBN: PB: 978-1-3994-2298-7;
ePub: 978-1-3994-2295-6;
ePDF: 978-1-3994-2296-3

10 9 8 7 6 5 4 3 2 1

Designed by Austin Taylor
Printed and bound in China by Toppan Leefung Printing, DongGuan, GuangDong

MIX
Paper | Supporting responsible forestry
FSC® C104723

To find out more about our authors and books visit www.bloomsbury.com and sign up for our newsletters

For product safety related questions contact productsafety@bloomsbury.com

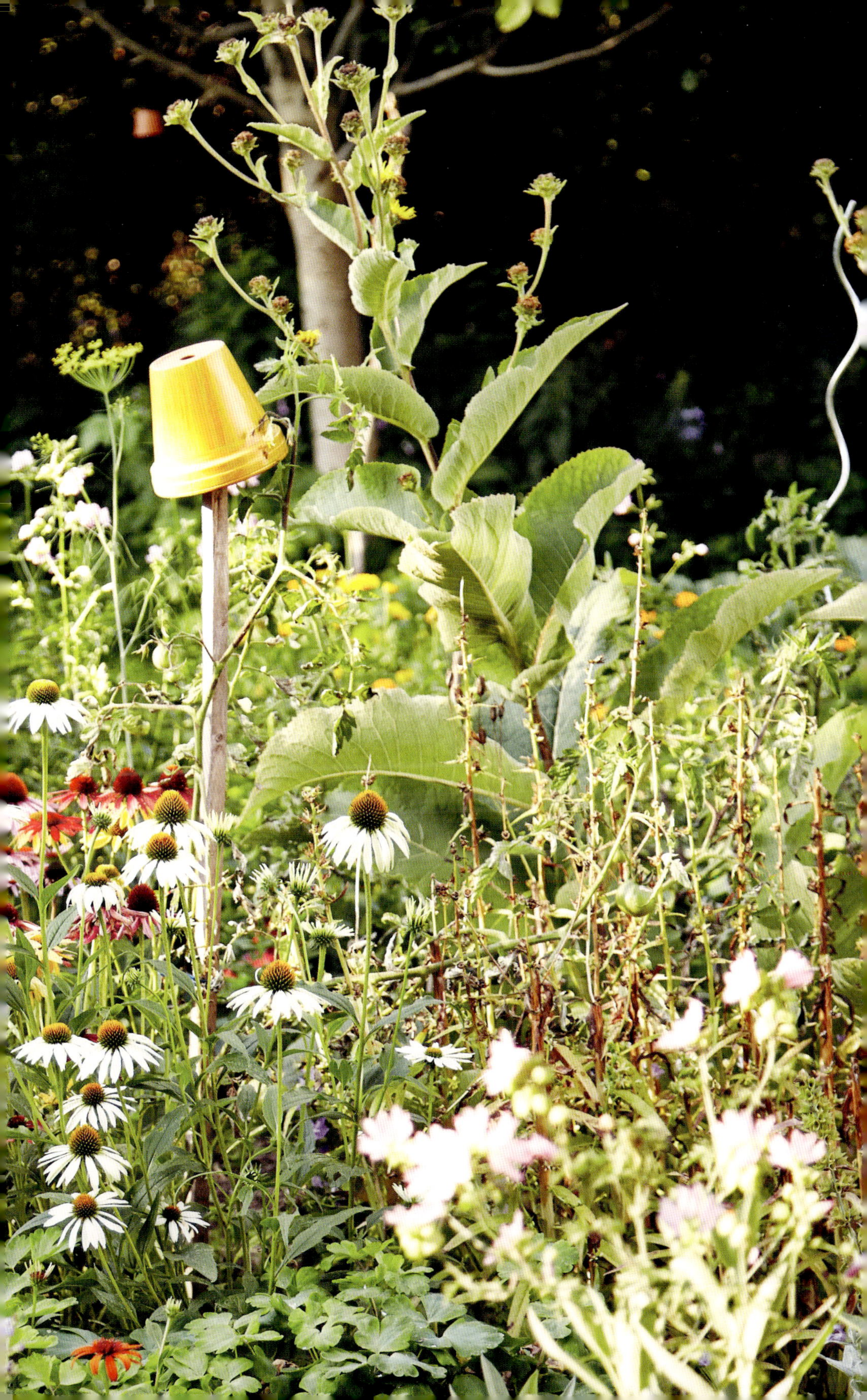

Contents

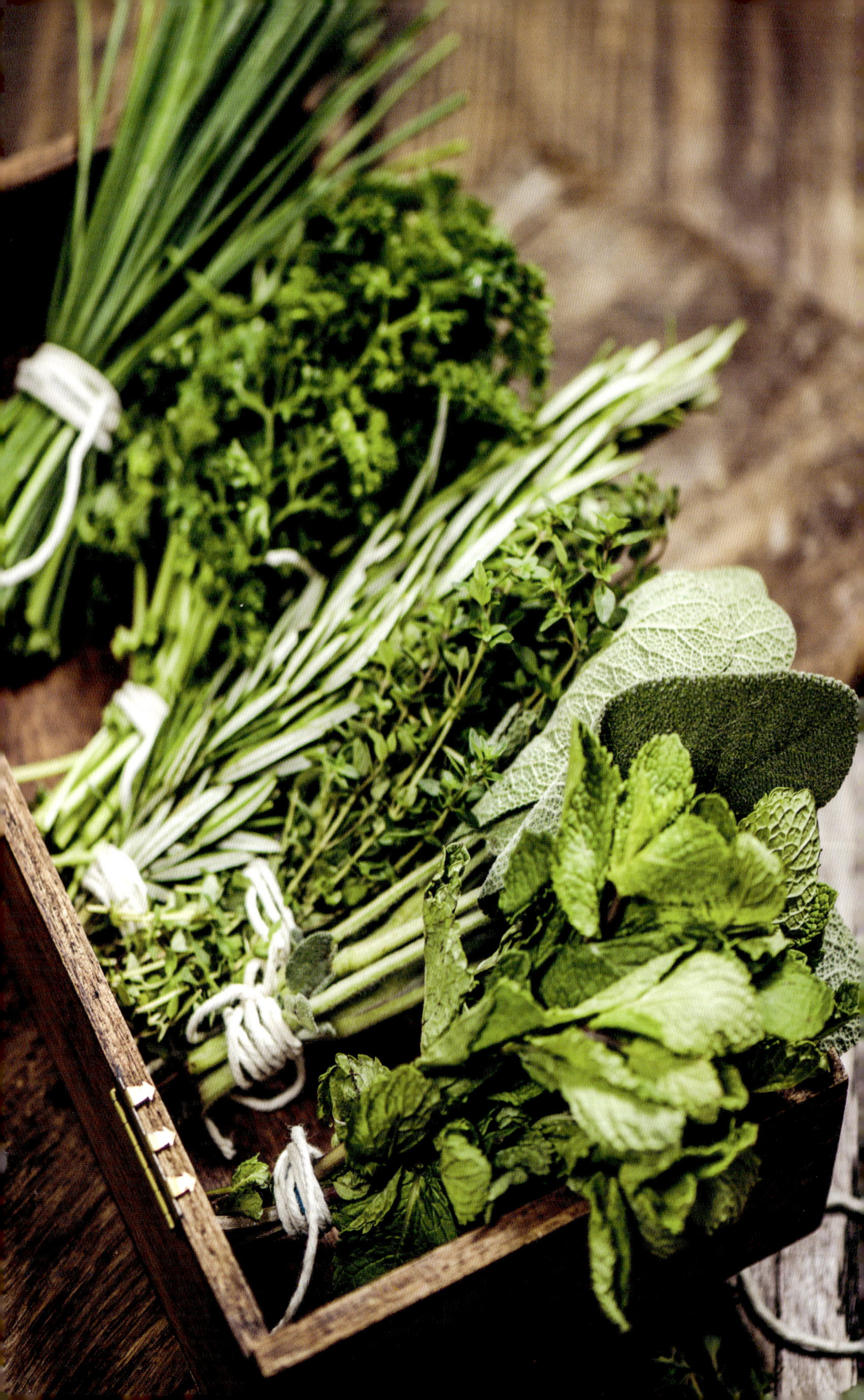

Introduction

This book is a simple guide to self-medicating with medicinal herbs. It deals with non-emergency first-aid situations and everyday ailments that people commonly treat with over-the-counter medicines. It focuses exclusively on using herbs as medicines, and is based on first-hand experience. I have been running a successful herbal medicine practice for 25 years after being awarded a degree in Phytotherapy (Herbal Medicine) by the University of Wales. All of the advice you will find in this book is a reflection of treatments that have been successfully used by me, my patients and members of my family on many occasions. The main purpose of this book is to share the practical knowledge and expertise that I have accumulated over the last 30 years.

My confidence in using herbs for self-treatment stems not only from my qualifications and experience as a practising medical herbalist, but also from the fact that I was brought up in Central Europe where herbal use was still commonplace, and by a mother who was very knowledgeable about medicinal plants and knew many home prescriptions for treating a variety of common problems. I have vivid memories of taking her remedies as a child – a bitter chamomile infusion for tummy ache, tasty comfrey syrup for coughs, or alder-leaf plaster to heal a cut finger. These simple remedies worked every time, and as I grew older I acquired a deep respect for the healing powers of plants.

Herbs are the most natural form of medicine. Our bodies have evolved to digest the majority of plant materials efficiently (with the exception of cellulose and other cell wall compounds) and absorb the nutrients. It follows that botanical remedies, being of plant origin, are easy for our digestive system to break down and assimilate. In fact, many food items found

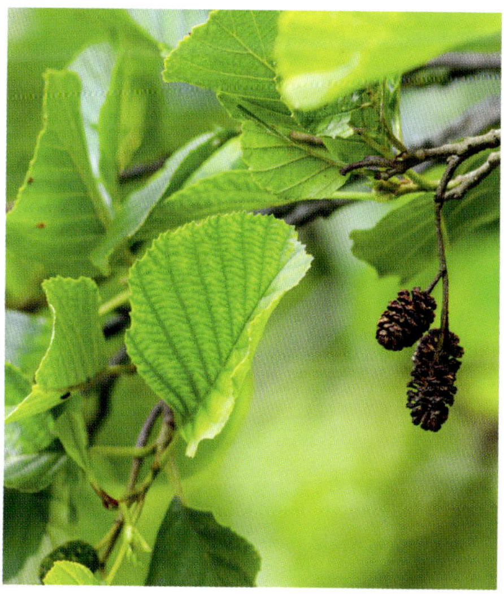

Right Alder is a native tree throughout Europe.

Opposite Many popular kitchen herbs have additional health benefits.

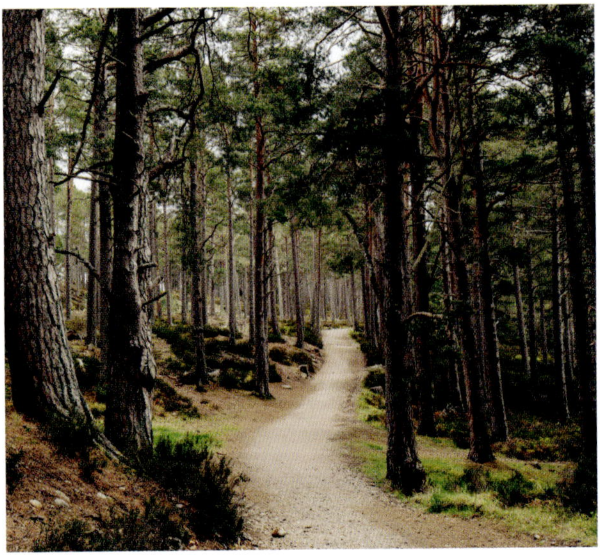

Left When walking somewhere remote, it is useful to know what plants can help you in an emergency.

in most kitchens (e.g. garlic or thyme) become effective medicines when used in appropriate amounts. Unlike modern pharmaceuticals, which are normally composed of a single synthetic chemical compound, herbs contain hundreds of different compounds. The biochemical complexity of plants matches the complexity of our bodies, which is one of the reasons why even comparatively low doses of whole-plant preparations can be very effective.

For centuries, herbal medicine has been based on long-established patterns of use derived from empirical observations. Nowadays there is also plenty of scientific research to back up traditional use, and you will find some useful references at the end of this book (see page 240).

There are a number of advantages to being able to medicate with herbs. You avoid the potential side effects of many common pharmaceuticals – for example, many people are allergic to paracetamol. Herbs are also cheap and readily available – you would be surprised by the medicinal potential of the average spice rack. Most important of all, you will be helping your body to heal itself in a safe, natural way, rather than just suppressing symptoms.

At home I use (as and when needed) around five medicinal herbal teas, two types of skin ointments, four essential oils and three specific blends made up from a few other tinctures. I do not need a full-blown apothecary to treat the majority of common health problems, and neither will you. The beauty of medicinal plants is that they are incredibly versatile, so the same herb can be used for a very diverse range of problems. For example, common chamomile can be used to treat morning sickness, infant colic, indigestion, toothache, puffy eyes and acne – and these are just a few of its potential uses. I have relied on botanical remedies on holidays in the UK and mainland Europe as well as in the remote areas of Bhutan and Mongolia. This book will help you to assemble your own personalised herbal medicine kit, depending on your family's specific needs, to use at home. It will also give you guidance on what herbs can be useful to grow outside in your own medicinal herb garden – also boosting biodiversity.

As I mentioned earlier, all of the remedies recommended in this book have been used by me, my patients and members of my immediate family on many occasions, and I do not advocate anything that I have not tried first hand. Each treatment is based on my own personal experience of administering it, and has repeatedly proved positive and successful. As a result, this well-tested selection of effective remedies will be appropriate for most families, though I always clarify when you should seek specialist advice, as some common conditions, such as eczema, irritable bowel syndrome or depression, are quite complex and tricky to treat by yourself.

The book is structured according to the various systems of the body and their associated ailments, and my advice focuses on a few select herbs that can be used for several different systems. You will come across the same herbs in many different chapters, but in each case a unique set of actions and uses is described, specific to the ailments of that particular system.

My aim is to give you confidence in using herbs rather than conventional over-the-counter medications. If you are a health-conscious person, concerned about the quality of the food you eat and the impact of the environment on your family's health, this simple guide will show you how to add another healthy option to your lifestyle – that of natural botanical medicine.

Below Dried herbs can be used for tinctures, ointments, infused oils and herbal syrups.

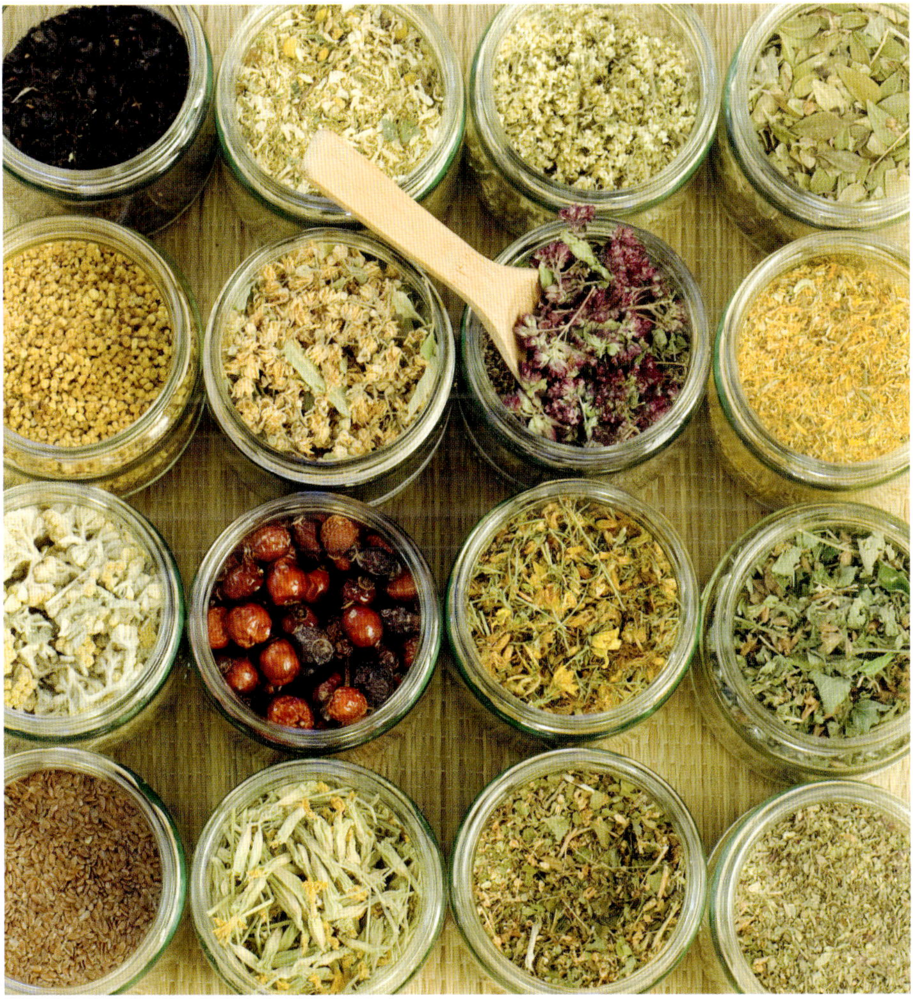

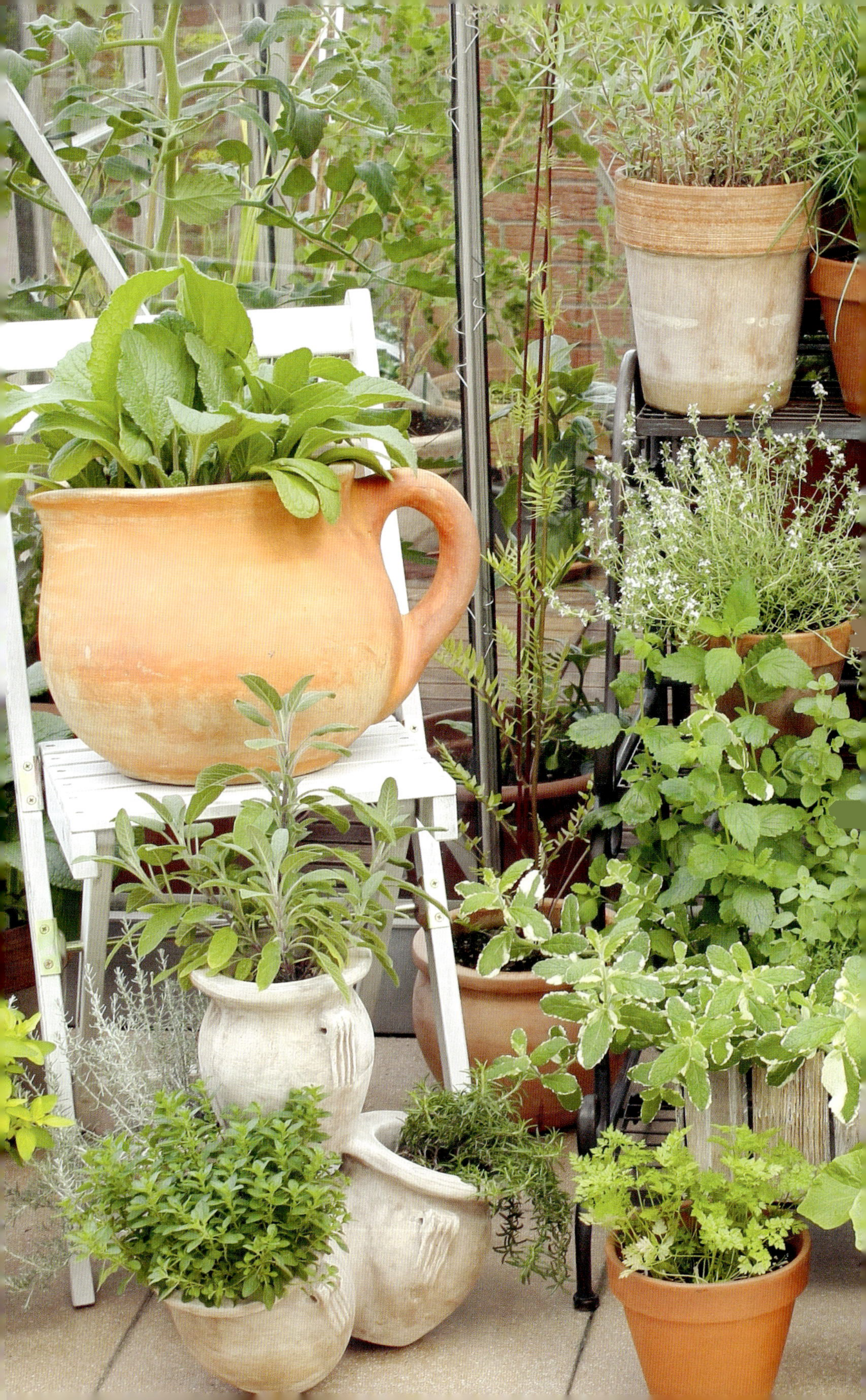

PART 1

Using herbs

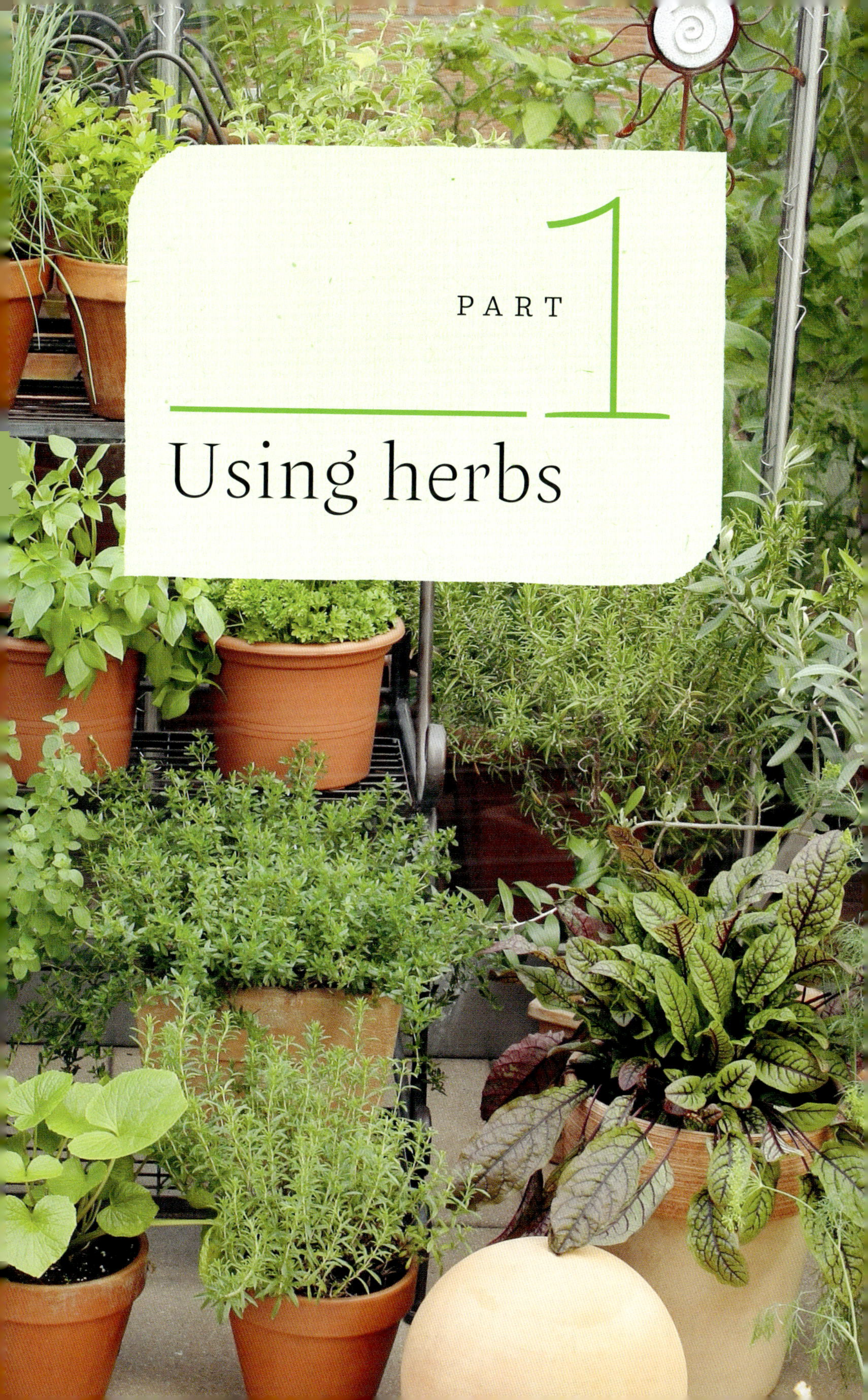

CHAPTER 1

Why herbs?

Specific plants have been used medicinally around the world for millennia – they were the original medicine in all cultures and major civilisations. Plants with medicinal properties are referred in this book as medicinal plants, botanicals, medicinal herbs or simply herbs. It is regrettable that in many Western countries the twentieth century saw herbal medicine being downgraded to a complementary or alternative therapy, as it deserves a place in mainstream health care. Indeed, Eastern countries such as China and Japan recognise the value of traditional medicine, and incorporate it into their health care alongside their orthodox medicine. In the West these traditional forms of medicine are referred to as traditional Chinese medicine (TCM) and Kampo (which is similar to TCM but adapted to the Japanese culture and traditions). The Indian subcontinent has its own system of traditional medicine known as Ayurveda. All of these use botanicals as the core of the treatment but also incorporate massage, acupuncture and dietary interventions.

Furthermore, humans are not unique in using plants as medicines. Many animals – for example, monkeys, horses, birds, cats and dogs – self-medicate with plants. Chimpanzees have been observed to use herbs both internally and externally to get rid of parasites, stomach ache and itchy skin; in 2024, a wild orangutan was observed to put a chewed-up plant directly on to its injury to promote fast healing. Presumably these animals have an instinct that guides them to the right plant for a specific situation. People who live very close to nature, such as the Amazonian Indians, claim that the plants themselves 'tell' them which disease they are for.[1] It is unlikely that people in Western countries have retained even a tiny vestige of that instinct, but we can learn from the knowledge accumulated by our predecessors as well as from modern scientific research into plant properties.

There are a number of reasons why we should go back to using herbs medicinally, and I shall discuss each of them in turn in this chapter.

Well-documented effectiveness

In many instances herbs are as effective as, and sometimes more effective than, conventional pharmaceuticals in the treatment of many common health problems. For instance, clinical trials have shown St John's wort to be more effective than selective serotonin reuptake inhibitors (SSRIs) in treating mild to moderate depression.[2] Medicinal plants can often successfully treat conditions that defy modern medicine, including the common cold and chronic fatigue syndrome.[3] They are equally effective for ailments that arise suddenly, such as heartburn, and for long-standing conditions, such as joint pain.

Herbs help the body to heal itself, rather than just suppressing the symptoms. A classic example is the treatment of high blood pressure. The appropriate herbal treatment can not only lower blood pressure but also restore the healthy function of the circulatory system. Similarly, taking echinacea will improve the function of your immune system, which will then be able to fight off disease more effectively.

Alongside the historical records we have from those who were skilled at treating everyday illnesses with herbs even when they did not understand the nature of the disease, the effectiveness of herbal treatment has been validated by many clinical trials and scientific studies.[4] Today, we have the enormous advantage of being able to benefit from the best of both worlds and combine modern understanding of what causes a particular ailment with traditional insight into which herbs best treat that ailment. A good example of this is the elderflower, which has been used for centuries by rural communities in Britain and Austria alike to treat the common cold, but has only relatively recently been shown to exhibit antiviral properties.[5]

Low risk of side effects

The majority of herbs carry an extremely low risk of side effects compared with conventional medicines. However, although all plant medicines are natural, it would be naive to assume that they are all equally safe. Some should be taken only with the guidance of a qualified medical herbalist. You should treat herbs with the same respect as you would show towards any medicine – stick to the recommended dose, and make sure that your information comes from suitably qualified professionals.

The medicinal herbs that I recommend in this book have an exceptionally good safety record, and so long as you follow the guidance on their use and pay attention to

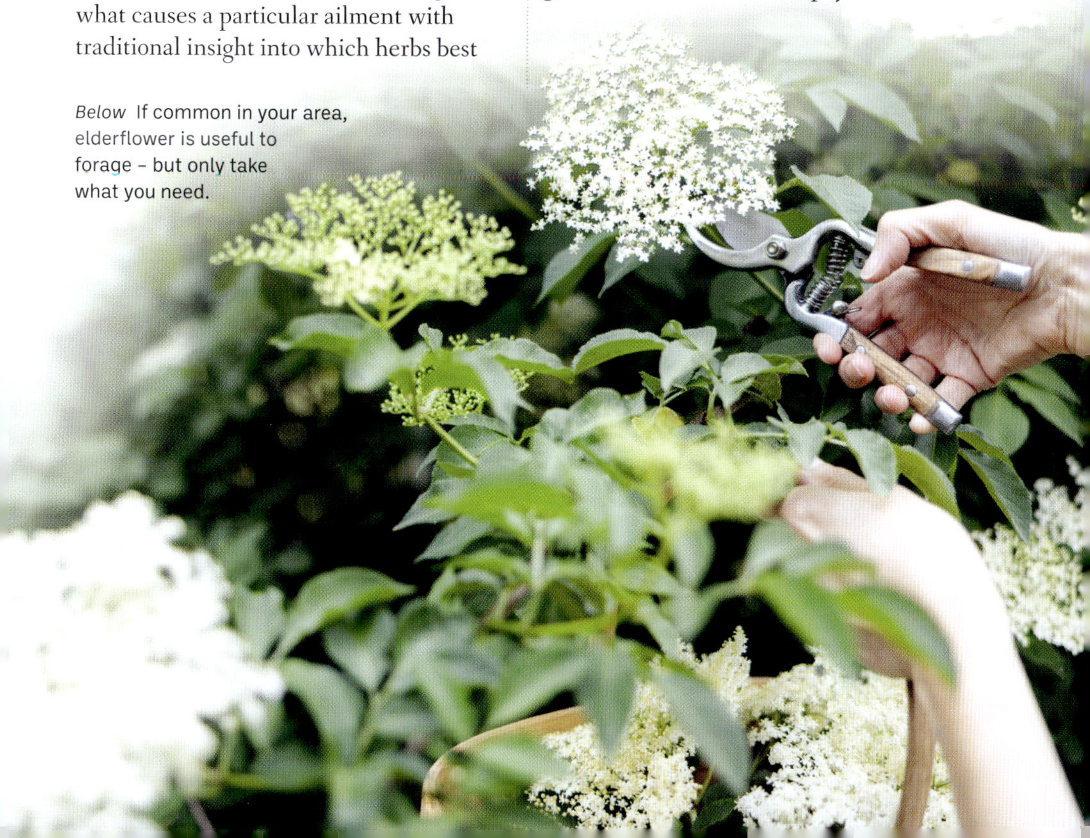

Below If common in your area, elderflower is useful to forage – but only take what you need.

the cautionary advice, you are unlikely to experience any serious problems. Many herbs carry warnings, which normally state that they are not suitable for a very small proportion of people. For instance, in my practice I have come across one person who is allergic to echinacea and one person who is allergic to chamomile, yet these herbs are commonly used by many people every day without any problems.

The fact that some people may experience an allergic reaction to certain herbs is no different to being allergic to certain foods or to conventional medicines, and on very rare occasions some individuals may experience a headache or digestive upset. For safety reasons it is important to obtain herbs from reputable suppliers and as far as possible to use native herbs, as some imported rare herbs have been shown to be adulterated with potentially harmful species.

I would like to point out that the low risk of side effects applies to herbal products that have undergone minimal processing. This category includes dry herbs and ordinary-strength tinctures. However, *highly concentrated products, such as essential oils, are not safe to be used internally and should be reserved solely for external treatment.* All highly concentrated herbal extracts, which greatly exceed the concentrations historically used in traditional herbal medicine, should be treated with circumspection (for more information on the safety of specific preparations, see Chapter 5).

Herbs are non-addictive

Another important benefit is that herbs that are used medicinally are non-addictive – you can stop using them at any time without risking the onset of withdrawal symptoms. This is especially important for people who suffer from anxiety, depression or insomnia, as they often become dependent on conventional medications. Most herbs can also be used alongside orthodox medication, although this is best done under the supervision of a trained medical herbalist.

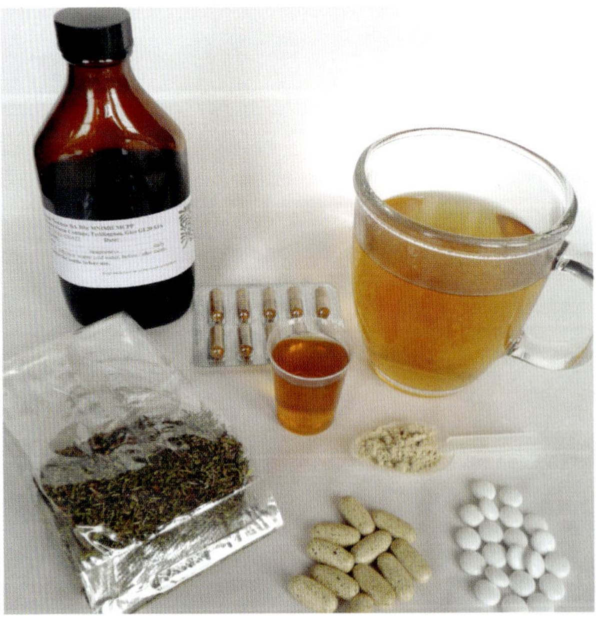

Left There are many herbal preparations to consider.

Complex medicine for complex bodies

Medicinal herbs are complex mixtures of many constituents, which mirror the complexity of our bodies. Many of these constituents improve the function of a specific organ or bodily system so that the body can fight disease more effectively. Herbs can harness our natural ability to heal – working along with our immune system, they gently nudge our bodies towards recovery. The constituents of herbs also have high bioavailability, which means that we absorb them well and therefore do not need large doses. Our bodies are adapted to digest and absorb plant material, and many of the constituents of herbs are similar to those of fruit and vegetables – and just as beneficial for our health.

Plants that are used medicinally can be viewed as a category of healing substances that sit somewhere between pharmaceuticals and food. Many have proven medicinal properties but are akin to food in their biochemical composition and the way in which they are absorbed. Some herbs are very familiar in the kitchen – for example, garlic and thyme. Most are strictly medicinal yet gentle enough to be taken every day. However, modern lifestyles have meant that people often become so detached from nature that they can sometimes perceive even the most natural medicine to be alien and hazardous.

The complexity of the biochemical composition of each medicinal herb is crucial to its effectiveness and safety. A modern view favoured by many scientists is that a single substance is a more effective medicine than a complex mixture. Certainly it is easier to study, but is it really better for our health?

Botanicals are often referred to as crude medicines, and many of the individual components have been isolated with a view to converting them into pharmaceuticals. Many medicinal plants have yielded or inspired the development of useful drugs such as ephedrine, digoxin or aspirin. However, by comparison with the huge number of medicinal plants that are known, the number of single-component pharmaceuticals that have been derived from plants is relatively small. It seems that the active constituents of herbs rarely perform better in isolation. The reason for this is that plant constituents work in a synergistic way – that is, the combined effect of several different components is greater than the sum of the effects of the individual components. Moreover, medicinal plants often display a curious combination of strong-acting constituents, which have potential side effects, and protective constituents, which moderate the potential for side effects. For instance, the use of dandelion leaf tea as a diuretic could lead to depleted potassium levels in the body if it wasn't for the fact that dandelion leaf contains enough potassium to compensate for this loss.

Herbs are affordable

Herbs have the advantage of being cheap and easily available – you can grow some for domestic use either in your garden or in plant pots. Growing your own medicine is immensely satisfying, as it gives you a real sense of self-sufficiency. Whether you decide to grow your own herbs or buy them over the counter, you will be taking a positive step towards maintaining optimal health. You will be choosing an effective, safe and natural option, and one that has been tested over many previous generations.

It is worth remembering that many culinary herbs, spices and food items have medicinal properties, so you can raid your kitchen in an emergency. For instance, if you are developing a cold you can use garlic and ginger to fend it off. Any inflammation would benefit from turmeric in your diet. Thyme tea can ease a cough. The seeds of many spices, such as fennel, caraway and aniseed, when brewed as tea can help to relieve bloating and indigestion. Onions can be used to make a very effective and

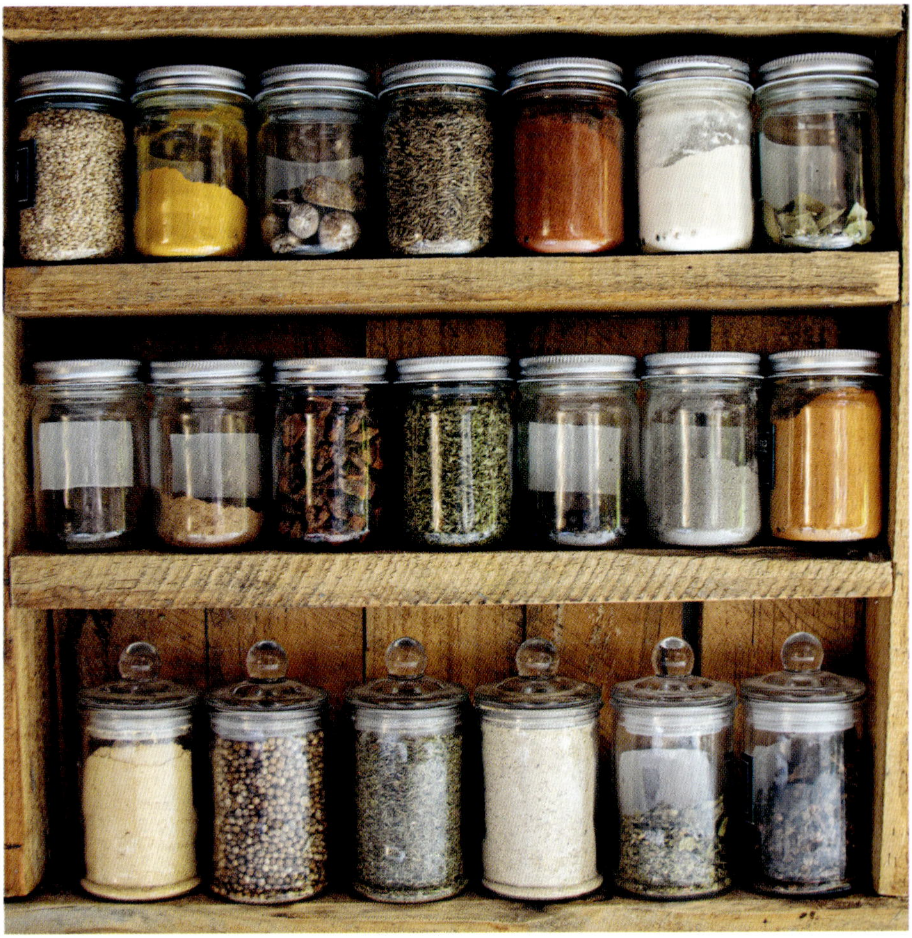

Above Eating lots of herbs and spices is a great way to boost your immune system.

surprisingly tasty cough syrup. This overlap between a food item and a medicine further supports the view that botanical medicine is the most natural way of treating disease. Our bodies naturally process plant material and deal with a multitude of constituents that they contain.

Seeking professional help

Of course, there are limits to what conditions can be treated with herbs, and there are situations where self-medicating with medicinal plants is not the best choice. Throughout the book I make it clear when it is advisable to seek professional help. Although every care has been taken when compiling the information presented in this book, ultimately the responsibility for deciding whether to use these treatments must be taken by you, after assessing the risks and your medical history and allergies, and seeking professional advice if necessary.

CHAPTER 2

How to get the most from this book

This book is designed to be a quick reference source. If you have a specific health problem, look it up either in the index or in the contents list. For example, if you have a cold, refer to Chapter 11 on the respiratory system, or if you have stomach ache, refer to Chapter 8 on the digestive system.

Before you commence any treatment, I would strongly recommend that you read all of the introductory chapters in Part One of the book, paying particular attention to the information on herbs and the environment (Chapter 3) and the advice on dosage (Chapter 5). The advice that follows in Part Two will then make much more sense, as you will already be familiar with the terminology and basic concepts, and you will understand why it is better to use some herbs than others. This is particularly important if you have never used herbs as medicines before, but even seasoned herb users should familiarise themselves with the contents of Chapter 5 to ensure that they use the botanicals in a responsible way.

If you are a complete novice, I would recommend that you stick to one herb at a time for self-treatment initially, and only later progress to mixing different herbs together. This will mean that you will minimise the risk of allergic reactions, and you will learn to observe the effects of individual herbs on your body. Once you are confident in the use of single herbs, read Chapter 6 on combining herbs. Then you can start mixing and matching different herbs to suit your particular situation.

Before you buy any herbs, refer to the Useful resources chapter where there is a list of reliable suppliers (see page 246). Not only is this really important from a safety point of view, but it will also make a difference to your pocket!

Below A cup of peppermint tea is good for digestion.

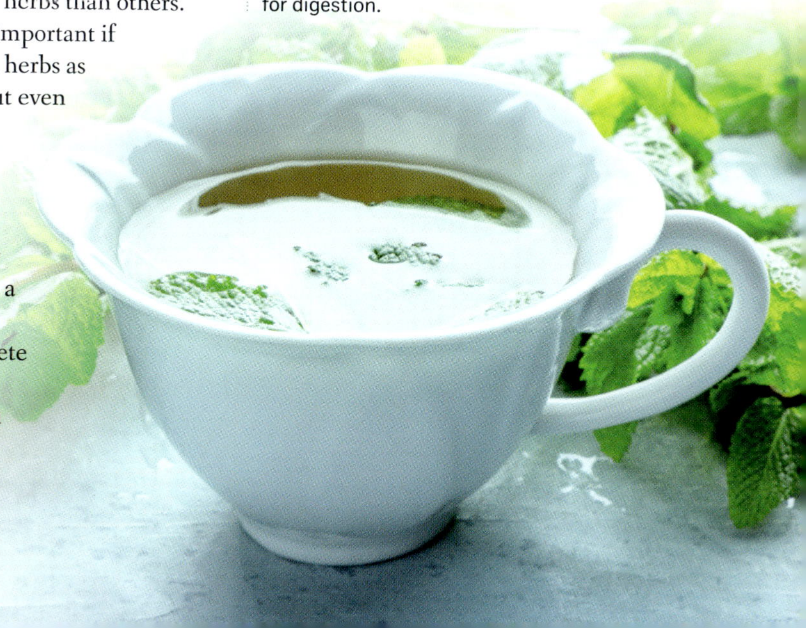

General precautions

The herbs recommended for self-treatment in this book are extremely safe, but you must follow the guidelines on dosage as strictly as you would with conventional medicine. Do not take higher doses than those recommended, and only use the herbs on adults, unless otherwise specified. Please take extra care if you are over 70, pregnant or are taking other medicines. In addition to the general dosage advice given in Chapter 5, more specific advice is given in the descriptions of particular treatments.

Specific precautions

Please pay attention to the specific precautions highlighted throughout the book, as some herbs are not suitable, for example, for women who are pregnant or breastfeeding, or for young children, or people who are taking conventional medications, including the contraceptive pill. Epilepsy is a special consideration, as even small amounts of medicinal herbs can interact with the medication, and you should seek professional advice before using them if you suffer from this condition.

Throughout this book, the following icons are used:

Practitioner treatment is strongly recommended.

Take caution if the specified allergies or conditions apply to you. Speak with a professional if unsure.

Do not take this treatment if the specified allergies or conditions apply to you.

Treating infants and young children

With one or two exceptions I would recommend that you always consult a qualified medical herbalist before treating children with medicinal herbs. I also advise that you always consult a trained aromatherapist or herbalist before using essential oils in skin preparations for infants, young children or pregnant women.

Seek professional help if necessary

Self-diagnosis and self-treatment are safe as long as you can recognise situations where you need to seek professional help. Use your common sense – if you or another person show any of the following symptoms, seek prompt attention from a doctor or other healthcare professional:

- prolonged severe pain, including constant head pain, whether or not the pain has resulted from injury
- high fever of over 39°C (102°F) (invest in a digital thermometer, as these are easy to use and read)
- prolonged vomiting and diarrhoea, especially in young children
- marked changes in normal behaviour, especially in young children and the elderly.

You should also seek professional medical help if:

- you are unsure about the treatment
- you are concerned about any symptoms, even those that seem benign
- you are not getting better despite the treatment – you should normally expect to see an improvement within a few hours to a few days, depending on the condition that is being treated
- the condition is long-standing
- the condition is a complex one with many symptoms.

Drug-herb interactions

In rare cases, certain herbs can interact with certain drugs, so if you are taking medication prescribed by your doctor or hospital you should first check with

Right Dandelion root stimulates the liver, whereas dandelion leaves are primarily a diuretic.

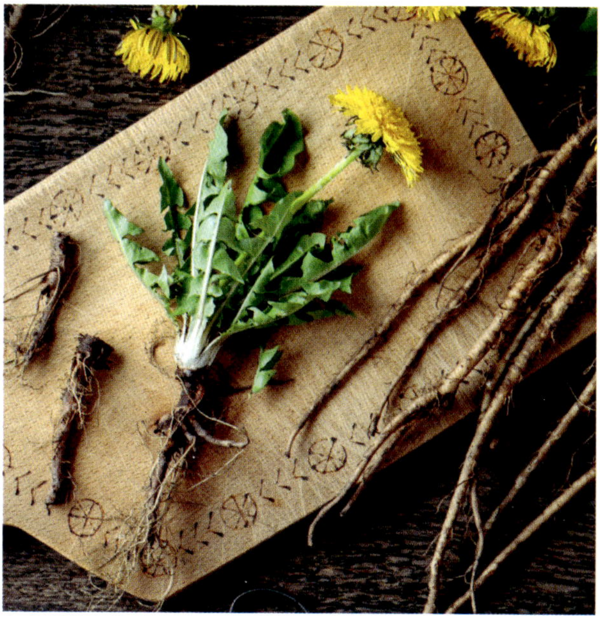

a medical herbalist whether it is safe to use herbal treatments. You should also check with your GP as even though they may not be trained in herbal medicine they are likely to be aware of the most important drug–herb interactions. In most instances it is safe to use herbs alongside conventional medicines, but it is always best to double check, as some herbs can reduce the efficacy of such medicines. The warnings in this book are based on specific references that carefully assess the risk of any interactions in the light of the available scientific evidence.[6] If you are about to undergo an operation or medical investigation it is also important to tell the medical staff that you are using medicinal herbs. To be on the safe side, stop taking any herbs at least a week before the procedure. Throughout this book I shall alert you to possible drug interactions with specific herbs.

Possibility of allergy

Very occasionally, herbs can cause allergic reactions. If you develop any rash, itchiness, headache or stomach upset while taking a particular herb, stop using it immediately.

If you are prone to allergies, watch out for herbs belonging to the daisy family (the Asteraceae, formerly known as the Compositae), such as yarrow, chamomile and echinacea, and use them only in very small amounts initially.

Rules for safe herb use

It is sensible to follow a few basic rules to maximise safety when using herbs:

- Make sure you have the right species – refer to the scientific names and common names that are given in this book (also see pages 230–237). Anything that you buy over the counter must be labelled with the full scientific name of the plant.
- Make sure that you are using the right part of the herb – there are often distinct differences in the actions of different parts of the same plant.
- Always buy herbs from a reputable supplier and use reliable sources of information (see the Useful resources chapter for further details).
- Always follow the advice on dosage and check whether there are any contraindications to use of the herb.

CHAPTER 3

Herbs and the environment

If you want to use herbs in a way that does not harm the environment, the rules are simple – try to use native species or species that can be cultivated in your country, buy herbs grown locally and organically, grow your own herbs, do not collect from the wild and never buy any endangered species.

Loss of wild plants

It is very disheartening for a committed herbalist like me to learn how many herbs have become endangered and rare as a result of indiscriminate harvesting from the wild and loss of habitat. For example, in the UK we have lost the lady's slipper orchid and sundew from the herbal repertoire, as both herbs are only just surviving in a few isolated spots. Worldwide, Korean ginseng and *Echinacea angustifolia* are thought to be close to extinction in the wild, false unicorn and golden seal have become rare, and slippery elm is now considered to be at risk. The destruction has been driven by demand, and although all of the above-mentioned species are extremely useful herbs, they can all be substituted with other herbs possessing similar properties that either occur naturally in Britain or can be easily cultivated.

Below Pick-your-own fields are a great way to ethically gather herbs such as lavender.

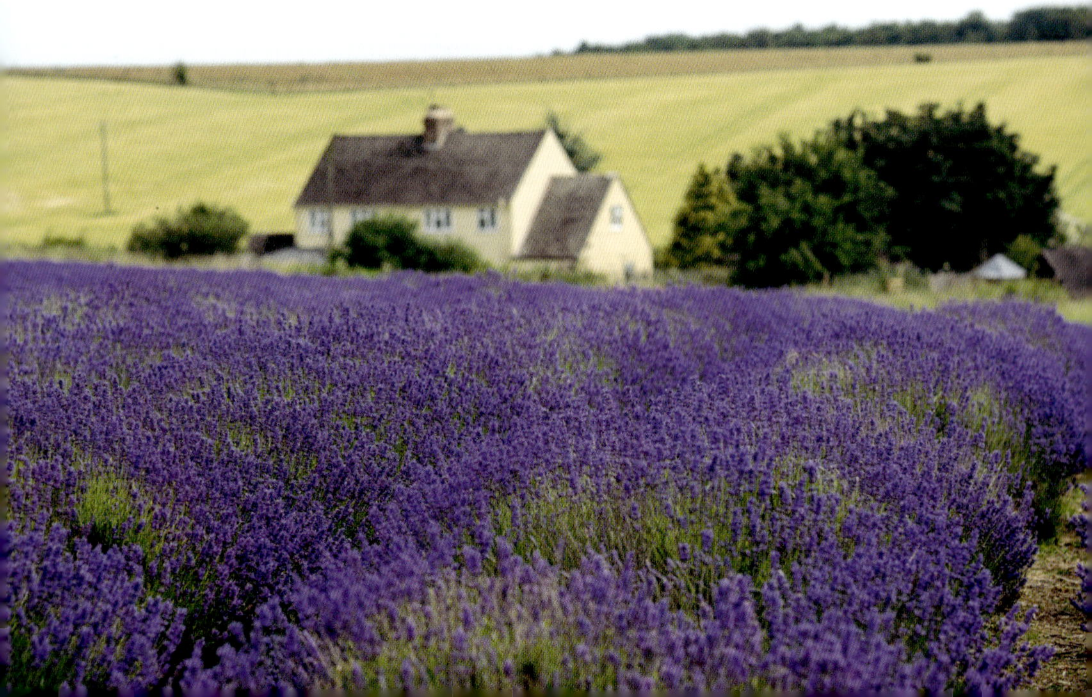

Local or imported herbs?

The fact is that our native flora provides enough options to treat most problems, so there is rarely a true need to resort to exotic, imported plants. By limiting yourself to herbs that are cultivated in your own country you will also be reducing the carbon footprint associated with their transportation. Furthermore, quite a few herbs that are not native to the UK can be successfully grown in this country, and this can even result in improved properties. For example, although lavender is native to the Mediterranean region, British-grown lavender has a higher concentration of volatile constituents than lavender grown in France.

However, as always, there is another side to the story. Some herbs can be grown only in specific climatic conditions, and such cultivation, assuming that it is organic, provides a livelihood for many people in developing countries. Similarly, some herbs are difficult to cultivate and can be collected only from the wild, and so long as such harvesting is sustainable it is a useful source of income for local communities. Some environmentalists even argue that careful harvesting from the wild can lead to the protection of the environment, as it is in the interest of harvesters to look after the habitats of specific plants so as not to destroy their source of income.

A significant number of herbal product manufacturers are highly ethical and actively pursue a policy of minimal environmental impact, either through encouraging organic cultivation or by ensuring sustainable harvesting by indigenous communities.

Sometimes it is more energy efficient to grow and dry herbs in countries with a warm climate and then transport them than to cultivate such herbs locally, especially if they need to be grown in hothouses.

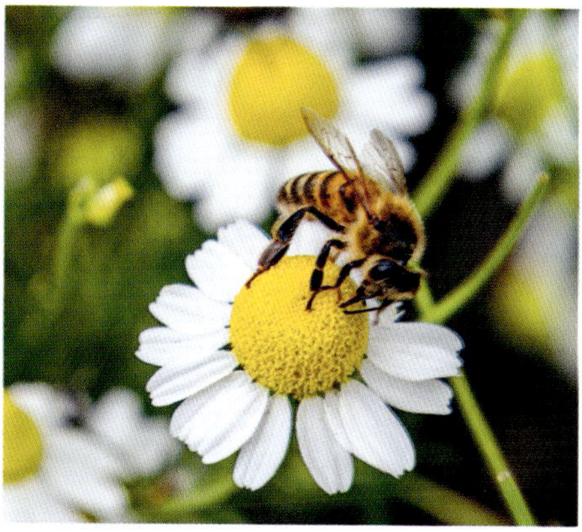

Above Growing medicinal plants is also good for pollinators.

You need to balance all of these arguments carefully. In my view, a sensible compromise is to use native and locally produced herbs whenever possible, and to use imported ones only on the rare occasions when you cannot find a suitable local substitute. Always check that imported herbs come from sustainable sources or have been grown organically.

I would generally avoid fads for foreign herbs that occasionally pop up seemingly from nowhere and claim to be a cure-all. Exotic herbs are rarely unique in their effectiveness, and you can usually find a perfectly adequate local equivalent of such a herb.

Only organic

It goes without saying that medicinal herbs that are being cultivated for sale should be grown organically or, even better, biodynamically. This is better for the environment, for the plants and for you. A healing plant that contains pesticide residues is a contradiction in terms and should never be used.

Similarly, if you decide to grow herbs yourself you should always do so in a completely organic way (for information on growing your own herbs, see Chapter

22). At this point it is worth mentioning that by growing herbs in your garden or allotment you will be encouraging a wide range of insects and other wildlife. Wild herbs often have less showy flowers than garden cultivars but are a magnet for bees and butterflies, while the seeds are popular with birds. Like wild flowers, many herbs attract natural predators and discourage pests, so they make excellent companion plants. As a result, not only will you be healthier as a result of using herbs, but also your garden will be healthier if you grow them there.

Collecting from the wild

Worldwide, many herbs are collected from the wild. This practice, often called wild harvesting, is not without effects on the environment. Wild harvesting is not the same as foraging, when you gather small amounts of a particular plant for your own use. Harvesting from the wild, as the name implies, involves taking a substantial amount of a particular plant for the purpose of selling it on. In many countries the native flora is already under threat due to the disappearance of its natural habitat. Therefore any collecting from the wild on a commercial scale is best done in a regulated, sustainable way by professional, contracted collectors who know how, what and when to collect in order to have minimal impact on the environment. At present there is very little of this kind of regulation in most parts of the world, although there are many initiatives in individual countries to protect medicinal plants from over-harvesting.

It is also worth bearing in mind that some herbs grow in proximity to intensely farmed crops and so are likely to be accidentally sprayed with pesticides and other chemicals. Others grow near busy roads and will therefore accumulate air pollutants.

In my view it is better not to collect from the wild at all, but instead either to grow your own or to buy ready-dried or processed herbs from an ethical supplier. Unless you are absolutely certain that a particular plant is so abundant that what you take will make little difference, please do not collect from the wild. Wild habitats have become so fragile that even collecting seemingly common plants such as elderflower or nettle may be harmful to the local environment.

I suggest that you ask your local wildlife trust about the plants you wish to collect. If you are given the green light by them, collect a small amount just for your own use, and do not destroy whole plants. Make sure that you have identified the plant correctly – there is no margin for error here, as some poisonous plants can look similar to non-

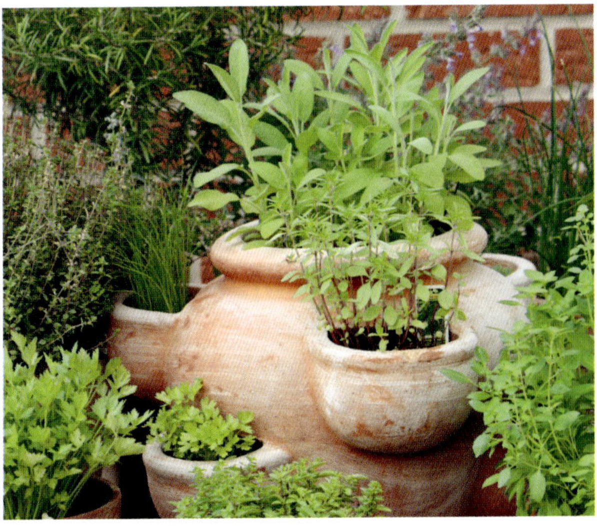

Left Even a small pot can grow lots of different herbs.

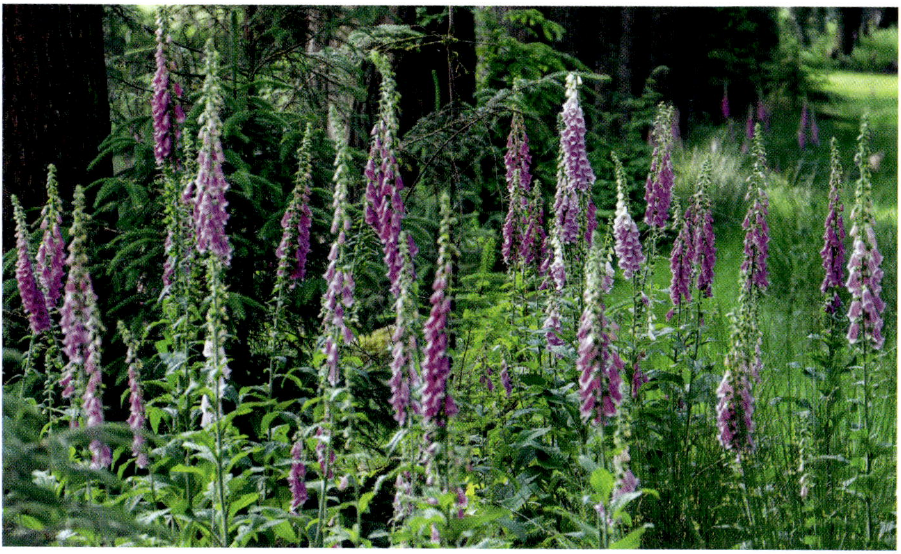

Above Comfrey leaves are commonly confused with the leaves of alkanet or foxglove, and alkanet leaves are often mistaken for those of borage.

poisonous ones. For example, comfrey leaves are commonly confused with the leaves of alkanet or foxglove, and alkanet leaves are often mistaken for those of borage.

Currently endangered herbs

Below is a list of some commonly used medicinal plants that are currently either endangered or threatened. The list is likely to be updated in the future as continual efforts are made to ensure the conservation of specific plants, and some wild plants are also beginning to be cultivated. A number of international organisations monitor the status of plants (including medicinal species) in the wild, such as the Convention on International Trade in Endangered Species of Wild Fauna and Flora (CITES), the World Wide Fund for Nature (WWF), Plantlife International, the Wildlife Trade Monitoring Network (TRAFFIC), United Plant Savers and the United States Department of Agriculture (USDA). You can search online to obtain the most up-to-date lists reported by these organisations.

Please refrain from using the following plants, unless you are certain that they are cultivated products:

Arctostaphylos uva-ursi (bearberry)
Caulophyllum thalictroides (blue cohosh)
Chamaelirium luteum (false unicorn)
Cinchona calisaya (Jesuit's bark)
Echinacea pallida (pale purple coneflower)
Hydrastis canadensis (golden seal)
Panax ginseng (wild Korean ginseng)
Ulmus fulva (slippery elm)
Uncaria tomentosa (cat's claw).

Choose the right supplier

If you care about the environment, buy only from suppliers who will not sell endangered species and who adhere to strict standards for sustainable wild harvesting. A list of such retailers can be found in the Useful resources chapter. Your local practising herbal clinician will also be able to recommend reputable suppliers.

CHAPTER 4

Tea, tincture or tablets?

Botanical medicines come in many different forms, and you will probably find some of them more convenient to use than others, or you may have a personal preference for a particular type of preparation. Throughout this book I usually recommend tinctures and teas (infusions) because they work quickly and you can easily mix two or more ingredients together, but there will be situations where a powdered herb or a syrup is more suitable. Good-quality capsules or tablets can also work well. You can take different forms of preparation together – for instance, garlic tablets and herbal tea. Tablets are best for travelling, as there is no risk of spillage. The preparations most commonly used are described below, with an explanation of how to take them. I assume that most readers will buy ready-made tinctures, creams and syrups, but instructions on how to make your own at home can be found in Chapter 23.

Tincture

A tincture is an extract that results from steeping herbs in alcohol for a period of time. During the steeping process active constituents from the plant dissolve in the alcohol. Specific proportions of herbs and alcohol are used to produce different tincture strengths or ratios. Typical proportions are 1:5, 1:3, 1:2 or 1:1, but occasionally you may come across different ratios, such as 1:8, 1:10 or 2:1. Tinctures are also sometimes referred to as herbal extracts, liquid extracts, fluid extracts or glycerite (based on glycerine instead of ethyl alcohol).

Tinctures are easy to use, well absorbed and versatile in application. The amount of alcohol in each dose is negligible, which means that they can be used for all age groups except for babies, and during pregnancy.

I have adopted a traditional approach to making tinctures[7] where, for example, a 1:5 (one in five) tincture is made with one part of plant material and five parts of alcohol, both expressed in terms of weight (for the sake of simplicity you can assume that 1ml of alcohol is equivalent to 1g). If you buy a ready-made tincture, the strength of alcohol used for making it will be indicated on the label, and is expressed as a percentage, which can range from 25% to 90%. It is important to realise that the term 'tincture strength' refers only to the concentration of plant constituents in a given tincture, and must not be confused with the strength of alcohol used for the extraction process. Tincture strength determines the dosage of a particular tincture, whereas the strength of alcohol is relevant to the process of extraction and the quality of the product.

Concentrated and standardised tinctures

Avoid any tinctures that are highly concentrated (i.e. more than 2:1), as these have not been used traditionally and little is known about their safety. For the same reason I would generally advise against using standardised tinctures, although there are some exceptions. Standardised tinctures usually focus on one specific constituent of a particular herb and are guaranteed to contain a particular amount of that constituent. Traditional herbal preparations use the whole spectrum of phytochemicals in a given plant without focusing on any specific compound and it seems that the synergy between various compounds of the whole plant extracts contributes to its potency. Some tinctures may be standardised for a specific constituent that has been wrongly assumed to be the most active one, or they can contain an artificially high proportion of a particular compound, which does not occur naturally at that level. However, some extracts will not work very well unless a particular constituent or a set of constituents are at the right level. A good example is garlic tincture/capsules, which should be standardised to have high allicin content in order to have the right activity.

How to take tinctures

A dose of tincture must be mixed with water before drinking. Never take tinctures neat (undiluted)!

The amount of water used to dilute a dose of tincture can be as little as 30ml or as much as a full cup. This is a matter of personal preference – if you dilute with a small amount of water you will have less to drink but the taste is strong, whereas if you dilute with more water the taste is better but there is more to drink. Some people choose the former option and then follow it with a cup of plain water. Although water is preferable, you can also use fruit juice to dilute tinctures.

If you want to make your own tinctures instead of buying ready-made ones, instructions can be found in Chapter 23.

Infusion

Otherwise known as tea or tisane, an infusion is a hot-water extract of a particular herb or herb mix. I recommend that you brew a fresh infusion each time it is required. In theory you can store an infusion for 24 hours in the fridge, and gently reheat it when you need it, but freshly brewed herbs taste much better. You can use herbs available in tea bags, but for medicinal use brew them stronger than usual (two tea bags per cup). Infusions are the best way of administering herbal medicines for the digestive system.

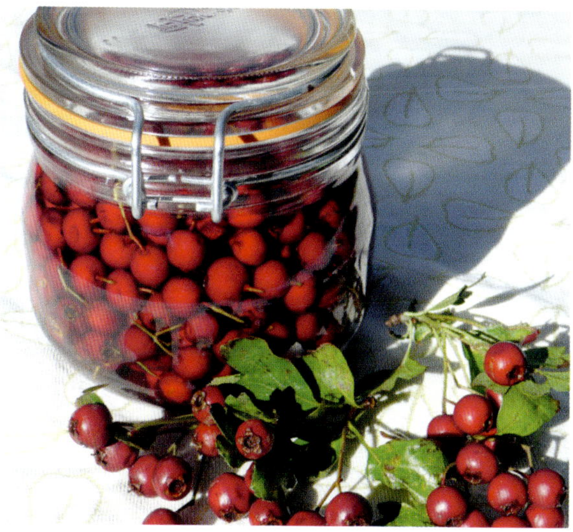

Left Hawthorn tincture.

How to make an infusion

1. Take 2 teaspoonsful of dry herbs, two herbal tea bags or 3–4 teaspoonsful of roughly chopped fresh herbs.
2. Put them in an average-sized tea mug or small teapot (you should be able to fill it with approximately 300ml of water).
3. Pour boiling water over the herbs, stir and cover with a lid or small saucer.
4. Leave to infuse for 10–15 minutes. Strain and drink while still warm.

Right Herbal infusion.

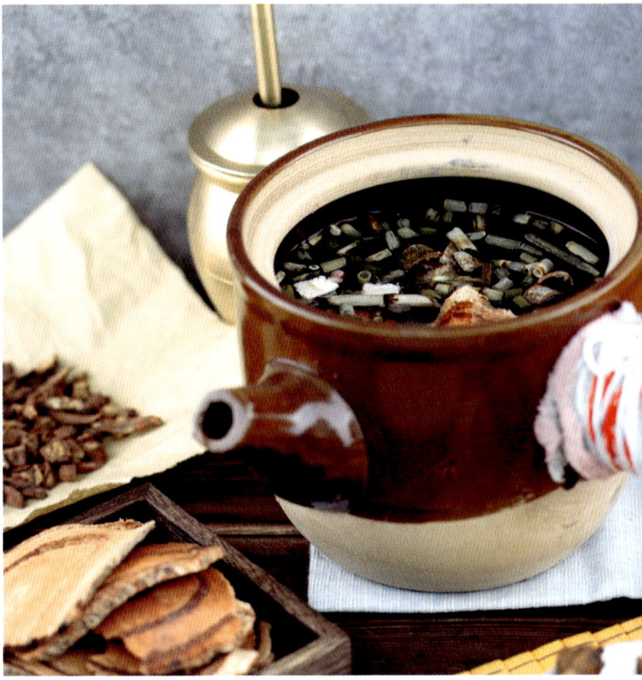

Decoction

A decoction is also a hot-water extract of herbs, but it requires 15 minutes of gentle boiling. This method is used for dried roots and bark. I generally recommend that you use tinctures of such herbs, but there may be some situations in which alcoholic extracts are undesirable, in which case you may need to resort to a decoction. You can make a greater quantity of decoction in one batch by using multiples of the same proportions, and then store the strained liquid for up to 48 hours in the fridge. Most decoctions have a strong and bitter taste, and are not for the fainthearted!

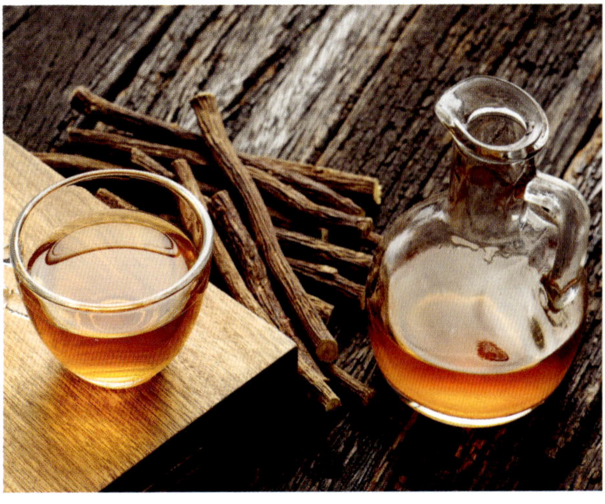

How to make a decoction

1. Put 2 teaspoonsful of dry root or bark in a small saucepan.
2. Pour about 400ml of water over the herbs.
3. Bring to the boil and simmer uncovered for 15 minutes.

Left Liquorice root decoction.

Capsules and tablets

These are very convenient to use. They usually contain either a finely powdered herb or freeze-dried extract. The quality is very variable, so use only well-known brands or purchase them directly from a herbal practitioner.

Powder

Powdered herbs can be taken mixed with water to create a protective coating for the digestive system. Powders of marshmallow root, slippery elm bark or liquorice are most commonly used, and they are great natural substitutes for over-the-counter antacids.

Creams and ointments

These are used mainly for skin conditions, and for muscle and joint aches. Herbalists make their own creams that combine base creams with tinctures, essential oils, infused oils, aromatic waters and infusions. Nowadays it is easy to obtain good-quality herbal creams, but if you want to make your own, instructions can be found in Chapter 23.

Essential oils

Never use essential oils internally unless you are doing so under the guidance of a health professional, as many essential oils can be harmful even in small quantities if ingested. Some essential oils are not suitable for babies or pregnant women.

Essential oils are highly concentrated products usually made by steam distillation of plants rich in volatile substances, and they should not be equated with the plants they come from in terms of actions or safety. Essential oils are obtained from plants with a strong scent, such as rosemary, peppermint, lavender or pine. They should *always* be diluted in a carrier oil or in a cream/ointment for external application.

With one or two exceptions that are specifically mentioned in this book, I do not recommend the use of essential oils for children under the age of three or for pregnant women, except under the guidance of a professional aromatherapist or medical herbalist. Many components of essential oils are absorbed through the skin, and if the dilution is too strong they can be potentially harmful, especially to babies or a developing foetus.

Below Marshmallow root powder.

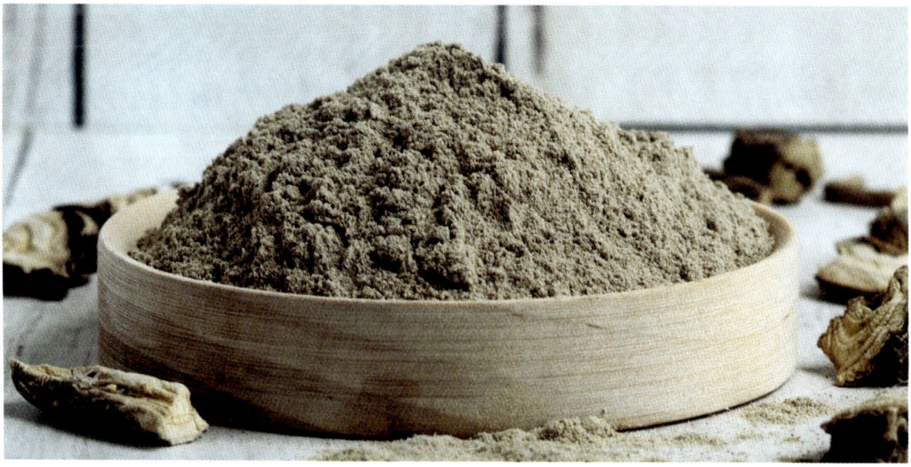

Compresses

For a compress you can use cotton wool, a clean cloth or a flannel soaked in very warm (almost hot) herbal tea. I have found cotton wool to be best, as it can hold more liquid without dripping than a cloth or flannel. Place it against the painful area and keep re-soaking it every few minutes, as the compress works best when it is warm. If you want the compress to remain in place for longer, cover the cotton wool or cloth with a plastic bag or some cling film, and then secure it in the required position with an elastic bandage. The idea is to trap the heat as well as the moisture, so you should use a very warm infusion – as warm as you can bear, but being careful not to burn yourself – for that purpose.

Herbal tea bags (or ordinary black tea bags) can be used directly as eye compresses, but make sure that they are warm and not hot, as the eyelids are very sensitive.

Poultices

Poultices involve direct contact of herbs with the skin. In my experience they work better than compresses, but are a bit messy. They can be made in two ways.

1. You can mix herb powder with hot water to form a thick paste. Put it on a clean cloth (lint or gauze) and apply it directly to the skin (provided that the skin is not broken). Marshmallow root powder or slippery elm bark powder can be used in this way to draw splinters out.
2. You can use fresh herbs that have been quickly scalded with hot water and drained, or dry herbs that are brewed to make a very strong tea (use twice the amount of herbs you would use for normal brewing, and infuse for 10 minutes). Squeeze the herbs lightly while they are still almost hot to remove the excess liquid, spread on to a clean cloth and apply to the sore area. This method can be a little messy, but the direct contact between herbs and skin is extremely soothing and effective, especially for painful joints or muscles and for swellings of various origins.

Syrups

These are strong herbal infusions that are mixed with sugar syrup or honey and used to treat coughs. You can buy ready-made herbal syrups from some suppliers, but if you want to make your own you can find a generic recipe in Chapter 23.

Below Thyme syrup.

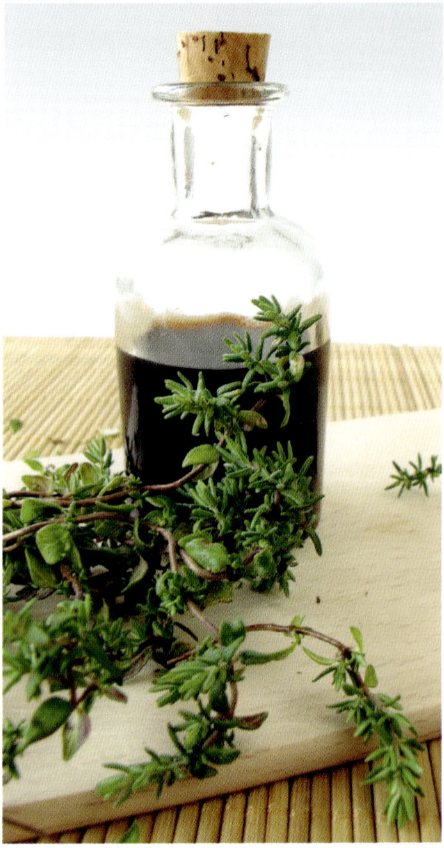

CHAPTER 5

Dosage

Dosage is normally specific to a herb and its preparation. Therefore you must follow the manufacturer's instructions if you buy a ready-made product.

Tinctures

The recommended tincture dosages in this book refer to particular tincture strengths. Each dosage recommendation follows the same pattern throughout the book – for example, 1–2ml, one to three times a day, 1:2 tincture strength.

Adjusting the dosage to the situation

As you can see from the dosage example above, a single dose can range from a minimum (1ml in this case) to a maximum (2ml in this case). If you have mild symptoms you should use the minimum dose at the minimal daily frequency (usually just once a day), but if the symptoms are severe you should use the maximum dose (three times a day). If you are of slight build you should opt for low doses, but if you are of large build you will need doses close to the recommended maximum.

If you are not getting the desired effect using the minimum dose, increase it gradually, but do not take more than the recommended maximum. There is wide variation in the doses that people need as individuals, and it may take you some time to work out your own optimal dose. Sometimes I recommend a specific dose for specific circumstances, which will differ from the usual dose range (such instances will be clearly indicated in the text).

Different tincture strengths

Because the dosage depends on the tincture strength and varies from herb to herb, it is not possible to give general guidance on the amount of tincture you should take. I suggest that you obtain the exact tincture strengths recommended in this book, so that you can follow the advice on the dosage directly. If you have a different tincture strength from the one recommended in this book you must use the tincture according to the manufacturer's instructions.

Measuring out the dose

For practical purposes, 5ml is equivalent to an average teaspoonful, but if you want to be exact you can buy measuring spoons or beakers from the chemist. Sometimes it is easier to measure out a dose in drops. In this book I assume that 1ml of a tincture is equivalent to ten drops. This means that any dosage below 1ml can be easily converted into drops. For example, 0.4ml is equivalent to four drops. Use a glass dropper to measure out the drops. You may find that other sources assume that 1ml is equivalent to 20 drops. This variation results from differences in the viscosity of the liquids and the size of the dropper. I have tested many droppers and tinctures and have found that 1ml is close to ten drops in most cases.

Teas

Herbal teas are not as concentrated as tinctures, so you do not need to be as precise about the dosage. On average, an adult dose is 1 cup of herbal tea, one to three times a day. This dosage refers to the method of brewing described earlier. However, sometimes I recommend a strong infusion, which means that you add an extra teaspoonful or two to the normal amount and brew it for 5–10 minutes longer than usual. Conversely, if a weak infusion is recommended, use one teaspoonful of herbs and brew it for only 2–3 minutes.

Adjusting the dosage to the situation

As with tinctures, the daily dosage depends on how severe your symptoms are. 1 cup a day constitutes a minimum dosage, and 3 cups a day is the usual maximum. Occasionally the maximum dosage goes up to four to five cups a day, and again such instances are clearly indicated in the text.

Essential oils

I do not recommend using essential oils in external preparations for infants or children under three years old, or for pregnant women, without first talking to a qualified aromatherapist or medical herbalist.

Essential oils should be used only for external applications. You can use almond, sunflower or hemp oil as carrier oils and dilute 5–20 drops of essential oil per 50ml of the carrier oil or 50g of the cream base. I generally recommend using essential oils in a bath, varying the amount according to age:

- children aged 3–4 years: one drop in a bath

Below A delicious cup of herbal tea.

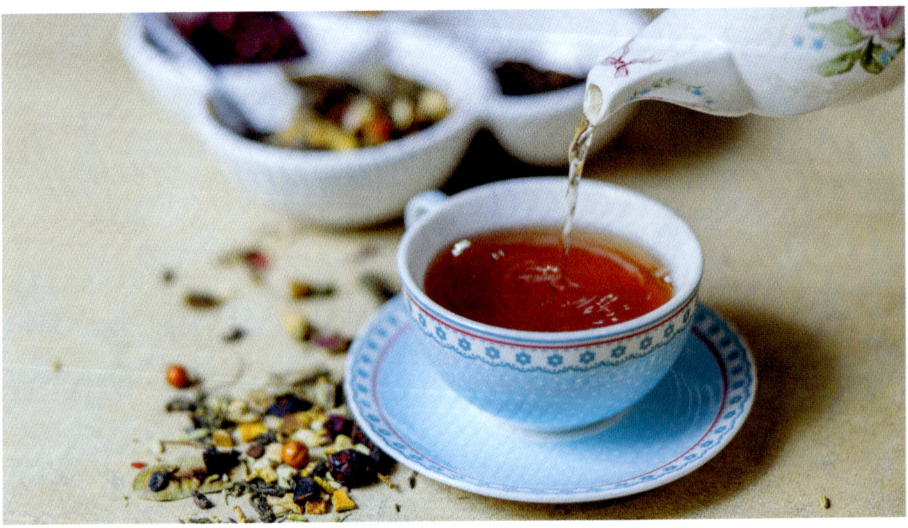

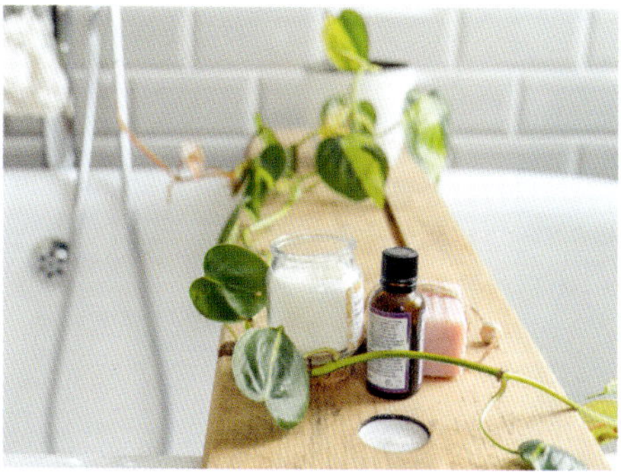

Above Essential oils are best when added to a bath.

- children aged 5–6 years: one to two drops in a bath
- children aged 7–12 years: two to three drops in a bath
- children aged 13–16 years: three to four drops in a bath
- adults: five drops in a bath.

Swish the water around well to disperse the oil.

Remember that many components of essential oils are absorbed through the skin, and if the dilution is too strong and too much of the essential oil is absorbed it can cause harm, especially to babies or a developing foetus.

Adjusting the dosage for specific users

Children and teenagers

I do not recommend giving herbal preparations to infants or children under three years old without first seeking advice from a qualified medical herbalist.

In general, I advise against treating babies with medicinal herbs at home because they need tiny doses and some herbs are not suitable. Having said that, a few common problems in infants can be safely treated with herbs, and I give precise dosages for specific situations throughout this book. Similarly, I advise that you do not treat children or even teenagers without first consulting a herbal clinician. In this book I recommend only adult dosages, with the exception of a few very safe herbs that are specifically effective for children's problems.

However, for the majority of the herbs described in this book you can use the following formula to calculate the dosage for young people over 12 years old (it is based on body weight rather than age). Divide the body weight of the teenager by 60 (for kilograms) or 132 (for pounds) to find the fraction of the adult dose that would be appropriate to use.[8]

Pregnancy and breastfeeding

Caution is advised with regard to the use of many herbs in pregnancy, and some herbs should be avoided altogether. If you are pregnant or breastfeeding, do not use any essential oils for external applications without first consulting a specialist.

During pregnancy it is wise to avoid taking any medicines, including herbal ones, and to be extra cautious in the first trimester of pregnancy.

However, some herbs are quite safe and can help to relieve conditions associated with pregnancy, such as morning sickness. Again, I indicate clearly which herbs should not be taken during pregnancy. The dosage for herbs that are safe when taken in pregnancy may differ from the standard adult dose, so double check the recommendations for each herb.

Breastfeeding mothers can take the standard adult dose, but some herbs (e.g. sage, peppermint) should be avoided. This is because the active constituents of the herbs will be present in the mother's milk and ingested by the infant. Such herbs are clearly indicated throughout the text.

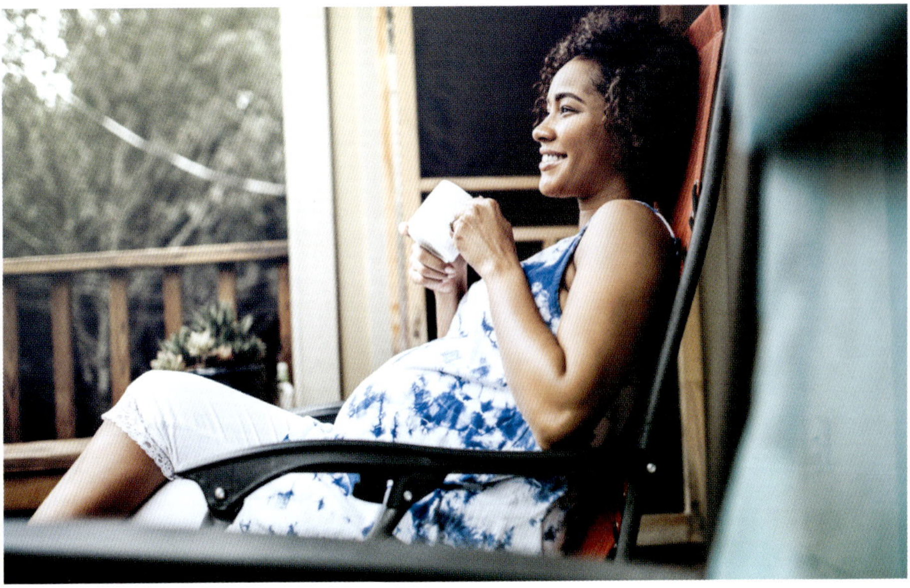

Above If pregnant, check with a professional before taking any medicine.

Older people

People over 70 years of age or those who are frail or of slight build should take half the adult dose.

People with epilepsy

In my experience people with epilepsy need to be extra cautious when taking herbs as even very gentle herbs used in small amounts can alter the blood levels of their medication and cause an epileptic episode. Therefore I strongly advise anyone with epilepsy to consult a herbal clinician before self-medicating with medicinal botanicals.

When to take herbs

Some herbs are best taken before food, and others should be taken after meals. For example, to improve your liver function or increase your appetite you need to sip your (quite bitter) medicine at least 15 minutes before the meal, but if you experience heartburn you should take a soothing tea after the meal. Unless specifically advised otherwise, you should assume that the herbs should be taken before food.

How long to take herbs for

An issue related to dosage is the length of time necessary to achieve an improvement in your condition. Most treatments recommended in this book are intended to be short term – for example, one or two doses to get rid of stomach pain, two to four days of treatment to get rid of a cold, or a few months of treatment to keep hot flushes at bay. The general principle is that you take the herbal medicine until your symptoms disappear, and the longer you have had a problem, the longer it will take to get rid of it. If the length of time for which a particular herb is taken is important, specific information is provided in the book.

If you are unsure about the dosage, or how long you need to take the herb, contact your local medical herbalist.

CHAPTER 6

Herb selection

Choosing an optimal herb or herb selection for a particular health problem experienced by a particular person is quite an art. Not all stomach aches will be cured by meadowsweet, nor will all colds be cured by elderflower. If you don't match the appropriate herb(s) to the specific situation you will obtain poor results.

Below Among its many benefits, garlic lowers blood pressure and cholesterol levels.

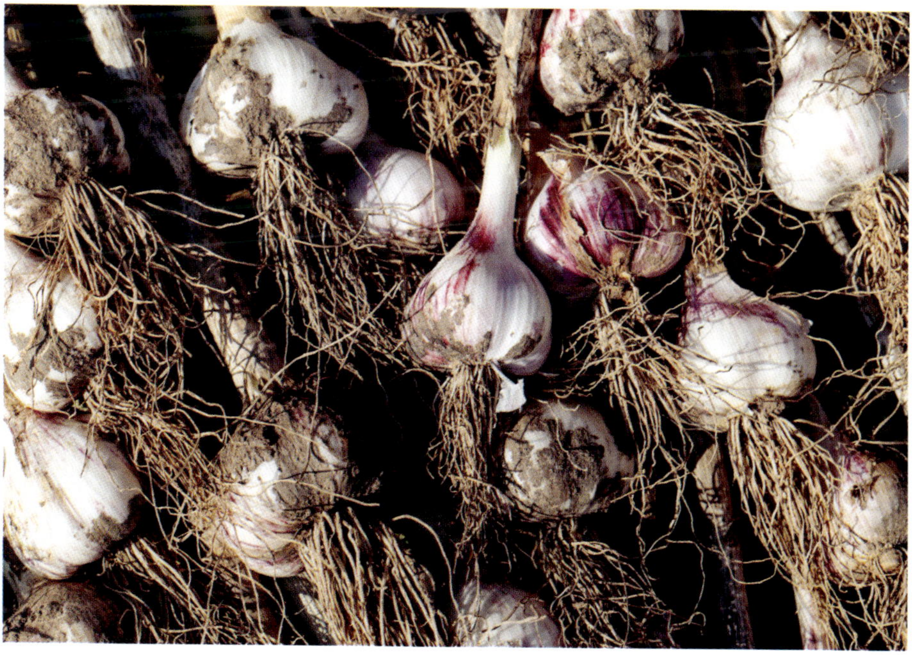

Conversely, a good match of a medicinal herb to an illness will usually result in quick improvement.

Choosing the right herbs for the situation

Using herbs successfully is not a matter of using fixed prescriptions, but rather you need to learn to make considered choices for individual problems and individual people. It is not difficult – this book does not require you to learn about hundreds of herbs. On the contrary, I suggest that you rely on as few herbs as possible.

However, even when faced with a small choice it is important that you select the best possible herb(s) for a given situation. You need to take a number of criteria into account, including the range of symptoms, their severity, the age of the ill person and any other medication and/or supplements that they are taking. Also remember to check whether they have any allergies that might make them react badly to the herbs.

Symptoms

First, assess the symptoms carefully. For instance, if you have a cold, is it predominantly a runny nose, a sore throat

Below Preparing dried herbs for medicinal recipes.

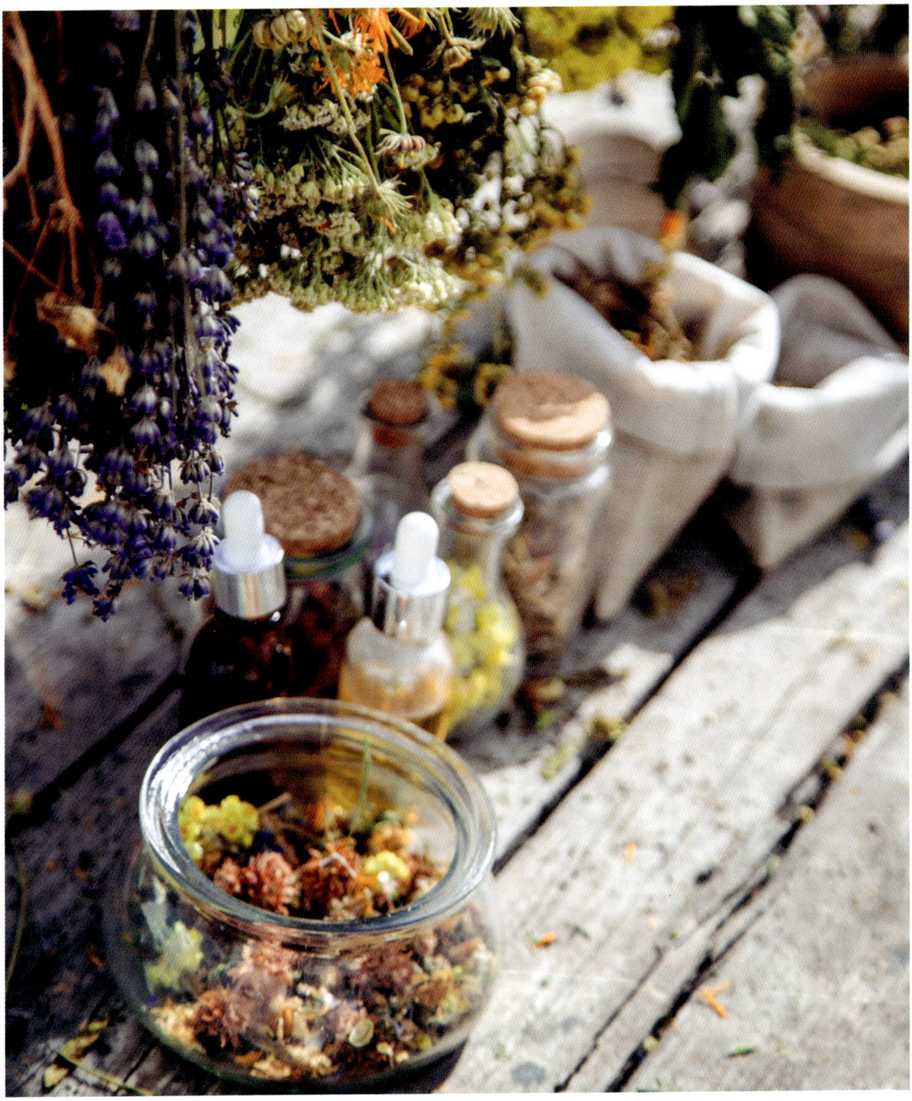

or a cough, or any combination of these three symptoms? Are you running a high temperature or do your muscles ache? If you have a stomach ache, is it related to something you have eaten or drunk recently, or is it a condition you suffer from regularly when you are stressed? Do you feel bloated or nauseous? Try to identify as many characteristics of your problem as possible. Decide which system of the body your ailment relates to and refer to the appropriate chapter in the book.

Matching the treatment to your ailment

Look up your illness and individual symptoms and familiarise yourself with the treatment options. Read the descriptions of the must-have herbs at the beginning of the chapter, as most treatments are based solely on these.

Choose one herb that would treat the condition as a whole, but consider adding one or two more herbs with specific actions if particular symptoms are very pronounced.

Returning to the examples given at the beginning of this chapter, elderflower would be good for a cold with just a runny nose, but for a cold with a bad cough you will need additional herbs – perhaps a thyme and liquorice syrup. A cold with a very sore throat may require garlic or propolis as well as elderflower. Similarly, if you have a stomach ache resulting from possible food poisoning you may have to use garlic, charcoal and barberry, but if it is simply indigestion a meadowsweet tea will do the trick. The structure of the book will help you to choose the right herbs for a given situation, and if you read the descriptions of individual herbs and indications for their most appropriate uses, deciding on the right treatment should not be difficult.

Special considerations

If you are treating a child, check whether any of the herbs are specifically recommended for children and make these your first choice. If you are treating pregnant women or people on conventional medication, double check whether the herbs you have chosen are suitable for them – if they are not, look for alternatives among the herbs suggested in 'optional herbs' section. If you are already taking a herbal supplement long term, do not include the same herbs in your self-prescription. For instance, if you are taking St John's wort for mild depression and need to treat a cold, do not include St John's wort in your anti-cold prescription as the combined dosage might be too high.

How to combine herbs

Some combinations of medicinal plants work better than others. I usually advise people to start using herbs individually in order to get to know them well, and then to proceed to combinations or mixes. However, if you are feeling adventurous you may want to combine a few herbs straight away.

In general, you should combine herbs based on their individual actions and on how well they work together. I have made suggestions for good combinations throughout the book, based on my experience. To begin with you can copy my prescriptions exactly as you learn the underlying principles of mixing different herbs together. However, in the longer term, after you have followed my suggestions for good combinations that are included in the herb descriptions, you can try making your own herb mixes or combinations to match your individual needs.

Combining different forms of herbs

As well as combining different herbs you can also combine different forms of botanicals together. Tablets of one herb can be taken at the same time as a tea, tincture or syrup of another herb. Any combination of these is fine as long as you don't take too many herbs at any one time – stick to a maximum of five for any one ailment. Some herbs work better in the form of a tea whereas others are more effective in the form of a tincture, so it makes sense to use the best form for each herb, even if you are using them together. You can drink herbal tea to allow you to swallow herbal capsules or tablets, or you can add tincture to the tea (not a great taste improver!), or you can take different forms of herbs at different times if you wish. Throughout the book I suggest many useful combinations of different forms of herbs – you will notice that a tincture-and-tea combination is a common one, but if you favour tablets over tinctures, follow your preference.

Rules for herb mixing and dosage

There are a few basic rules that you need to follow for successful herb mixing and for calculating the dosage of the mix.

- Keep it simple. To begin with, stick to one herb for a particular problem.
- Add one herb at a time to your combination unless I specifically advise that more should be included.
- Start by mixing the exact replicas of the herb combinations recommended in this book before trying your own.
- Don't combine herbs that have opposite effects – for example, relaxing and stimulating herbs don't mix well, and neither do warming and cooling herbs.
- Two herbs with similar properties can often be combined successfully – for example, two relaxing herbs or two cough herbs will mix well.
- Try to put together herbs that will deal with different aspects of your particular problem, but use no more than five herbs at any one time.
- When combining herbs in tincture form, use the minimum recommended dose of each individual herb.
- If you have combined several herbs in a single tincture, your single dose should be a teaspoonful (5ml).
- Always label the mixed tinctures with the ingredients and the date – you can keep the multiple compound tincture for up to a year.
- When combining teas, use roughly the same weight of each herb and then brew the blend in the same manner as for a single herb.
- The dosage for herbal tea that is made up using a few different herbs is similar to that for a single herb tea – that is, 1–3 cups a day for an adult.
- Do not make more than 50–100g of a dry herb mix, as dry herbs do not keep as well as a tincture mix. Make sure that you label the mixture with the ingredients and the date, and keep it for no longer than six months.

What if it doesn't work?

You may sometimes find that the herbs you have used to treat a particular health problem do not produce the desired effect. Don't be discouraged, but consider carefully the possible causes of the problem.

- Your choice of herb(s) might not have been right for this particular illness. For example, if you were to treat a bacterial throat infection with antiviral herbs, you would not have much success.
- The herbs that you used may have been of poor quality. This is an important issue, so please refer to the Useful

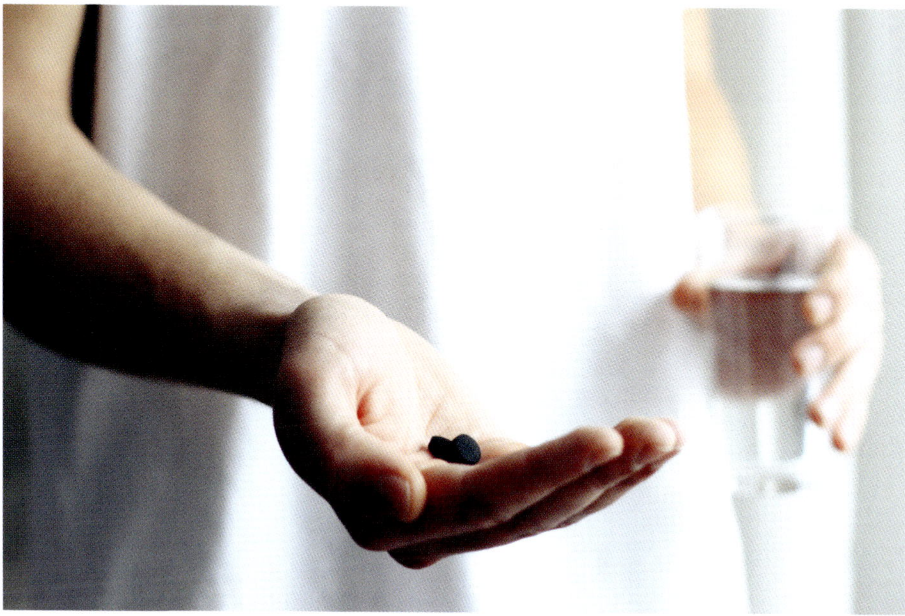

resources chapter for a list of suppliers of the best-quality herbs.

- You may have purchased the wrong herb or the wrong part of a herb – double check the scientific name and the herb part (see pages 230–237).
- You may have used an inappropriate dose (see Chapter 5).
- Your self-diagnosis may have been incorrect. Read up again on the distinguishing features of different diseases, or consult a health professional to have your diagnosis confirmed.

Successful treatment with herbs requires some experimenting. We are all genetically unique, so we all vary in our individual response to herbs. Some people will need larger doses than others, and some people will react well to a particular herb that has little effect on others. If you tried a particular herb selection from the 'must-have herbs' section and this did not resolve the problem, try some herbs from the 'optional herbs' section, as these may suit you better. Observe your reaction to a particular herb carefully – for most conditions described in this book I would expect to see results within a few hours to a few days. Once you have found a reliable herb that works for you in a particular situation, stick to it.

Above Medicinal charcoal tablets can be useful after food poisoning.

One of the reasons why I encourage people to try herbs singly to begin with is to see whether a particular herb does have a positive effect on the individual's body in the context of a particular disease. If you experiment with a lot of different herbs at any one time you may not be able to see the wood for the trees. Remember that the botanicals recommended in this book are exceptionally safe, so you are very unlikely to encounter any problems while trying out different options with them. The more you use medicinal herbs, the more easily you will be able to tell whether a particular herb suits your particular body type, and you will start to get consistently good results.

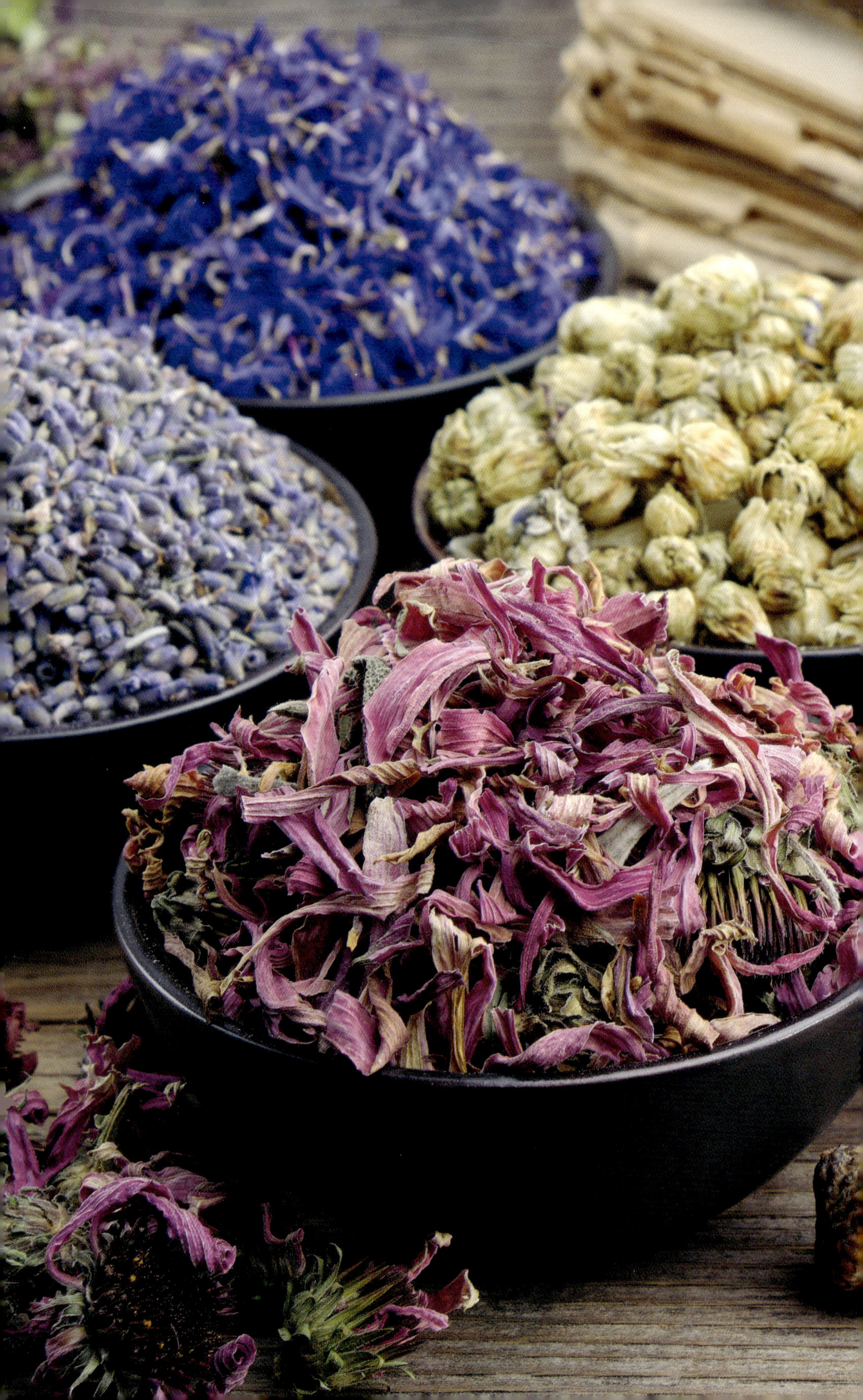

PART 2

Ailments and treatments

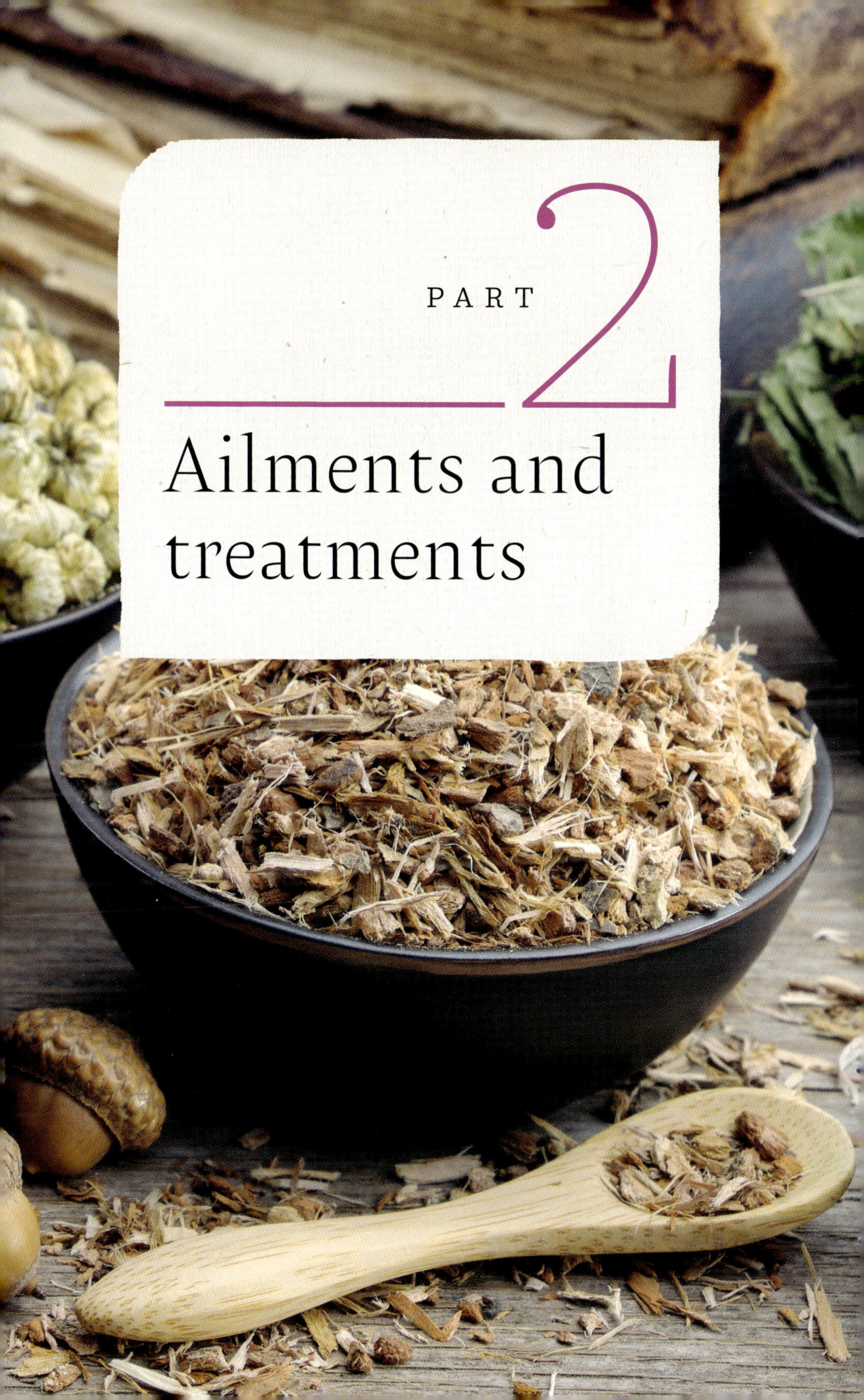

CHAPTER 7

The circulatory system

The circulatory system comprises the heart and all of the blood vessels in the body – arteries, veins and small capillaries. Blood is of course a vital part of the circulatory system!

Disorders that affect the circulation are very common. Mild problems such as chilblains can be easily treated at home, but potentially serious problems such as irregular heartbeat require professional help.

Many spices, such as ginger, chillies, turmeric, cinnamon and horseradish, are beneficial for the circulatory system. They all have a mild stimulatory effect, which becomes obvious when you eat any of these items – the feeling of warmth that is experienced after having a hot curry is a direct result of more blood flowing through the capillaries! Using spices regularly (ideally on a daily basis) in your cooking will be enough to provide a sustained benefit.

When to seek help

If you are already taking medication prescribed by your doctor for a heart or circulation problem, I would not recommend that you try out any herbal remedies yourself. However, a professional may be able to advise you on remedies that can work alongside orthodox medication.

Many cases of mild heart disease can be successfully treated by herbal medicine, but this needs to be done under the supervision of a medical herbalist, especially in view of the fact that some of the more potent herbs are not available over the counter.

Looking after your heart

Diet and lifestyle have a huge effect on the health of the circulatory system, which thrives on exercise and plenty of fresh fruit and vegetables, but suffers badly if you smoke, take no exercise or eat too much junk food.

People are often confused about what constitutes a healthy diet for the heart and circulatory system, and there are many myths about what causes high cholesterol levels, which fats are good for you and how much red wine it is safe to drink. If there is a history of heart disease in your family, or you have been diagnosed with a circulatory disease, you should see a dietary or herbal practitioner who will be able to advise you on specific dietary requirements.

Must-have herbs

Hawthorn *Crataegus monogyna* (Common hawthorn) or *Crataegus laevigata* (Midland hawthorn)

Hawthorn is not recommended for people with low blood pressure. It is not always compatible with heart medication.

Uses

Hawthorn berries and flowering tops can be used to treat a wide range of problems associated with the circulatory system. This herb improves the function and health of the heart, increases the peripheral blood supply to the hands and feet, and slightly lowers the blood pressure. It can speed up recovery from a heart attack or stroke. Hawthorn can be taken alongside orthodox medication under the supervision of a herbalist, but it is not always compatible with medicines for heart conditions or high blood pressure. For the purpose of self-prescribing I would recommend using it for poor circulation and slightly raised blood pressure.

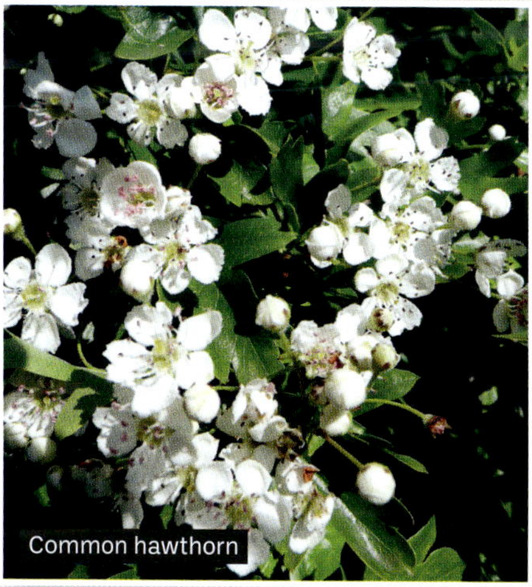
Common hawthorn

COMBINATIONS: Hawthorn combines well with yarrow or lime tree flowers.
HOW TO TAKE IT: Hawthorn should be taken as a tincture.
DOSAGE: **Adults:** 1–2ml, one to three times a day, tincture strength 1:2.

Garlic *Allium sativum*

Do not take large doses for prolonged periods of time, or when pregnant or breastfeeding.
Medicinal use of garlic is not recommended for children under six years of age.
Discontinue garlic 10 days before undergoing surgery.

Caution is needed if taking anticoagulant or antiplatelet medication.

Uses

Garlic is another botanical (as well as a common food item) that can be used to treat many different health problems. It greatly improves the circulation and can prevent the development of clogged-up arteries in people who are at high risk for this (e.g. due to having a family history of heart disease, being overweight, being a smoker or having a high-calorie diet). It can help to bring high blood pressure down and keep your cholesterol levels low, and it also reduces the risk of blood clotting.

HOW TO TAKE IT: To be effective for problems of the circulatory system, garlic should be eaten raw or taken as tablets made from freeze-dried extract or freeze-dried powder (the effect of garlic oil on the circulation is unclear). Raw garlic, finely chopped or crushed, can be added to food or each dose can be mixed with a teaspoonful of honey and swallowed.

You may need to take large amounts for specific ailments, and if you are receiving another treatment it is best to consult a health professional, as garlic can interact with some medications.

For garlic to be of benefit to the circulatory system you should use only preparations that state the content of alliin or allicin (the active constituents of garlic), and they should contain 5–12mg of alliin or allicin in a total daily dose. The tablets should also be enteric-coated to prevent the destruction of the active constituents in the stomach. Large doses of garlic taken for a long time can affect the digestion. To avoid this, either take garlic for a month and then have a month off, or reduce the dose to the minimum.

DOSAGE: **Adults:** one to three fresh cloves a day, or 0.5–1g of dried powder in tablets or capsules (the equivalent of approximately 5g of fresh garlic), or 1 teaspoonful of freshly squeezed juice a day.

It is possible to use tincture made from fresh garlic, but this is less effective than tablets. **Adults:** 2–4ml, one to three times a day, tincture strength 1:1.

I have found in my practice that a stabilised garlic juice is also a good option. You can buy this from some health food shops or online, or make your own (for the method and dosage, see pages 113–114).

Ginkgo *Ginkgo biloba*

Caution is needed if taking anticoagulant or antiplatelet medication, including aspirin. Discontinue ginkgo a week before undergoing surgery.

Uses

Ginkgo increases the circulation to the extremities and specifically improves the blood supply to the brain. Although it is generally a very safe herb to take, treat it with respect, as there are situations when it is best not to self-medicate with it – for instance, if you have high blood pressure, a history of strokes or are taking blood-thinning medicines (you may still benefit from ginkgo, but the dosage should be determined by a qualified herbalist).

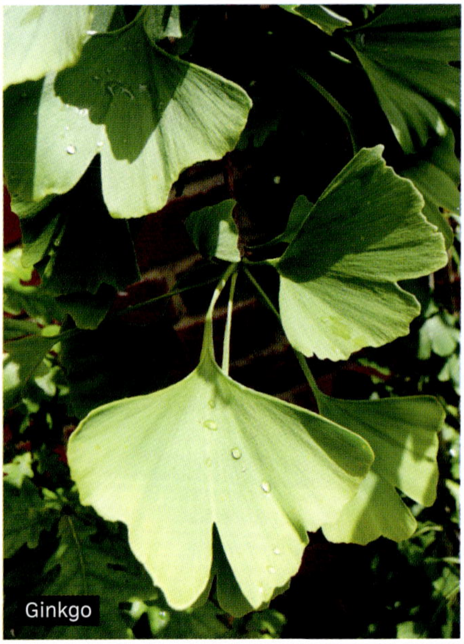
Ginkgo

If your health is generally good, ginkgo can be very useful for improving memory and concentration as well as general blood circulation. It should be your first-choice herb if you always have cold hands and feet and do not cope well with cold weather. It is very useful when mountaineering at high altitude.[9]

HOW TO TAKE IT: A tincture is the preferred form, though tea can be used instead. Make sure that the tincture strength is 2:1, as the benefits from other strengths are unclear.

DOSAGE: **Adults:** 1–2ml, one to three times a day, tincture strength 2:1, or 2–3g of dried leaf to make a cup of tisane, one to three times a day.

Optional herbs

Blueberries and bilberries *Vaccinium corymbosum* and *Vaccinium myrtillus*

Uses

Blueberries and bilberries (which are in the family Ericaceae and stain the tongue and fingers black) are another example of foods that are also medicinal herbs. These berries have an affinity for the so-called microcirculation (the very smallest blood vessels in the body), especially at the back of the eye. Blueberries and bilberries can help people who have sustained damage to the retina[10] because of high blood pressure, and they generally restore the health of the blood vessels within the body. Eating blueberries or bilberries will be of benefit for people with virtually any disease of the circulatory system, and it will also have a preventative effect. You can eat them daily if you wish, and frozen blueberries or bilberries are just as beneficial as fresh ones.

HOW TO TAKE THEM: Blueberries and bilberries are taken in the form of food, as either fresh or defrosted berries. You can also take a blueberry or bilberry supplement in the form of tablets or capsules.

DOSAGE: **Adults and children (over two years old)**: 50–100g of berries a day. The supplement should be taken according to the manufacturer's instructions.

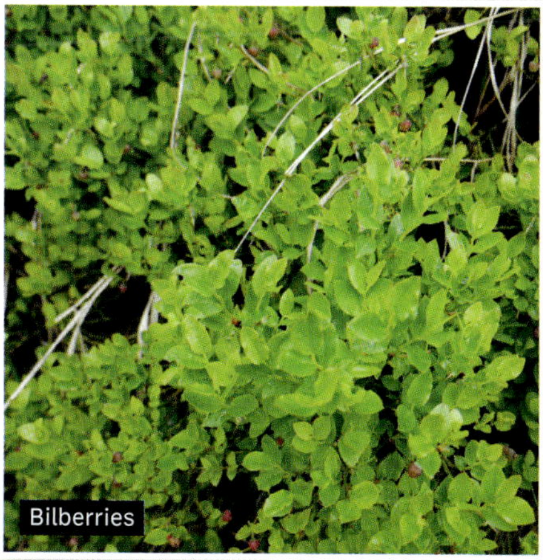
Bilberries

Ginger *Zingiber officinale*

Caution is needed when breastfeeding, in cases of stomach ulcer or gallstones, and if taking warfarin or other blood-thinning medicines. During pregnancy, intake should be limited to 2g/day of dried ginger.

Uses

This is a warming herb, which means that it improves the overall blood supply to all parts of the body, including the skin, hands and feet. If you have poor circulation, particularly in winter, adding ginger to your food or drinking ginger tea will have a beneficial effect.

HOW TO TAKE IT: As a tea made from fresh or dried rhizome, or use it in cooking. A tincture can be useful when added to multiple herb mixes.

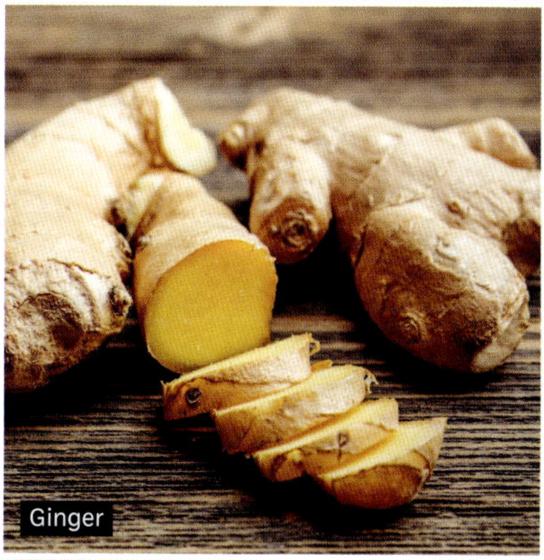
Ginger

DOSAGE: Adults: 1g of fresh or dried rhizome one to three times a day as an infusion, or 1–3 cups a day if you use tea bags, or 1–3g of fresh or dried rhizome used in cooking, or 0.2–0.7ml, one to three times a day, tincture strength 1:2.

Horse chestnut *Aesculus hippocastanum*

Do not take horse chestnut during pregnancy. Large doses can cause stomach irritation and reflux.

Uses

The fruit of the horse chestnut tree is used medicinally to improve the health of the veins. It has a reputation for being beneficial for varicose veins, though in my experience it mostly works as a preventative measure. However, people who suffer from varicose veins often have poor blood flow from the legs to the heart, and horse chestnut will help to treat the resulting tendency to swelling. This herb is also useful for inflamed haemorrhoids and leg ulcers, as well as acne rosacea.

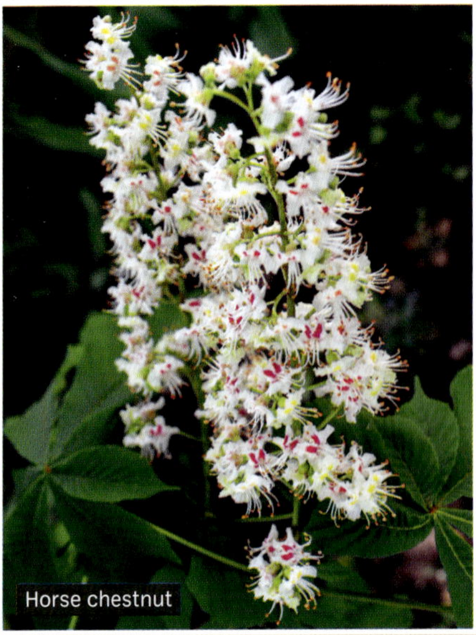
Horse chestnut

HOW TO TAKE IT: As a tincture.
DOSAGE: Adults: 0.7–1.7ml, one to three times a day, tincture strength 1:2.

Lime tree flowers *Tilia cordata, Tilia platyphyllos* and *Tilia × europaea*

Lime tree (also known as linden) flowers should be avoided in people with known allergy, and should not be taken at the same time as iron supplements.

Uses

Lime tree flowers can help to lower mildly raised blood pressure. They are suitable for people who are tense and stressed, as they are a gentle relaxant.

COMBINATIONS: Lime tree flowers combine well with hawthorn and yarrow.
HOW TO TAKE IT: Either as a tea made from the dried flowers, or as a tincture.
DOSAGE: Adults: 1 cup of tea, one to three times a day, or 0.7–1.4ml, one to three times a day, tincture strength 1:2.

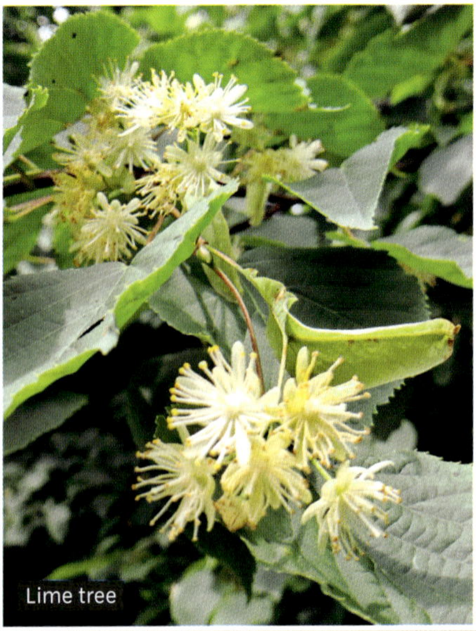
Lime tree

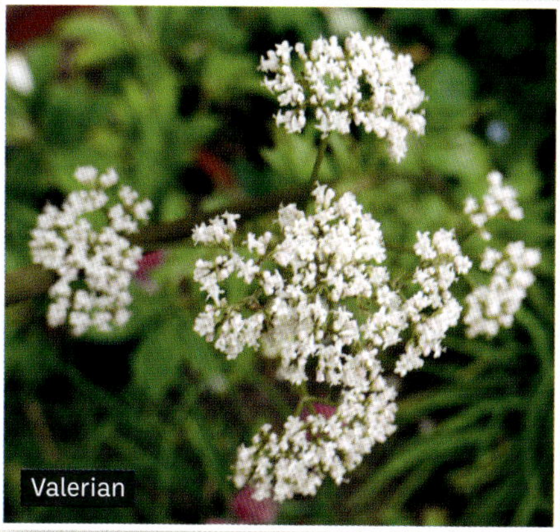

Valerian

Valerian *Valeriana officinalis*

Large doses of valerian can cause drowsiness or tiredness.

Uses

Valerian is primarily a relaxant for the nervous system, and as such it will help with disorders of the circulatory system that are caused by stress, anxiety and tension. The range of problems that valerian can be used to treat includes raised pulse rate, heart palpitations caused by stress, and mildly raised blood pressure.

COMBINATIONS: Valerian combines well with hawthorn and/or lime tree flowers for the above-mentioned problems.
HOW TO TAKE IT: As a tincture.
DOSAGE: **Adults:** 0.7–2ml, one to three times a day, tincture strength 1:2. It is advisable to start with minimal doses and gradually increase the dose if necessary.

Yarrow *Achillea millefolium*

Do not take yarrow during pregnancy.

Caution is needed in people who are allergic to plants belonging to the daisy family (the Asteraceae, formerly known as the Compositae).

Uses

Yarrow has many medicinal actions, one of the more significant ones being the ability to improve blood circulation. It can be used in many conditions where circulation is a problem, such as cold hands and feet, general sensitivity to cold, susceptibility to chilblains, nosebleeds, bruising easily, varicose veins and bleeding haemorrhoids. Yarrow improves the blood flow to the extremities and reduces the tendency to excessive bleeding (so is useful in menstrual disorders). It can be used directly on cuts to staunch bleeding. It is also helpful for reducing mildly elevated blood pressure, although it is best to have an individual dosage determined by a herbalist who can check your blood pressure on a regular basis.

COMBINATIONS: Yarrow combines well with hawthorn.
HOW TO TAKE IT: Either as a tincture or as a tea.
DOSAGE: **Adults:** 0.7–2ml, one to three times a day, tincture strength 1:2, or 1 cup of tea, one to three times a day.

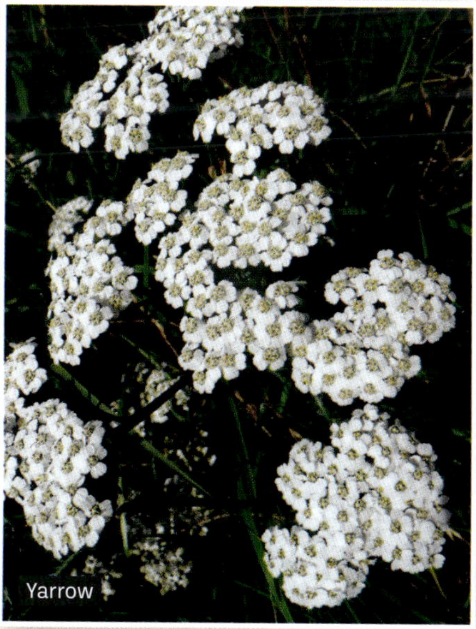

Yarrow

Specific ailments affecting the circulatory system, and herbs that can help

Anaemia

Practitioner treatment is recommended for this condition.

Anaemia means that your blood is deficient in haemoglobin, which transports oxygen round the body in red blood cells. Usually anaemia results from blood loss due to injury, surgery or excessive menstrual bleeding. It can also develop if your diet is not providing enough iron, or if the iron is not being absorbed from the ingested food. There may be other rarer causes of anaemia, and it is important to identify the underlying problem and treat it.

The main symptoms of anaemia are tiredness and shortness of breath on exertion, and many people do not realise they are anaemic until their symptoms become severe. The measures described below will provide good sources of easily absorbable iron that are free from the side effects associated with iron supplements. If you are vegetarian or vegan the following foods are good sources of iron: tofu, beans, lentils, green leafy vegetables, nuts and seeds. Breakfast cereals are often fortified with iron, but do choose the least processed ones. If you are not vegetarian, black pudding is the best food source for iron, liver being the second-best source.

Below A bowl of dried fruit and seeds makes a healthy cereal.

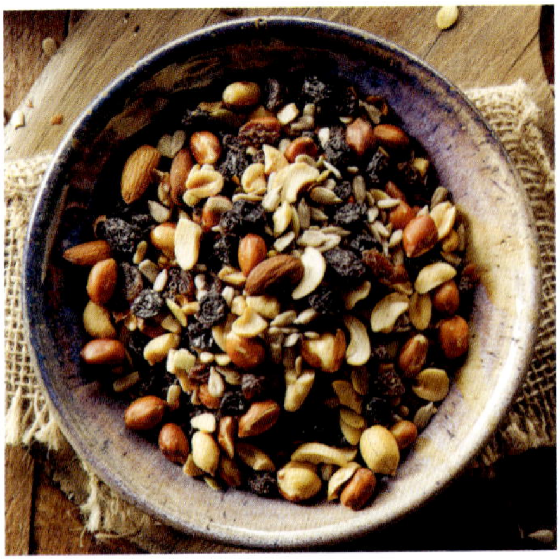

Treatment options

- Take an iron tonic, such as Floradix – this is a concentrated syrup made from yeast and herb and fruit extracts that are naturally high in iron (take it according to the manufacturer's instructions).
- Eat a variety of dried fruits and seeds daily (e.g. figs, apricots, prunes, raisins, pumpkin seeds, sunflower seeds, nuts).
- Drinking certain herbal teas will help, although this is not normally sufficient as herbs contain only small amounts of iron (useful herbs include nettles, couch grass, wild strawberry leaves).

Adults: 1 cup of tea, two to three times a day.

Bleeding (cuts, small wounds)

Here I am referring to domestic accidents such as cutting your finger with a knife while chopping vegetables (large cuts may need stitching), scraped knees or nipping your skin when shaving. The treatment options described below will help to arrest the bleeding, but if the cut is dirty you will need to clean and disinfect it, and then apply a suitable dressing if necessary. For details of how to treat cuts and wounds, see Chapter 12.

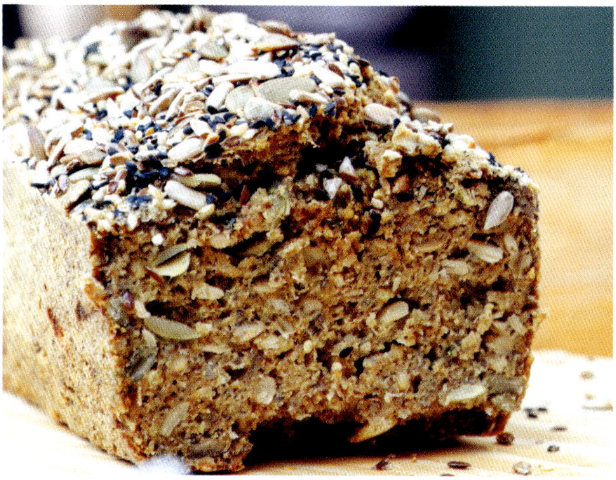

Above Buckwheat bread is a great way to boost rutin levels.

Treatment options

- Use yarrow tincture diluted with cold water to reduce bleeding. Either dab the cut or press gently on the area with cotton wool soaked in dilute yarrow tincture until the bleeding subsides (do not use neat tincture, as it will sting). **Application for adults and children:** dilute 10ml of tincture in half a cup of clean water, as a one-off use which can be repeated if necessary.
- Use yarrow tea instead of the yarrow tincture (use either fresh or dried herbs). **Application for adults and children:** make a strong yarrow tea with 2 teaspoonsful of herbs per half cup of water, and use it in the same way as diluted yarrow tincture.
- Use freshly squeezed yarrow juice instead of tea or tincture. **Application for adults and children:** juice fresh yarrow plants to obtain a few teaspoonsful of yarrow juice, and use in the same way as diluted yarrow tincture.

Bruising

Bruising happens when small blood vessels leak blood into the surrounding tissues. It is normal to develop a bruise after bumping into something or falling over. However, some people show bruising after minimal pressure has been applied to their skin, and this indicates that the walls of their blood vessels are particularly fragile.

The first measure listed below is applicable to all types of bruising and is a first-aid item, whereas the others relate to an excessive tendency to bruise, and constitute long-term treatment. See page 89 for more on bruising.

Treatment options

- If you apply arnica ointment as soon as you have had an accident you may prevent the bruise from forming altogether. Do not use arnica on open wounds or cuts (although you can apply the ointment near the periphery of the cut, about 2.5cm away from the edge). **Application for adults and children:** apply generously only once on small bruises; larger bruises will benefit from two to three applications a few hours apart.
- Take a rutin supplement daily for a few months (follow the manufacturer's instructions).
- Eat buckwheat or buckwheat flour on a regular basis, as this is a good source of rutin.
- Eat 50–100g of blueberries every day, or as often as you can.
- Make sure you include plenty of vitamin C in your diet by eating at least five helpings of fresh fruit or vegetables daily.

Chilblains

Chilblains appear on fingers or toes if you try to warm up very cold hands or feet too quickly – for instance, in front of a fire or by getting into a very hot bath. They affect people whose circulation to the extremities is inadequate, resulting in very cold fingers and toes. Chilblains can be quite sore and red to begin with, and as they heal they can start to itch as well. If you are prone to chilblains you should take warming herbs on a daily basis during the winter months.

Treatment options

Please see pages 135, 44 and 45 for herbal precautions.

- Use marigold cream on chilblains as soon as you are aware of them. **Application for adults and children:** apply the cream generously twice a day.
- Take ginkgo tincture during the winter months. **Adults:** 1–2ml diluted with some water, two to three times a day, tincture strength 2:1.
- Drink ginger tea regularly. **Adults:** 1–2 cups a day.
- Incorporate chillies into your diet (for precautions, see page 84).

High blood pressure

Practitioner treatment is strongly recommended for this condition.

Raised blood pressure is a common problem which, if left untreated, may have serious implications for your health. Many factors can contribute to high blood pressure, including diet, lifestyle, stress, genetic predisposition and level of exercise, so it is important to address all of the possible underlying causes. I do not advise treating high blood pressure at home, unless it is only slightly raised (no higher than 135/85). If you decide to treat it yourself you need to invest in a blood-pressure monitor so that you can check whether the treatment is working. If the results are not satisfactory, speak to your doctor and consult your local herbalist for an individual prescription.

Herbal treatment of raised blood pressure does not have to be lifelong. It will be long term (6–24 months), but it often results in sustained improvement after that. The treatment options below should give you a cumulative 10–15% reduction in your readings (the optimal readings are 120/70 for a healthy young adult). Remember that blood pressure fluctuates throughout the day, and will increase markedly after drinking coffee or alcohol (in the case of the latter, the rise often occurs the next day).

Mix for raised blood pressure

INGREDIENTS

- 30ml hawthorn (tincture strength 1:2)
- 20ml yarrow (tincture strength 1:2)
- 30ml lime tree flowers (tincture strength 1:2)
- 20ml valerian (tincture strength 1:2)

METHOD

1. Mix the ingredients together.
2. Pour the mixture into a clean, dark glass bottle.
3. Label the bottle with the contents and the date.
4. Store at room temperature for up to a year.

ADULT DOSE: 5ml, diluted with some water, two to three times a day.

Treatment options

Please see pages 43–47 for herbal precautions.

- Take hawthorn tincture, made from either flowering tops or fruits. **Adults:** 1–2 ml diluted with some water, one to three times a day, tincture strength 1:2.
- Take garlic, either fresh or as freeze-dried powder in capsules. **Adults:** one to two fresh cloves a day or the equivalent of 5g of the fresh plant in a dry form once or twice a day.
- Drink lime tree flower tea. **Adults:** 1–3 cups a day.
- Take yarrow tincture. **Adults:** 0.7–2ml diluted with some water, one to three times a day, tincture strength 1:2.
- Take valerian tincture, particularly if you are under a lot of continuous stress. **Adults:** 0.7–2ml one to three times a day, tincture strength 1:2.
- Take the mix for raised blood pressure (see opposite). This mix should be taken instead of single herbs, not in addition to them. However, garlic is not included in the mix, so you can add it to your regime if you wish.

High cholesterol

High cholesterol levels are considered to be one of the factors that contribute to atherosclerosis, which is the development of fatty deposits (plaques) on the inner walls of arteries. If these deposits obstruct an artery they can cause a heart attack or a stroke, so it is important to keep the cholesterol at optimal levels. You can do a lot by having a sensible diet (avoiding sugar and processed carbohydrates, having the healthy fats in your diet and including lots of garlic in your cooking – or even better eating garlic raw). Eating fresh, raw vegetables in a salad every day as well as a selection of fruit can also lower your cholesterol levels, as the cholesterol released in bile binds to fibre in your digestive tract, so less of it is reabsorbed. If these measures are not enough, I recommend that you see a herbal practitioner, who will recommend specific herbs and supplements that you can take to keep your cholesterol levels down.

Treatment options

Please see pages 43–47 for herbal precautions.

- Eat fresh garlic every day (see pages 113–114 for more information about garlic preparations). **Adults:** one clove a day, crushed and mixed with salad dressing or honey.
- Take garlic tablets or capsules. **Adults:** the equivalent of 5g of the fresh plant, once or twice a day.
- Drink lime tree flower tea. **Adults:** 1–3 cups a day.
- Eat artichokes as often as you like, as these can also lower your cholesterol levels.

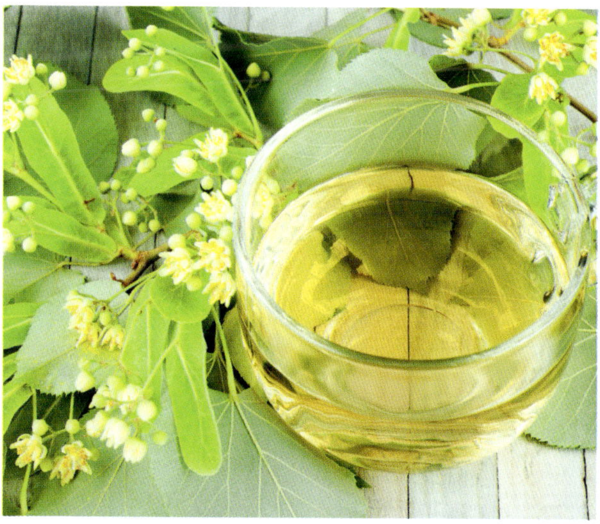

Right Lime tree flower tea.

Low blood pressure

Low blood pressure is not normally a problem. A small proportion of people with very low blood pressure may lack energy and feel the cold easily, or can faint occasionally or feel lightheaded and dizzy. People who have low blood pressure should avoid any herbs that can decrease it even further (e.g. hawthorn, yarrow, lime tree flowers), but herbs that stimulate the general circulation are perfectly safe.

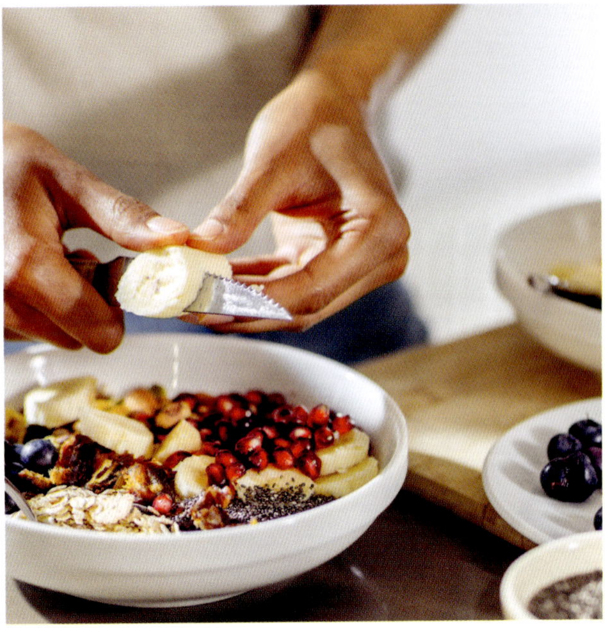

Above Blueberries can easily be incorporated into breakfast.

Treatment options

Please see pages 43–47 for herbal precautions.

- Drink ginger tea. **Adults**: 1–2 cups a day.
- Incorporate chillies into your diet.
- Take ginkgo tincture. **Adults:** 1–2ml diluted with some water, one to three times a day, tincture strength 2:1.
- Eat horseradish as a condiment on a regular basis.

Nose bleed

Frequent nose bleeds can be a sign of specific nutritional deficiencies, so if your diet is not as healthy as it could be it may be worth consulting a specialist for advice on improvements or supplements. However, nose bleeds sometimes occur due to a fragile blood vessel, or exposure to dry air or high altitude. The measures listed below apply to people who have frequent nose bleeds and who need to know how to stop a nose bleed quickly as well as how to prevent it from happening again.

Treatment options

Please see pages 43–47 for herbal precautions.

- Apply yarrow tea (or fresh juice) to the nostril in which bleeding is occurring. Soak a piece of cotton wool in the yarrow tea, squeeze out the excess liquid, shape the cotton wool into a thin cylinder and push it gently into the nostril. Keep it there for a few minutes and then replace it with another piece if necessary.
- Drink yarrow tea for a month. **Adults**: 1–2 cups a day.
- Take yarrow tincture for a month. **Adults**: 0.7–2 ml diluted with some water, two to three times a day, tincture strength 1:2.
- Include blueberries in your diet on a regular basis.
- Take a rutin supplement according to the manufacturer's instructions.
- Eat buckwheat or buckwheat flour (a good source of rutin) on a regular basis.

Poor circulation

There are several signs of poor circulation – your hands and feet always feel cold or look blue in cold weather, you get chilblains easily or you find yourself dressed in twice as many clothes as everyone else around you! Energetic regular exercise improves circulation considerably, as does eating spicy food, especially chillies and ginger.

Treatment options

Please see pages 43–47 for herbal precautions.

- Take ginkgo tincture. **Adults**: 1–1.3ml diluted with some water, one to three times a day, tincture strength 2:1.
- Take yarrow tincture. **Adults**: 0.7–2ml diluted with some water, two to three times a day, tincture strength 1:2.
- Take hawthorn tincture, made from either flowers or fruits. **Adults**: 1–2ml diluted with some water, one to three times a day, tincture strength 1:2.

Varicose veins and haemorrhoids

Although these two problems have quite different causes, they can both improve with a similar herbal treatment. If you are not getting satisfactory results using the measures outlined below, you may need more specific herbs that are best taken after consultation with a medical herbalist.

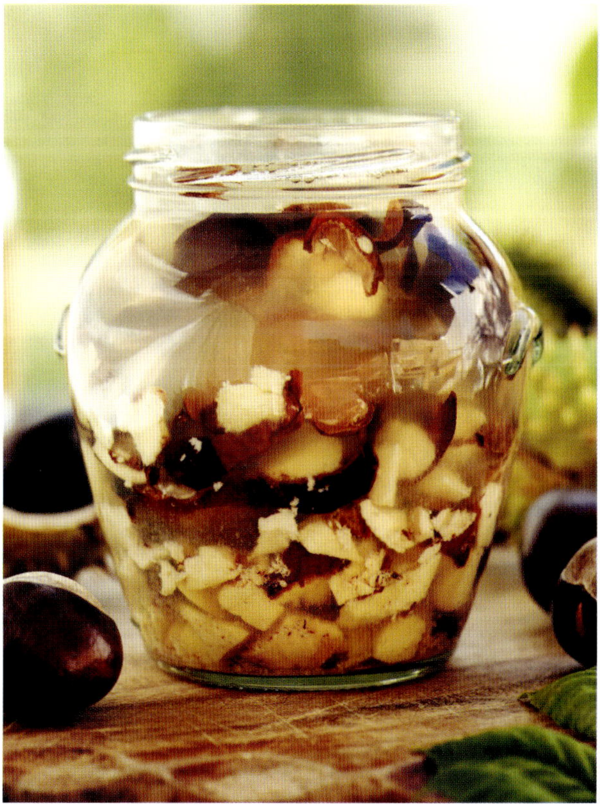

Right Horse chestnut tincture.

Treatment options

Please see pages 43–47 for herbal precautions.

- Take yarrow tincture. **Adults**: 0.7–2ml diluted with some water, one to three times a day, tincture strength 1:2.
- Drink yarrow tea for two to three weeks and for 3–12 months if the problem has been long-standing. **Adults**: 1–2 cups a day.
- Apply witch hazel ointment to the affected areas one to three times a day.
- Take horse chestnut tincture. For haemorrhoids you can take it until there is an improvement. For varicose veins you can take it continually to slow down the worsening of the condition. **Adults**: 0.7–1.7ml, one to three times a day, tincture strength 1:2.

Conditions for which home treatment is not recommended

- Leg ulcers: these usually affect older people or those with diabetes (see your GP for a diagnosis). An integrated herbal treatment is needed, which comprises an individual mix for internal use to improve the blood supply to the leg area, and a special dressing to apply externally.
- High blood pressure (significantly raised blood pressure): this is not suitable for home treatment, as it requires regular monitoring and adjustment of the prescription depending on the results.
- Minor heart problems (e.g. palpitations, stable angina): these respond very well to herbal treatment, but often require the use of herbs that are in the practitioner-only category.
- Very high cholesterol levels: you will need high doses of specific herbs, so this is best done under supervision.
- Frequent swelling of the legs and/or feet: this can indicate serious problems with the circulation, so it is best to see a health professional to establish the root cause of the problem.

When to seek medical attention

- If you experience chest pain, especially during exertion.
- If you have sudden, extremely painful headache and/or visual disturbances.
- If you have cellulitis, which is an inflammation of the skin due to a bacterial infection, usually somewhere on a limb. Symptoms include red, shiny skin, swelling, a lot of pain in the affected area and high temperature.

CHAPTER 8

The digestive system

The digestive system includes the mouth, oesophagus (gullet), stomach, small intestine (small bowel), large intestine (large bowel) and rectum. The liver and pancreas are two organs that are intimately connected to the digestive system and contribute vital secretions that enable proper digestion, but these organs are also involved in other functions. The liver is primarily a detoxifier in the body, but it has many functions – for example, it stores quite a few nutrients, it synthesises cholesterol, it produces essential plasma proteins and it removes worn-out red blood cells and some bacteria, to name just a few. The pancreas releases two important hormones into the bloodstream – insulin and glucagon – that regulate the glucose levels in your blood. Most diseases of the liver and pancreas tend to be of a serious nature, and I would advise you to seek professional help and not to attempt home treatment of these.

However, the rest of the digestive system is, in my experience, the easiest system to treat with herbs. The four herbs described below can treat most of the common stomach problems, such as ordinary indigestion, heartburn and bloating. They can be combined with each other or with other, more specific herbs. You can view these herbs as non-specific digestive aids – they bring almost immediate relief.

Nutrition

Herbal treatment of the digestive system is more successful if combined with a temporary change to your normal diet. Detailed advice on different diets for different ailments is beyond the scope of this book, but the general principle for

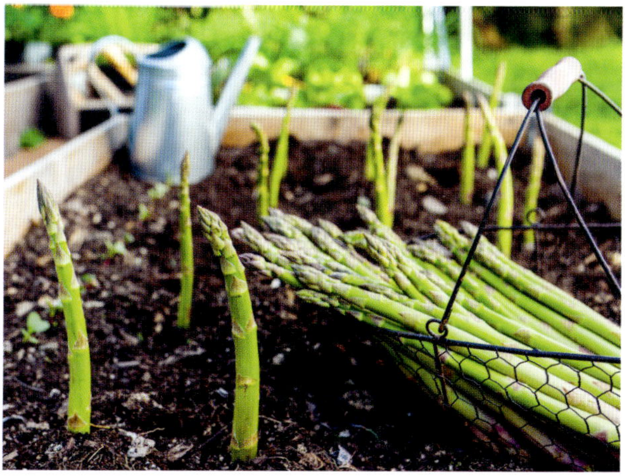

Right Asparagus is a good source of prebiotics and an easy, perennial crop to grow.

any digestive problem is to eat foods that are easily digestible, such as plain white rice, simple vegetable soup, plain semolina cooked with water, plain couscous, weak black tea, steamed vegetables, poached fish or chicken. It is also advisable to avoid stimulants such as coffee, fizzy drinks, strong tea and alcohol. You need to maintain a plain diet only for short periods of time, sometimes a day or two, until your digestive function returns to normal.

It goes without saying that a healthy diet is the foundation of a healthy digestive system, and that an unhealthy diet will sooner or later cause digestive problems.

The importance of a good microbiome

The microbes that live in your digestive system form a complex, diverse and ever-changing collection of many different species of bacteria. Nowadays they are called a microbiome or microbiota, and they are also often referred to simply as 'gut bacteria'. Some of these bacteria are more desirable than others, and the actual composition of the microbiome varies hugely from one individual to another. Most of the microbiome is thought to be acquired by the age of three, but the actual balance of the individual bacterial populations can vary depending on the environmental influences throughout a person's life, especially their diet. We now know that the greater the diversity of bacteria in your microbiome the healthier you will be and, conversely, the lower the diversity of bacteria the more likely you are to develop health problems.

Many digestive problems stem from having the wrong balance of bacteria in the gut. This can be an overgrowth or absence of specific species in your large intestine, or the presence of too many bacteria in your small intestine, known as small intestinal bacterial overgrowth (SIBO). Such an imbalance can be caused by having repeated courses of strong antibiotics, by ingesting unfamiliar bacteria when travelling abroad or by having an unhealthy diet. If you suspect that your bowel flora is not balanced, you can supplement your diet with probiotics or prebiotics. Probiotics are actual bacteria, usually the rod-shaped *Lactobacillus* or *Bifidobacterium* species. Prebiotics are the specific foods for the desirable species of bacteria, which if ingested can boost these bacterial populations. They can be taken in the form of supplements (e.g. partially hydrolysed guar gum or inulin) or you can increase your intake of foods containing prebiotics (e.g. onion, asparagus, all berries, green tea, dark chocolate, wholegrains).

According to current research we should aim to eat about 30 different varieties of plant food per week to maintain a good diversity of gut microbes.[11] Avoiding processed foods and instead cooking from scratch using organic and seasonal vegetables and fruit is a simple way to improve the diversity of your microbes. Looking after your microbiome will translate into benefits not only for your digestive system but also for your immune system, cardiovascular system and even your mental health.

Drink herbal teas

The digestive system responds well to remedies that come into direct contact with its mucous membrane lining. As the digestive tract has a large surface area, it is logical to use remedies that are available in large volumes in order to maximise such contact. Therefore teas are preferable to tinctures for stomach or bowel problems. *If you use a tincture for digestive ailments, dilute it with a full glass of lukewarm or warm water.*

Must-have herbs

The herbs in this section are arranged in order of usefulness.

Meadowsweet
Filipendula ulmaria

Caution is needed if you are allergic to salicylates. Seek professional advice if you are asthmatic, pregnant or breastfeeding.

Uses

You use the aerial parts of this herb: leaves, flowers and stems. Meadowsweet is extremely soothing for an irritated stomach or bowel, or for any inflammation of the digestive tract. Digestive discomfort is often relieved within minutes of drinking it. It is the tea to take after a late meal that is sitting too heavily, or to drink regularly if you suffer from acid reflux (heartburn), hiatus hernia or stomach over-acidity, and also if you are recovering from a stomach ulcer. It has antacid, astringent and anti-inflammatory properties. It can be used for virtually any digestive problem, and I strongly recommend that you include it among your home remedies.

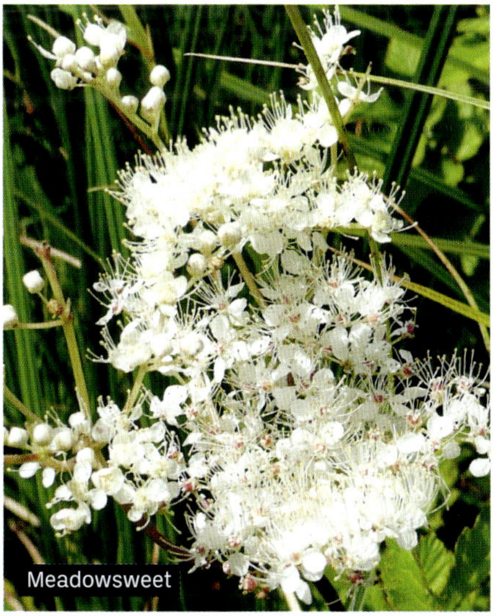
Meadowsweet

COMBINATIONS: Meadowsweet combines well with marshmallow root or with chamomile, either as a dried herb or as a tincture.

HOW TO TAKE IT: Meadowsweet is best taken as a tea and consumed after mealtimes. Brew fresh tea each time you need it and drink it warm. Fresh or dried herbs can be used. The tincture works almost as well as the tea, so long as you dilute each dose with a full glass of warm water.

DOSAGE: **Adults:** 1 cup of tea one to four times a day, or 1–2ml of tincture, one to three times a day diluted with some water, tincture strength 1:2.

Chamomile (German)
Matricaria recutita
(syn. *Chamomilla recutita*)

Caution is needed in people who are allergic to plants belonging to the daisy family (the Asteraceae, formerly known as the Compositae).

Uses

Also known as Hungarian chamomile (kamilla), wild chamomile, blue chamomile or scented mayweed, German chamomile is normally sold under the name of 'chamomile' or 'camomile' in shops and supermarkets, usually as tea bags. Chamomile is an excellent herb for soothing painful conditions of the digestive tract, reducing bloating and relaxing tension in the bowel. It is most useful for conditions associated with anxiety and stress – so-called 'nervous indigestion'.

For this reason it is often helpful for people with irritable bowel syndrome (IBS). Chamomile is very effective for children's tummy aches and for morning sickness in pregnant women.

COMBINATIONS: Chamomile combines well with peppermint, either as a dried herb or as a tincture.

HOW TO TAKE IT: Chamomile is best taken as an infusion. You can use either fresh or dried herbs to make the tea. If you decide to use a tincture, each dose should be diluted with a full glass of warm water.

DOSAGE: **Adults:** 1 cup of infusion two to three times a day, or 1–2ml diluted with some water, one to three times a day, tincture strength 1:2.

Children: It is safe to give chamomile tea to children over three years old so long as they are not prone to allergies. Young children need only a few teaspoonsful of the chamomile tea (3–5 years old), whereas older ones (6–9 years old) can have a quarter or half a cup. From 10 years old a full cup of chamomile tea can be drunk once or twice a day. You can improve the taste by adding a little honey.

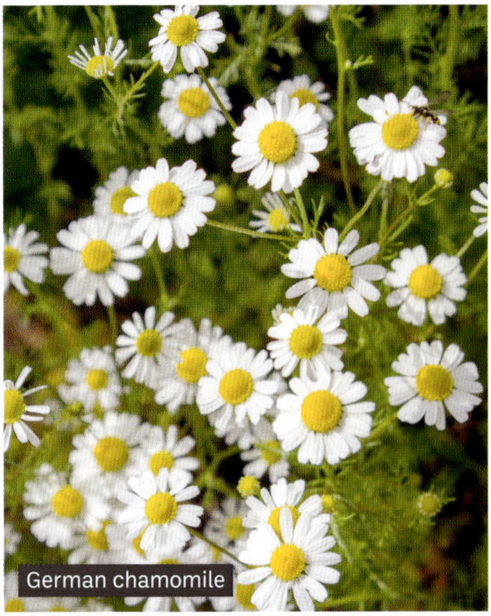

German chamomile

Peppermint *Mentha × piperita*

Peppermint essential oil should never be used internally.

Peppermint tea is not advised for children under four years.

Caution is needed if using peppermint tea or oil while breastfeeding.

Uses

This herb has a stimulating effect on the digestive process as well as a relaxing effect on the digestive tract. It will ease bloating and painful cramps caused by indigestion. Although peppermint helps to digest your food, it is easy to have too much of it, so in my view 2 cups of tea a day should be the limit. Peppermint tea can be too stimulating if you suffer from stomach overacidity, hiatus hernia, reflux or heartburn, but it often helps people with IBS by relaxing the smooth muscles of the intestines. Peppermint also makes a refreshing and cooling drink on a hot day.

COMBINATIONS: Peppermint combines well with chamomile, either as a tea or as a tincture.

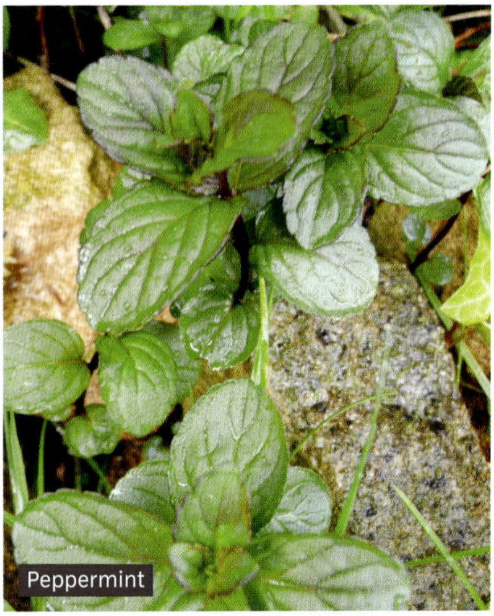

Peppermint

HOW TO TAKE IT: Peppermint works best as an after-dinner tea, but it can be taken before meals to improve the appetite. I would recommend using fresh leaves if these are available (use 5–10 leaves, torn into smaller pieces, per cup). Tincture can be used instead of tea, but remember to dilute each dose with a glass of warm water.
DOSAGE: **Adults:** 1 cup of infusion once or twice a day, or 0.5–1.4ml, one to three times a day, tincture strength 1:2.
Children (4–16 years): small amounts of peppermint tea can be given to children. Use just a few teaspoonful for 4- to 5-year-olds, and a quarter of a cup for 7- to 10-year-olds, but 11- to 16-year-olds can have a full cup. I suggest that you give this as just one dose to treat an occasional stomach ache, and not as a regular drink.

Marshmallow root powder *Althaea officinalis*

Marshmallow root powder can be taken with any conventional medication, but not at the same time – leave a two-hour gap between the two.

Uses

Marshmallow root powder provides a protective coating for the lining of the gut, as it releases its mucilage (a slippery, gluey substance) when mixed with water. This powder is a great option in any situation involving irritation or inflammation of the digestive tract, such as gastritis, heartburn, burning diarrhoea, diverticular disease, peptic ulcer, IBS or inflammatory bowel disease. I use marshmallow root powder instead of the powder from slippery elm bark, because the latter is seriously threatened in the wild.

HOW TO TAKE IT: You must always take marshmallow root powder with plenty of water (half a glass of water per teaspoonful

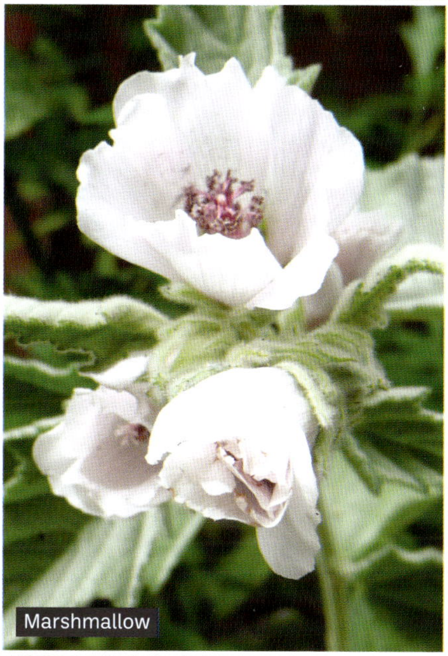

Marshmallow

of powder). Mix a teaspoonful of the powder with some water, and then add more water gradually until the mixture has the consistency of runny custard. Drink it quickly, and then drink a little more water to get rid of the taste. You can also mix a dose of marshmallow root powder with some yoghurt. Take the powder between meals for maximum effectiveness, and remember to leave a gap of two hours between taking it and any prescribed medication.
DOSAGE: **Adults:** 1 teaspoonful of powder, one to four times a day.

Medicinal charcoal tablets

Do not take charcoal tablets or charcoal biscuits habitually for indigestion or flatulence, as their long-term use may be harmful. Reserve them for emergencies.

Strictly speaking this is not a herbal product, but charcoal does come from plants – it is produced by heating wood with very little oxygen.

Uses

Charcoal tablets provide a very effective treatment for mild food poisoning and diarrhoea related to eating contaminated food. Charcoal works by binding to the bacterial toxins that cause the symptoms of food poisoning. This inactivates the toxins and reduces the symptoms while giving your body a chance to mount an immune response, which will get rid of the troublesome bacteria. Charcoal is not absorbed by the body but passes through the digestive tract unchanged, which means that it will stain the contents of your stomach black – so don't be alarmed if you happen to be sick! Your stools will also become very dark for a while.

COMBINATIONS: Charcoal tablets can be combined with any other herbal treatment for food poisoning or diarrhoea.
HOW TO TAKE IT: You can either swallow whole tablets with water or herbal tea, or you can crush the tablets into powder, mix this with some water and swallow the mixture. It is best to leave a short gap between taking the charcoal and herbs.
DOSAGE: **Adults:** Take 2 tablets with some water up to four times a day.

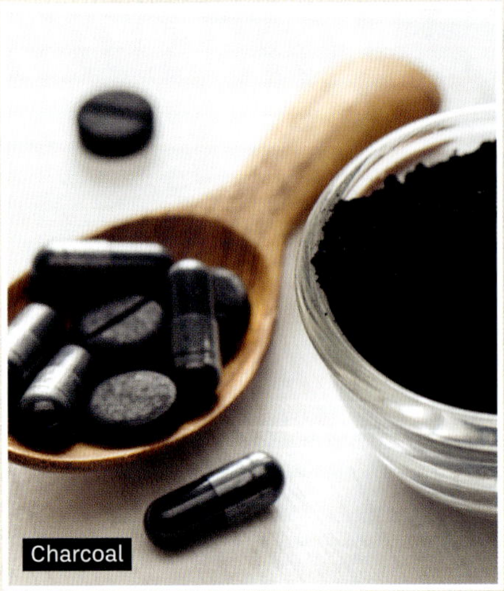
Charcoal

Optional herbs

Aniseed *Pimpinella anisum*

Caution is needed if you suffer from reflux or oestrogen-related conditions.

Uses

Also known as anise (but not to be confused with star anise), aniseed is an excellent remedy for bloating and sluggish digestion. It is a gentle stimulant for the digestive system as well as a carminative – that is, a herb that deals with excessive wind (too much gas caused by specific foods). It is a good alternative to peppermint for adults.

HOW TO TAKE IT: The best way to use this herb is to add a few drops of aniseed tincture to water or any other herbal tea and drink it after a meal. You can chew a few aniseed seeds directly if you like their liquorice-like flavour – this is a common habit in some curry houses, and it greatly aids digestion. I recommend occasional rather than habitual use.

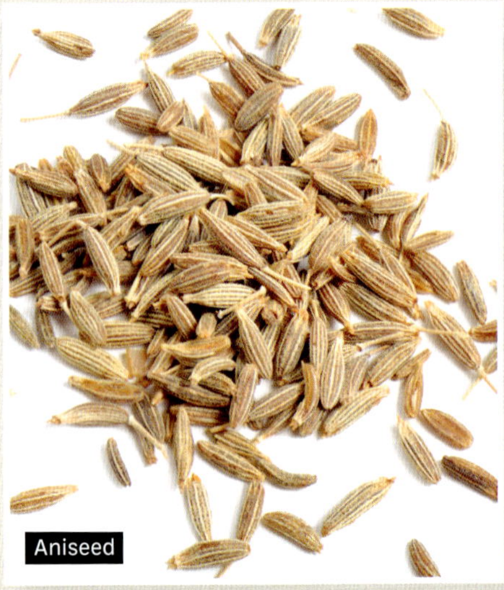
Aniseed

DOSAGE: Adults: 1–2ml diluted with some water, one to three times a day, tincture strength 1:2.

Barberry *Berberis vulgaris*

Do not ingest barberry when pregnant or breastfeeding. Care is needed if you have high blood pressure.

Uses

Otherwise known as berberis, this herb is an effective antimicrobial agent for infections of the digestive tract. It can be used to treat gastritis, food poisoning and diarrhoea of various origins.

COMBINATIONS: Barberry works well in combination with chamomile and witch hazel (see Diarrhoea entry on page 69).
HOW TO TAKE IT: A tincture is preferable to a tea. Take it either by itself or in combination with other herbs.
DOSAGE: Adults: 1–2ml diluted with some water, one to three times a day, tincture strength 1:2.

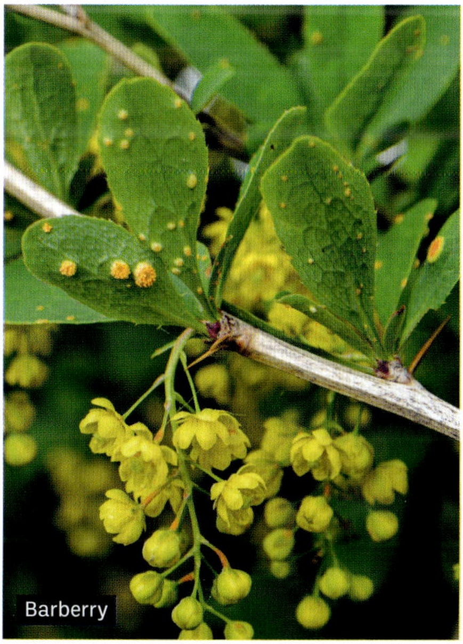
Barberry

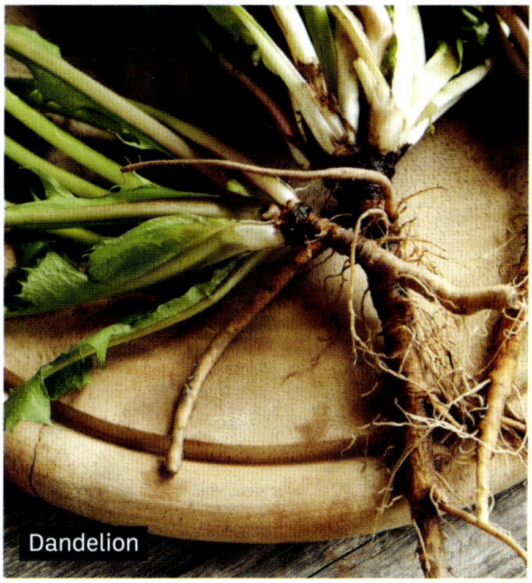
Dandelion

Dandelion root *Taraxacum officinale*

Caution is needed in people who are allergic to plants belonging to the daisy family (the Asteraceae, formerly known as the Compositae), and in those who have gall-bladder problems.

Uses

Both the root and leaves of dandelion are used medicinally, but for digestive complaints the root is the part that you need. Dandelion root stimulates the liver to produce more bile, which in turn improves digestion of fatty food. If you find that fatty food, such as bacon or full-fat cheese, makes you feel heavy and bloated, taking dandelion root will help. Olive oil is the healthiest of all fats and rarely causes digestive problems. The bitter taste of dandelion root is good for the whole digestive process, and may be used as a general digestive aid.

HOW TO TAKE IT: Dandelion root can be taken as an infusion, a decoction (stronger in taste and action than an infusion), dandelion coffee or a tincture. All of these have a bitter taste.

DOSAGE: Adults: 1 cup of decoction once or twice a day, or 1 cup of infusion once or twice a day, or 1 cup of dandelion coffee once or twice a day, or 1–2ml diluted with water, one to three times a day, tincture strength 1:2.

Fennel *Foeniculum vulgare*

Caution is needed if you are prone to heartburn (reflux). Women who are breastfeeding may experience an increase in milk production.

Uses

Fennel seeds (or aerial parts of the plant) help to relieve digestive problems that stem from bloating or excess gas. Fennel tea can be used for colicky pain, including baby colic. It is one of the options for IBS, as it has antispasmodic action. It is also useful in cases of poor appetite and nausea.

HOW TO TAKE IT: Fennel can be taken as an infusion or as a tincture. For infant colic it is best for the mother to drink a cup or two of fennel tea per day, as a small amount of the tea will find its way into the breast milk and then help with the baby colic. If the baby is on formula milk you can add 5–10 drops of freshly brewed and cooled fennel tea to a bottle.

DOSAGE: Adults: 1 cup of infusion once or twice a day, or 2–4ml diluted with water, one to three times a day, tincture strength 1:2.

Garlic *Allium sativum*

Do not take large doses for prolonged periods of time, or when pregnant or breastfeeding. Discontinue garlic 10 days before undergoing surgery. Garlic is not suitable for children under six.

Caution is needed in people who are taking anticoagulant or antiplatelet medication.

Uses

Garlic acts against a wide spectrum of bacteria that can cause digestive upsets. It can be used for mild food poisoning, traveller's diarrhoea, or as a preventative treatment when travelling in tropical countries. It can also be helpful for some worm infestations (see page 78).

HOW TO TAKE IT: Either fresh or processed garlic can be used for the treatment of digestive problems. Fresh garlic should be crushed or juiced, whereas processed garlic can be used in the form

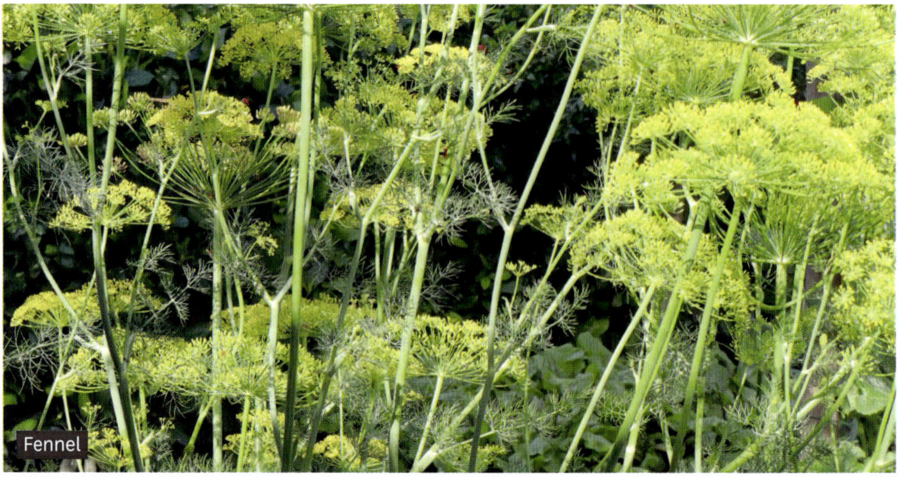
Fennel

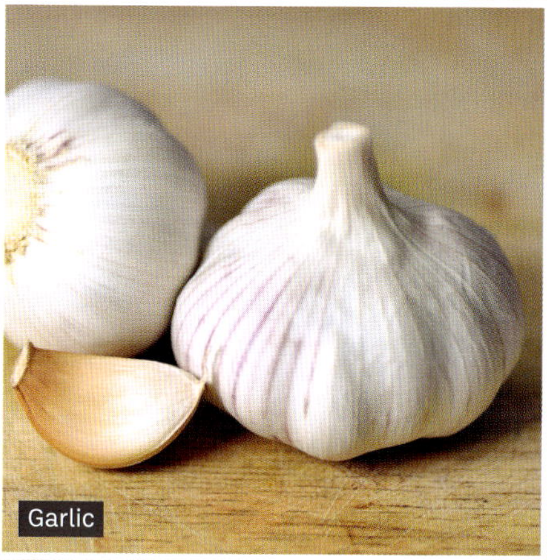

of a tincture, preserved juice, tablets or capsules.

Some people do not tolerate fresh garlic very well, so try a small amount if you have never taken it before. Young garlic is more likely to cause an adverse reaction. You can take garlic at the same time as demulcent (anti-irritant) herbs, such as marshmallow or linseed, to reduce the risk of irritation.
DOSAGE: **Adults**: 0.5–1g of dry powder equivalent in tablets or capsules, one to three times a day, or one crushed clove, one to three times a day, with plenty of water, or 2–4ml diluted with water, one to three times a day, tincture strength 1:1, or 1 teaspoonful of garlic juice diluted with water, one to three times a day.

Ginger *Zingiber officinale*

Caution is needed when breastfeeding, and in people with peptic ulceration or gallstones, or who are taking blood-thinning medications such as warfarin.
During pregnancy, intake should be limited to 2g/day of dried ginger.

Uses

Ginger is a warming herb that gently stimulates digestion. It also helps with nausea, including morning sickness and car or sea sickness.

COMBINATIONS: If you suffer from reflux, ginger tea may be slightly irritating for the inflamed gullet, so mix it with marshmallow leaf; otherwise drink it by itself or with a slice of lemon. You can add a slice of fresh ginger to green or black tea (with no milk).
HOW TO TAKE IT: Ginger is best taken as a tea, made with either a slice of fresh ginger (1g) or a teaspoonful of dried ginger powder (1g). Ginger tea bags are also very effective.
DOSAGE: **Adults**: 1 cup of infusion one to three times a day.

Lemon balm *Melissa officinalis*

Uses

Lemon balm makes a superb digestive tea that also has a relaxing effect and ensures good sleep. When it starts growing fresh in my garden in the spring and summer I often give it to my dinner guests at the end of the evening to aid their digestion, and many have commented on how well they slept afterwards. Lemon balm infusion, made from fresh leaves, has a wonderful green colour, a zesty scent and a fresh lemony taste. This tea, whether made from the fresh or dried herb, is good for people

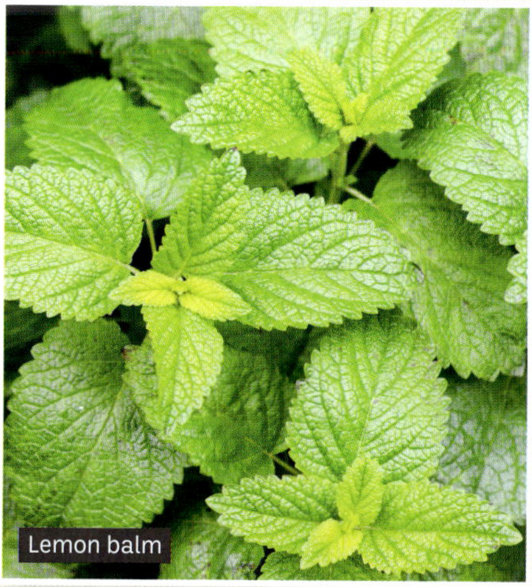

whose digestive problems stem from anxiety, as it is both a digestive aid and a relaxant to the nervous system.

COMBINATIONS: Lemon balm combines well with chamomile and/or meadowsweet, either fresh or dried.
HOW TO TAKE IT: Use a good handful of fresh leaves and young twigs, shredded into small pieces, per pint-sized teapot. You can add honey to this tea, or even a slice of lemon to enhance the natural taste. Dried lemon balm can be used to make tea outside the growing season, but is nowhere near as tasty. It is very hard to get a good-quality lemon balm tincture; tincture made from fresh herbs is preferable to that made from dried herbs.
DOSAGE: **Adults:** 1 cup of infusion one to three times a day, or 1–2ml diluted with some water, one to three times a day, tincture strength 1:2. I recommend using a lemon balm tincture made from a fresh plant.
Children: Lemon balm as tea can be given to children over four years old. Use just a few teaspoonful of tea for small children, a quarter of a cup for older children and a full cup for teenagers. I recommend this as an occasional treatment, but not as a regular drink.

Linseed *Linum usitatissimum*

Uses

I recommend using linseed to improve digestion in quite a range of situations. As a general rule you can use it when bowel movements are not regular, or when there is inflammation in any part of the digestive tract. Examples of ailments that will benefit from the daily use of linseed include constipation, diarrhoea, diverticular disease, IBS, gastritis and peptic ulcers. When using linseed for children it is best to strain the seeds and just use the liquid resulting from soaking (see below).

HOW TO TAKE IT: If you want to get the full benefit from linseed, you must soak it before use. The simplest way to do this is to put a tablespoonful of linseed in a cup, fill it with lukewarm water and leave it to stand overnight. Stir it well in the morning and drink both the liquid and the seeds. Eating dry linseed (many people sprinkle linseed on their cereal or salad) will be less effective, as the seeds will not have enough time to release the beneficial mucilage before they are excreted.
DOSAGE: **Adults:** 1–2 tablespoonful of soaked seeds, once a day.

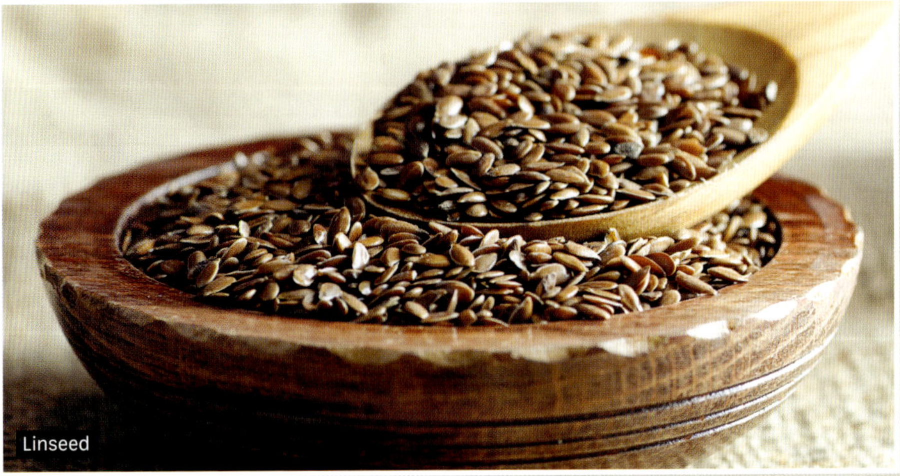

Linseed

Liquorice *Glycyrrhiza glabra*

Liquorice should not be taken during pregnancy, or by the elderly.
Do not take liquorice for a prolonged period if you have high blood pressure, low potassium levels, problems with your heart, kidneys or liver, or water retention.

Uses

Liquorice (or licorice) soothes the lining of the digestive tract and is therefore suitable for any condition that causes irritation of the intestinal lining. As such it is similar to marshmallow, but it also has a pronounced anti-inflammatory action. It is especially suitable for people who suffer from digestive problems due to stress, so long as they do not have high blood pressure (see below).

HOW TO TAKE IT: You can take liquorice either as a tincture or as a powder. The powder needs to be mixed with half a cup of water before it is swallowed. If you suffer from slightly raised blood pressure you can still use liquorice, but only in small doses and for short periods of time (half the normal dose for no longer than a week).
DOSAGE. **Adults**: 0.5–2ml diluted with some water, one to three times a day, tincture strength 1:1, or 1g of powder one to three times a day.

Milk thistle *Silybum marianum* (syn. *Carduus marianus*)

Milk thistle can have a hypoglycaemic effect (i.e. it can lower blood sugar), so its use is not recommended in people with type 2 diabetes on hypoglycaemic medication.

Caution is needed in people who are allergic to plants belonging to the daisy family (the Asteraceae, formerly known as the Compositae).

Uses

Milk thistle (also known as St Mary's thistle) is a very specific medicinal herb – the seeds are used mainly for liver and gall-bladder problems. It helps the liver to regenerate if it has been damaged by disease, and is appropriate for the liver that needs support in many situations. Its hepatoprotective capacity means that it can be used as a preventative measure to protect the liver cells (hepatocytes) from substances that can cause liver toxicity (e.g. some chemotherapy drugs and chemical toxins). It increases the production of bile and is therefore suitable for prevention of formation of gallstones, and it improves the cholesterol levels. It also has a reputation for helping to ameliorate a hangover.

HOW TO TAKE IT: As a tincture.
DOSAGE: **Adults**: 1.4–2.8ml diluted with some water, one to three times a day, tincture strength 1:1.

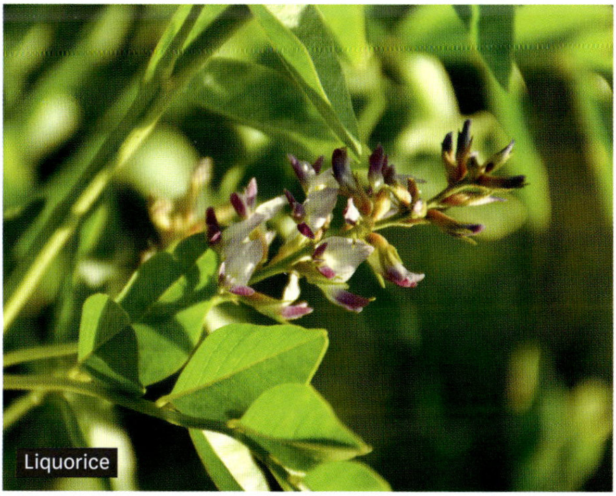
Liquorice

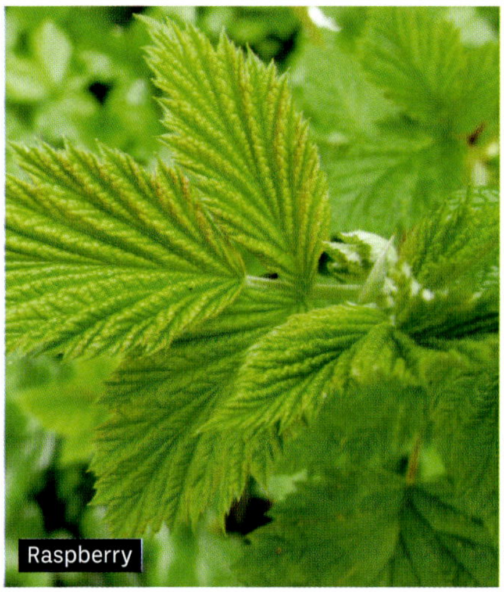

Raspberry

Raspberry leaf *Rubus idaeus*

Raspberry leaf is not recommended in the first trimester of pregnancy.

Uses

Raspberry leaf is a gentle astringent for the digestive system and provides a very pleasant-tasting tea that can be used to relieve diarrhoea of various origins. Generally it is not astringent enough to treat diarrhoea caused by food poisoning, but it is effective enough for a stomach bug (viral infection of the digestive tract), mild traveller's diarrhoea, children's diarrhoea, diarrhoea caused by antibiotics (in which case it is a good idea to take a probiotic supplement as well), some forms of IBS and even some cases of inflammatory bowel disease.

COMBINATIONS: It is best to mix raspberry leaf with meadowsweet and chamomile in equal quantities for the above purposes. You can use fresh or dried leaves, and although wild raspberry leaves are preferable, any garden variety can also be used, so long as it has not been sprayed with pesticides.

HOW TO TAKE IT: As a tea, either by itself or in a combination with meadowsweet and chamomile.
DOSAGE: **Adults:** 1 cup of an infusion, one to three times a day.

Witch hazel leaf *Hamamelis virginiana*

Uses

The primary use of witch hazel is for severe diarrhoea that results from eating or drinking something suspect. It is a very astringent herb and should therefore be reserved for extreme situations. Witch hazel is also used externally to treat haemorrhoids (see page 53).

COMBINATIONS: Witch hazel can be combined with an antimicrobial herb (barberry or garlic) and an anti-inflammatory herb (chamomile or liquorice) for the treatment of diarrhoea (see page 70 for details of mixing and dosage).
HOW TO TAKE IT: Witch hazel is best taken as a tincture.
DOSAGE: **Adults:** 1–2ml diluted with some water, one to three times a day, tincture strength 1:2.

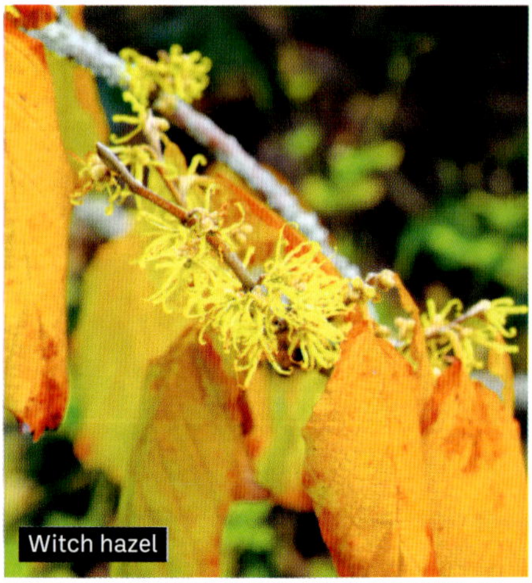

Witch hazel

Specific ailments affecting the digestive system, and herbs that can help

Appetite, lack of

Lack of appetite can be the result of an illness (including depression) or poor liver function. Bitter herbs can help to restore appetite and improve the general digestion. These herbs must be taken about 15–30 minutes before eating, and the bitter flavour needs to be 'tasted', which means that slow sipping is required rather than quick gulping. Many herbs have a bitter taste, and the degree of bitterness often depends on how long the herb is steeped for when making a tisane.

For the purpose of stimulating appetite, tinctures work as well as teas, so long as they taste bitter. If an illness is causing the appetite problem, try to treat that condition in the first place. If you are suffering from liver or gall-bladder disease, consult a herbalist before taking bitter herbs.

Below A simple non-herbal measure for improving the appetite is to increase your levels of exercise, especially swimming.

Treatment options

Please see pages 57–66 for herbal precautions.

- Drink strong chamomile tea.
  Adults: 1–2 cups a day, before meals.
- Take dandelion root tincture, diluted in half a cup of room-temperature water, and sip it slowly before meals.
  Adults: 1–2ml diluted with some water, three times a day, tincture strength 1:2.
- Drink dandelion root infusion.
  Adults: 1–2 cups a day.
- Take barberry tincture, diluted in half a cup of room-temperature water, and sip it slowly before meals.
  Adults: 1–2ml diluted with some water, three times a day, tincture strength 1:2.
- Add some warming herbs such as ginger or cinnamon powder to the bitter tea or tincture; put a pinch of either of the powders in the cup before brewing.

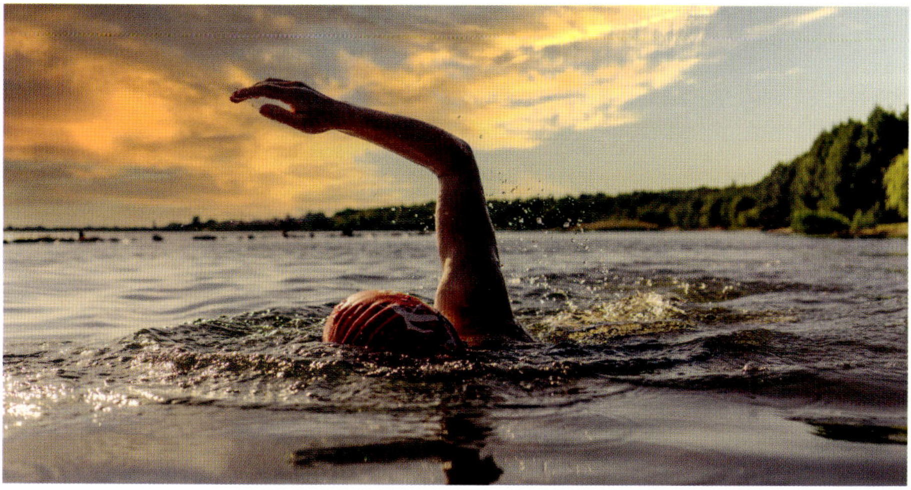

Bloating

Bloating is a subjective feeling of fullness in your abdomen that is not necessarily related to the actual expansion of your waistline or the amount of gas produced. It usually indicates poor digestive function and a shortage of 'gut-friendly' bacteria in your bowels. Sometimes people suffer from sensitivities to common foods such as wheat, yeast or cow's milk, so you could try removing such products from your diet for a while. Modern bread seems to cause bloating in many people, so try yeast-free breads based on sourdough. There are some foods, such as cabbage, beans and lentils, that almost everyone finds hard to digest – it is a good idea to add caraway seeds to these during cooking, to aid digestion. If you suffer from IBS, bloating will be one of the symptoms, and you will find that the herbs listed below offer relief. However, as IBS is a complex condition you will get much better overall results from treatment that is designed specifically for your particular symptoms.

Treatment options

Please see pages 57–66 for herbal precautions.

- Drink chamomile tea. **Adults:** 1 cup after each meal.
- Drink peppermint tea. **Adults:** 1 cup after lunch and 1 cup after dinner.
- Drink combined peppermint and chamomile tea. **Adults:** 1 cup after each meal.
- Supplement with probiotics for at least a month (follow the manufacturer's instructions); eating bio-yoghurts or kefir can be helpful as well.

Colic (baby colic)

Colic usually refers to baby colic – a painful condition that affects some babies. The treatment is either delivered through the mother's milk or added to formula milk. Use only tea – not a tincture – and only brew it for 2–3 minutes, so that it is not too strong.

Adults who experience a sudden colicky pain may be suffering from gallstones and must see a doctor. At times, both adults and children can experience colicky pain caused by trapped wind (see the treatment for excess wind on page 70).

Treatment options

- If you are breastfeeding, you can drink fennel tea, using one fennel tea bag per cup, and enough fennel will pass into the milk to get rid of your baby's colic – milk production may increase, too! **Breastfeeding mothers:** 1–2 cups a day.
- Add a tiny amount of fennel tea to the baby's formula milk. **Babies:** 5–10 drops per bottle.
- You can use chamomile tea in a similar way to fennel tea.

Constipation

Constipation is an extremely common condition that can have many different causes. It is often related to an unbalanced diet, lack of exercise and inadequate water intake. Soft fruit such as kiwis and plums will often resolve it, and you should also make sure that you consume about 2 litres of liquid every day (include all drinks and soup, but not coffee or alcohol, in that total). The herbs listed below can be used in pregnancy, unlike strong herbal laxatives, which should not be used.

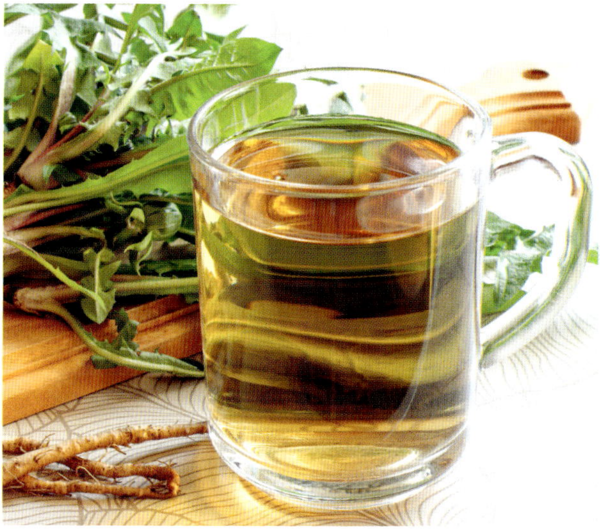

Above Dandelion root tea.

Treatment options

Please see pages 57–66 for herbal precautions.

- Take linseed. **Adults**: 1–2 tablespoonsful of linseed. Soak the seeds in a cup of warm water overnight, and drink both the liquid and the seeds in the morning. Strain the seeds if you are giving linseed to a child.
- Drink dandelion root tea – this herb stimulates the liver and improves overall digestion. **Adults**: 1–2 cups a day, or 1 cup during pregnancy.
- Take dandelion tincture. **Adults**: 1–2ml diluted with some water, one to three times a day, tincture strength 1:2.

Diarrhoea

Diarrhoea is a symptom of many different diseases. The recommendations for treatment included here refer to the simple, occasional looseness of stool that we all experience after a suspect meal or when eating unfamiliar food abroad. If your diarrhoea does not improve within 24 hours or is exceptionally watery you must seek medical help, as there is a danger of dehydration. This is especially important with small children, who can rapidly become dehydrated, so make sure that they have plenty to drink. Water with lemon juice and honey is suitable, or any diluted fruit juice.

Very strong black tea (with no milk or sugar) can be helpful for diarrhoea if you have no access to other medication. Oral rehydration powder (e.g. Dioralyte) available from the chemist should be taken if your diarrhoea is severe and lasts longer than a day.

Treatment options

Please see pages 57–66 for herbal precautions.

- Take a specific 'anti-diarrhoea tincture mix' (see box, below). In my own experience this mix has proved very effective on a number of occasions when I was travelling.
- It is a good idea to take charcoal tablets as well as the above tincture mix, as charcoal absorbs the toxins produced by the bacteria that cause diarrhoea. It is better to take the tincture first, and to follow it with the charcoal tablets about 10–15 minutes later, otherwise the charcoal may inactivate some of the herbal constituents of the tincture. **Adults**: 2 tablets up to four times a day (a maximum total of 8 tablets a day).
- Take marshmallow root powder, especially if there is a burning sensation associated with the diarrhoea.

Adults: 1 teaspoonful of powder mixed with water, one to three times a day.

- Meadowsweet or chamomile tea can be very effective for treating mild diarrhoea in children. **Adults:** 2–4 cups a day. **Children:** 3–5 years, 5–10 teaspoonsful a day; 6–12 years, 1–2 cups a day; older children, 2–4 cups a day.

Anti-diarrhoea tincture mix

Please see pages 57–66 for herbal precautions.

INGREDIENTS

- 30ml witch hazel leaf tincture (1:2)
- 40ml barberry tincture (1:2)
- 40ml chamomile tincture (1:2)

METHOD

1. Mix the ingredients together.
2. Pour the mixture into a clean, dark glass bottle.
3. Label the bottle with the contents and the date.
4. Store at room temperature for up to a year.

ADULT DOSE: 10ml diluted with some water, two to four times a day for 1–2 days; then reduce the dose to 5ml, one to three times a day until the symptoms improve.

Excess wind

Production of too much wind can be a result of diet, such as a vegetarian diet with a lot of lentils, or it can be related to having the wrong balance of bacteria in the gut, which may result from taking a lot of antibiotics. Occasionally, specific foods may need to be excluded from the diet. Flatulence is often accompanied by indigestion, and leads to bloating or colicky pain.

Treatment options

Please see pages 57–66 for herbal precautions.

- Drink fennel tea after meals. **Adults:** half a cup to 1 cup, one to three times a day.
- Drink peppermint tea. **Adults:** 1 cup twice a day.
- Take aniseed tincture. **Adults:** 1–2 ml diluted with some water, one to three times a day, tincture strength 1:2.
- Take probiotics for a month, according to the manufacturer's instructions.

Food intolerances

These are often incorrectly referred to as food allergies – true food allergies result in much more severe symptoms, including anaphylactic shock. Food intolerance leads to digestive discomfort after eating a particular food type, sometimes with headache and sometimes with skin rashes (eczema). Such food sensitivities seem to be very common nowadays.

Herbalists often recommend that you improve your digestive function and the condition of your intestines, rather than trying to exclude half the foods from your diet.

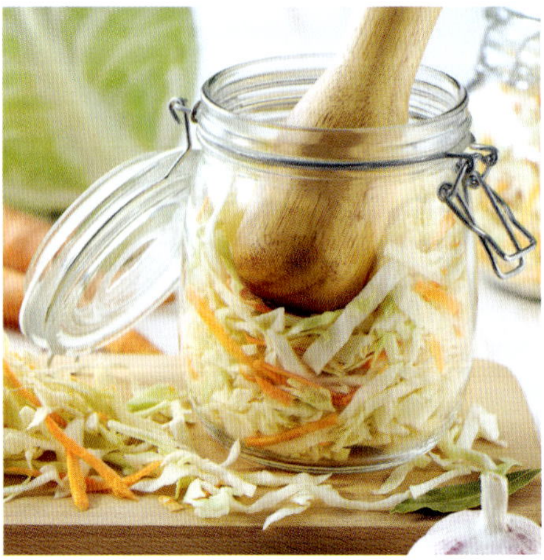

Right Fermented cabbage and carrots are a good probiotic.

Tea for reducing food intolerances (1)

Please see pages 57–66 and 135 for herbal precautions.

INGREDIENTS

- 50g dried meadowsweet aerial parts
- 50g dried marshmallow root
- 50g dried marigold flowers

METHOD

1. Mix the herbs thoroughly.
2. Infuse 2 teaspoonful of the mixture in a cup of freshly boiled water for 10 minutes.
3. Strain and drink while still warm. You can add honey to this tea.

ADULT DOSE: 1–2 cups a day, separately from meals.

Tea for reducing food intolerances (2)

Please see pages 57–66 for herbal precautions.

INGREDIENTS

- 50g dried barberry
- 50g dried chamomile
- 50g dried marshmallow root

METHOD

1. Mix the herbs thoroughly.
2. Infuse 2 teaspoonful of the mixture in a cup of freshly boiled water for 10 minutes.
3. Strain and drink while still warm. You can add honey to this tea.

ADULT DOSE: 1–2 cups a day, separately from meals.

Treatment options

- Take probiotics for at least a month, according to the manufacturer's instructions.
- Improve your digestive function by combining a bitter herb with a restorative and a demulcent herb in a tea and drinking it on a daily basis until the symptoms improve. Two examples are given above.

Food poisoning

Seek medical help if symptoms persist for more than a few hours or are very severe.

Food poisoning usually develops rapidly a few hours after eating a contaminated meal. The main symptoms include severe stomach ache, nausea, vomiting and, later on, diarrhoea.

Treatment options

Please see pages 57–66 for herbal precautions.

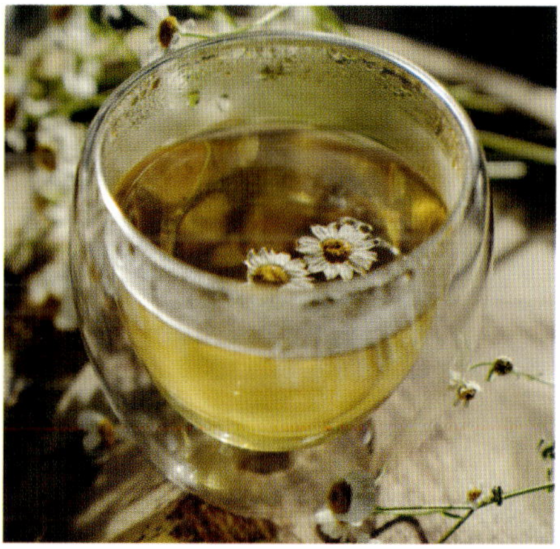

Above Chamomile tea.

- Take charcoal tablets with some water if you can manage to keep them down! **Adults**: 2 tablets every 2 hours, up to 8 tablets a day, with plenty of water.
- Drink strong chamomile tea to reduce the stomach irritation. **Adults**: 1–3 cups a day.
- Use the anti-diarrhoea mix (see page 70) if diarrhoea is a prominent feature.

Gall bladder, removed

If you have had your gall bladder removed because of gallstones, you may experience digestive problems for a while. There may be urgency of bowel movement, looseness of stools, and aches and pains in the abdomen. The symptoms are caused by the irritating effect of bile that is released into the digestive tract all the time, even in the absence of food. Make sure that you eat little and often, and that each meal includes a small amount of food that contains fat (e.g. cheese, meat, fish, salad with an olive oil dressing). The purpose of this is to make use of your bile to digest fat, thus reducing the amount of 'unused' bile which irritates the bowels. You can also use soothing, demulcent herbs as teas to reduce the irritation.

Treatment options

Please see pages 57–66 for herbal precautions.

- Drink chamomile tea. **Adults**: 1–2 cups a day.
- Drink marshmallow leaf tea. **Adults**: 1–2 cups a day.
- Take marshmallow root powder. **Adults**: 1 teaspoonful mixed with water, once or twice a day.
- Take linseed. **Adults**: pre-soak 1 tablespoonful of linseed in a cup of boiled water that has been allowed to cool; stir and drink the water with the seeds in the morning.

Gum problems

If your gums are inflamed or they bleed when you brush your teeth, these might be early signs of gum disease. A visit to a dentist is essential, and you may have to improve your oral hygiene routine. There may be nutritional deficiencies in your

Mouthwash mix (1)

Please see pages 57, 136 and 163 for herbal precautions.

INGREDIENTS

- 30ml sage (tincture strength 1:2)
- 40ml chamomile (tincture strength 1:2)
- 30ml thyme (tincture strength 1:2)

METHOD

1. Mix the ingredients together.
2. Pour the mixture into a clean, dark glass bottle.
3. Label the bottle with the contents and the date.
4. Store at room temperature for up to a year.

ADULTS: Dilute 1ml of the tincture mix with 40ml of water and swirl it around your mouth for about 1 minute, twice a day, after brushing your teeth.

Mouthwash mix (2)

Please see pages 116, 135 and 163 for herbal precautions.

INGREDIENTS

- 30ml propolis (tincture strength 1:5)
- 40ml sage (tincture strength 1:2)
- 30ml marigold (tincture strength 1:2)

METHOD

1. Mix the ingredients together.
2. Pour the mixture into a clean, dark glass bottle.
3. Label the bottle with the contents and the date.
4. Store at room temperature for up to a year.

ADULTS: Dilute 1ml of the tincture mix with 40ml of water and swirl it around your mouth for about 1 minute, twice a day, after brushing your teeth.

diet, and specific supplements may be suggested by a health practitioner. Recent research has demonstrated the importance of a good oral microbiome for the control of gum disease.

Treatment options

- Take propolis tablets/capsules for a few weeks, according to the manufacturer's instructions (see page 116 for precautions).
- Use a herbal mouthwash (see boxes opposite) on a daily basis until there is an improvement. You can use the same herbs (dried or fresh) to brew tea and use it as a mouthwash if you don't want to add any alcohol (omit the propolis, as it will not dissolve in water).

Haemorrhoids (piles)

Practitioner treatment is recommended for this condition.

Haemorrhoids are a troublesome problem at the very end of the digestive tract! Make sure that you do not get constipated, as this can make the problem worse. If the haemorrhoids don't improve quickly as a result of external application of the cream described below you may need an internal treatment from a herbalist.

Treatment options

Please see page 135 for herbal precautions.

- Apply a compress of warm marigold tea to the anus two to five times a day. Use small pieces of cotton wool rather than cloth – soak each one thoroughly, hold it pressed gently against the haemorrhoids until the tea cools down, and then use another piece to repeat the procedure.
- Apply plain marigold cream or ointment to the anus twice a day.
- Apply the cream described below to the anus two to three times a day.

Cream for haemorrhoids

Please see page 135 for herbal precautions.

INGREDIENTS

- 25g marigold cream
- 5ml witch hazel tincture or witch hazel distilled water

METHOD

1. Mix the cream and the tincture well.
2. Transfer the mixture to a clean, dark glass jar, and make sure that any air pockets are removed.
3. Store for up to 12 months.

ADULTS: Apply to the anus twice a day. Note: This cream may sting initially.

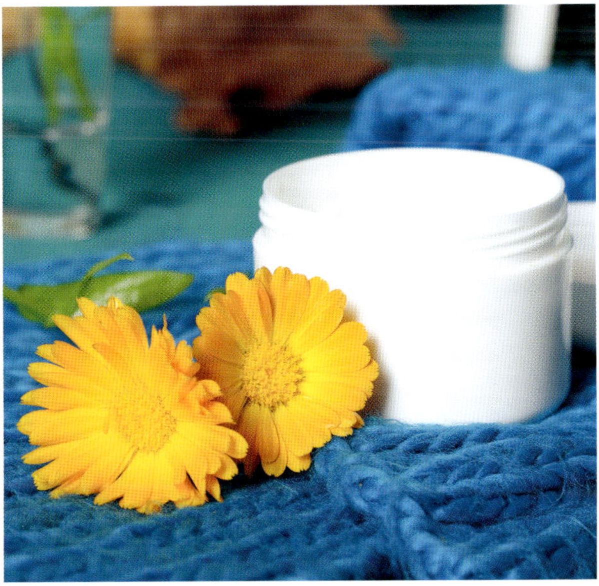

Right Marigold cream.

Heartburn, hiatus hernia and gastro-oesophageal reflux

Practitioner treatment is recommended for this condition.

If you are pregnant, or have high blood pressure or water retention, you can use liquorice on a one-off basis, but do not use it regularly.

Heartburn is a burning pain behind the sternum (breastbone) which results from hiatus hernia or acid reflux. The pain is caused by stomach acid entering the oesophagus (gullet or foodpipe) and irritating its surface. Sometimes this pain causes chest tightness and is similar to that of angina (a type of chest pain caused by a heart condition), so if you are not sure, check your symptoms with your GP. Heartburn is often related to diet, stress level, lifestyle or being overweight, or to a condition called hiatus hernia, which all need to be addressed to resolve the problem permanently.

Occasionally babies suffer from reflux, but I would not recommend treating this at home.

Treatment options

Please see pages 57–66 for herbal precautions.

- Take marshmallow root powder when you experience the symptoms. **Adults:** 1 teaspoonful of the powder mixed with enough lukewarm water to give it a 'runny custard' consistency; after you have swallowed it you can take a sip of water to get rid of the taste. Such a marshmallow 'meal' can bring almost instant relief. Repeat if necessary after about 20 minutes.
- Take liquorice root powder in a similar manner to the marshmallow root powder.
- Drink meadowsweet tea. **Adults:** 1–3 cups a day.
- Drink marshmallow root tea. **Adults:** 1–3 cups a day.
- Drink lemon balm tea regularly if your heartburn is related to stress. **Adults:** 1–2 cups a day.

Mouth ulcers

Mouth ulcers can have a number of different causes. Sometimes they can result from using a harsh detergent in the dishwasher, or not rinsing the dishes properly after washing up, or they may be due to a scratch caused by eating an abrasive food or by brushing your teeth too vigorously. However, the frequent presence of multiple mouth ulcers can indicate a weakened immune system or even a serious dysfunction of the digestive system, so in this case you should seek professional advice.

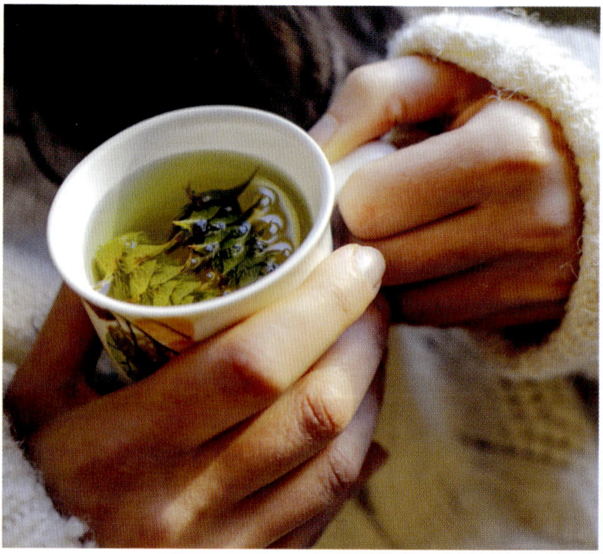

Right Sage tea.

Gargle with propolis tincture diluted in water

METHOD

1. Dilute 1ml of propolis tincture in 40ml of water (for precautions see page 116).
2. ADULTS: gargle two to five times a day for 30 seconds. The solution may sting initially.

Treatment options

Please see pages 57, 135 and 163 for herbal precautions. All of the tea gargles listed below are suitable for children over four years old. However, I do not recommend the propolis tincture as a gargle for children.

- Gargle with chamomile tea every hour for 1–2 minutes until you feel an improvement.
- Gargle with marigold tea every hour for 1–2 minutes until you feel an improvement.
- Gargle with sage tea every two hours for 1 minute until you feel an improvement.

Morning sickness

Morning sickness is nausea and vomiting that affects most women during the first three months of pregnancy. Eating something such as a sweet or savoury biscuit first thing in the morning, before getting up, can help a lot, as will a cup of warm herbal tea. The herbal teas recommended below should be fairly weak – either use tea bags or reduce the normal brewing time to 1–2 minutes if using dried herbs.

Nausea and vomiting that persist beyond the first three months of pregnancy need professional attention.

Treatment options

Please see pages 57–66 for herbal precautions.

- Drink ginger tea – use a ginger tea bag, half a teaspoonful of ginger powder or a slice of fresh ginger per cup of water, and add lemon and honey if you wish. Alternatively, simply add a slice of ginger to any weak tea without milk. **Adults**: 1–3 cups a day.
- Drink chamomile tea – use a chamomile tea bag or a teaspoonful of dried herbs per cup of water. **Adults**: 1–3 cups a day.

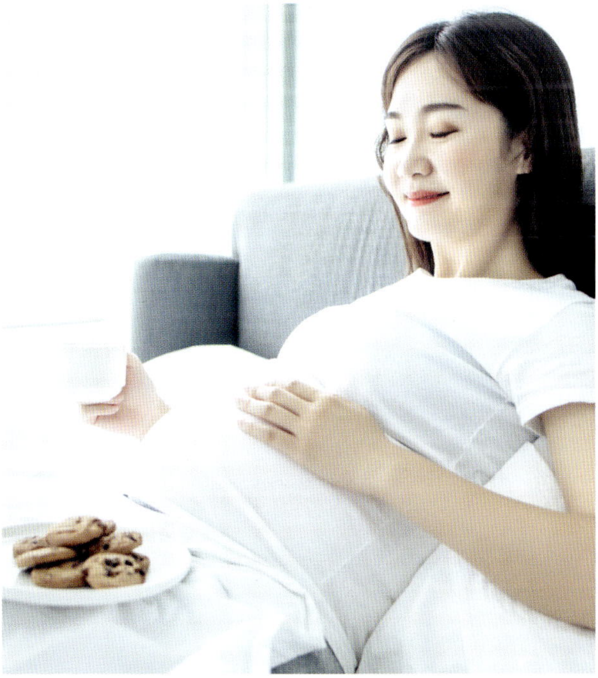

Right For morning sickness, you can make herbal tea the previous evening and store it in a thermos by your bed, so it's ready as soon as you wake up.

Nausea

Nausea can accompany many conditions that upset the digestive system. Sometimes it is not related to the digestive system at all – for instance, people with migraines often feel sick, as do people with inner-ear problems. The measures described refer to feeling sick after eating some suspect food or having a stomach bug.

Treatment options

Please see pages 57–66 for herbal precautions.

- Drink peppermint tea. **Adults:** 1–2 cups a day.
- Drink chamomile tea. **Adults:** 1–3 cups a day.

Prevention of digestive problems while on holiday

There are a few simple rules that will help you to avoid stomach problems when travelling abroad.

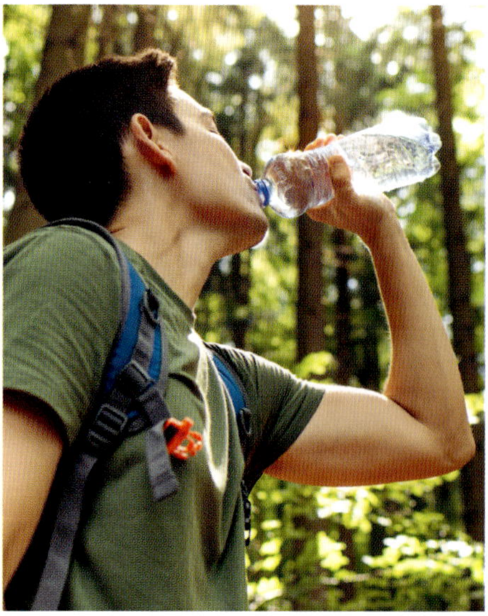

Above Bottled drinks reduce the risk of drinking contaminated water.

- Don't drink anything but boiled or bottled drinks.
- Don't have any ice in your drinks.
- Avoid salads and any fruit that cannot be peeled.
- Make sure that food is well cooked when eating out.
- Be fastidious about washing your hands after going to the toilet and before handling any food. Always use water and soap or a hand sanitiser.

If you are going somewhere exotic and remote you may want to take charcoal tablets and anti-diarrhoea mix (see page 70) with you, as a precaution.

Preventative measures

Please see pages 57–66 for herbal precautions.

- Eat fresh garlic every day. **Adults:** one clove of garlic, crushed and mixed with a teaspoonful of honey, once or twice a day.
- Take a single dose of charcoal tablets and anti-diarrhoea mix (see page 70) if you have eaten or drunk something that has the potential to cause a problem.

Stomach ache

A hot-water bottle applied to the stomach area can often relieve this symptom, especially if the pain is caused by trapped wind. Persistent and severe pain that does not improve in response to the measures listed below needs to be checked by a health professional.

Treatment options

Please see pages 57–66 for herbal precautions.

- Drink peppermint tea. **Adults:** 1–2 cups a day.

- Drink chamomile tea. **Adults**: 1–3 cups a day.
- Drink lemon balm tea if the stomach ache is caused by stress or anxiety. **Adults**: 1–3 cups a day.
- Take some marshmallow root powder or liquorice root powder if the pain has a burning quality (see Heartburn entry on page 74).

Stomach acidity, low

This condition is difficult to diagnose, as it may mimic other conditions. It is usually identified in association with other health problems, such as food sensitivities or skin disorders, so seek a professional opinion if you suspect low stomach acidity. It is more common in older people.

Herbalists treat low acidity by stimulating the production and release of stomach acid with bitter herbs. These must be taken 15–30 minutes before eating and the bitter flavour needs to be 'tasted', so you need to sip the herbs slowly. You can use either teas or tinctures so long as they taste bitter! Each of the tinctures listed below can be used by itself, or you can combine any two of them. Eating bitter foods such as chicory also helps.

Treatment options

Please see pages 57–66 for herbal precautions.

- Drink strong chamomile tea. **Adults**: 1–2 cups a day, before meals.
- Take dandelion root in a tincture form. **Adults**: 1–2ml, one to three times a day, tincture strength 1:2. Dilute each dose in half a cup of lukewarm water and sip slowly.
- Take barberry in a tincture form. **Adults**: 1–2ml, one to three times a day, tincture strength 1:2. Dilute each dose in half a cup of lukewarm water and sip slowly.

Stomach acidity, high

Practitioner treatment is recommended for this condition.

High stomach acidity is often related to stress. If this is the case, it may be worth taking relaxing herbs long term to deal with the effects of stress (see Chapter 10). There may also be other factors at play, such as diet or genetic predisposition. The most common symptoms include heartburn, bloating and stomach pain. Make sure that you get a proper diagnosis, rather than treating the condition on the basis of an assumption, as the symptoms of low stomach acidity may be remarkably similar. The measures listed below will make you more comfortable, but it may be challenging to get rid of the symptoms permanently by yourself.

Treatment options

Please see pages 57–66 for herbal precautions.

- Drink chamomile and meadowsweet tea, mixed in equal proportions. **Adults**: 3 cups a day, reducing this to 1 cup a day once the symptoms improve.
- Take marshmallow root powder, which will protect the stomach lining from possible damage. **Adults**: 1 teaspoonful mixed with half a cup of water, three times a day, between meals.

Vomiting

Vomiting is in one respect a healthy sign that your body is trying to get rid of something harmful. Therefore you should not try to suppress it, but allow yourself plenty of rest and take little sips of water, ordinary black tea or chamomile tea after you have been sick. The most common reasons for vomiting are food or alcohol poisoning or a 'tummy bug' (usually a viral infection). However, vomiting is not always directly linked to a problem in your stomach – it can be a sign of other conditions, such as migraine, concussion, meningitis or inner-ear problems. A baby or small child who keeps being violently sick should be taken to a doctor without delay, as there is a danger that they will rapidly become dehydrated.

Treatment options

- Drink weak chamomile tea in small amounts until the symptoms improve. You can give this tea to children over four years old, a teaspoonful at a time.
- Take charcoal tablets if you suspect food poisoning. Even if you are sick after taking the tablets, you will derive some benefit as the charcoal dissolves and acts rapidly once swallowed. **Adults**: 2 tablets up to four times a day.

Worms (intestinal parasites)

Practitioner treatment is recommended for this condition.

The most common worms are threadworms, and the treatment options described below refer to these. Try the recommended options for a couple of weeks. If they do not work, a pharmacy or medical herbalist may prescribe stronger worm-killing herbs.

Treatment options

- Take fresh garlic. **Adults:** one chopped clove mixed in a teaspoonful of honey, three times a day. **Children (6–16 years):** Raw garlic is not suitable for children under six years old, and for that age group I would suggest garlic capsules taken according to the manufacturer's instructions.
- Eat plenty of freshly grated carrots or drink carrot juice every day (do not continue this for more than two weeks). Note that the skin can become slightly yellow if you drink a lot of carrot juice – this is harmless and will disappear when you stop drinking the juice. **Adults:** 3–4 carrots a day. **Children (4–12 years):** 1–2 small carrots a day.
- Munch on pumpkin seeds during the day. **Adults:** a handful of seeds a day. **Children (4–12 years):** half a handful of seeds a day (you can add ground pumpkin seeds to yoghurt or cereal).

Below Carrot juice is useful for treating worm infestation.

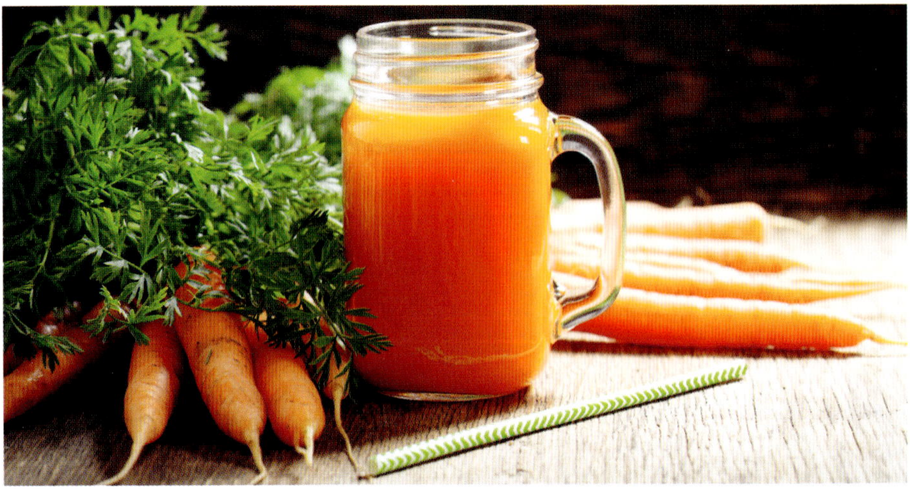

Conditions for which home treatment is not recommended

- Irritable bowel syndrome: herbalists recognise many variants of IBS, and the treatment will vary accordingly; this individualised approach leads to a very high rate of permanent relief from the symptoms.
- Ulcerative colitis and Crohn's disease: the treatment for both conditions requires specific protocols for diet and herbs, and as these patients are often on steroids the treatment needs to be supervised in collaboration with a GP or a consultant gastroenterologist.
- Stomach and duodenal ulcers: these are potentially dangerous conditions that respond remarkably well to herbal treatment; it is possible to combine orthodox and herbal treatment to improve the outcome.
- Liver disease: herbalists can help in many situations, but it is best to work in collaboration with your GP in order to monitor liver function.
- Gall-bladder disease (gallstones): treating gallstones with home remedies can be dangerous, as a gallstone can lodge in the duct that leads out of the gall bladder and cause serious complications.
- Diverticulitis: this requires a comprehensive review of diet and lifestyle as well as the use of individually appropriate herbs.
- Small intestinal bacterial overgrowth (SIBO): this requires appropriate testing for diagnosis, and a specific treatment protocol.
- Stomach or bowel cancer: herbalists are not allowed to treat cancer itself, but they can often offer treatments to reduce the side effects of the orthodox treatment.

When to seek medical attention

- If you experience persistent, intense pain in your abdomen, with or without fever.
- If you see blood in your stools (this will look red if the bleeding occurs from the lower digestive tract, but if the bleeding comes from the upper digestive tract it will look more like coffee grains in the stools, or the stools will become black).
- If you have stomach pain and/or diarrhoea and high temperature.
- If you notice a major change in your bowel habit without any obvious reason, and that change persists.
- If you become very weak or your child becomes 'floppy' after being repeatedly sick or having severe diarrhoea – this is a sign of dangerous levels of dehydration.

CHAPTER 9

The muscular and skeletal systems

The muscular system consists of all the muscles and ligaments in the body that are attached to the bones. The heart and the smooth muscles that are present in the digestive and circulatory systems are also muscle tissues, but cannot usually be voluntarily controlled. The skeletal system comprises all of the bones, including the skull and the spine, as well as all of the joints that articulate the bones. Because the muscular and skeletal systems are so intimately connected it makes sense to discuss them together.

Safety and compatibility

Many common problems associated with joints and muscles can be safely treated at home, and herbs have much to offer in terms of pain and inflammation control. However, some of the recommended remedies (e.g. arnica) need to be used in a specific way, otherwise they can be potentially harmful. Moreover, some herbal remedies may not be compatible with conventional medication for joint disorders. In such cases a professional herbal clinician will be able to advise you on alternative botanicals that can work alongside the orthodox medication – these can also offset the side effects of medication used for the treatment of advanced arthritis, and help you to recover from orthopaedic procedures, for instance, a hip replacement.

Other therapies

There are many complementary therapies (e.g. osteopathy) that can relieve joint and muscle problems, especially back problems. Herbal medicine works extremely well in conjunction with such therapies, and I would encourage you to combine herbs with another therapy of your choice to deal with problems that are mechanical in nature, such as strain injuries, misalignment and bad posture, among others.

Supplements

Both the muscular system and the skeletal system often benefit from specific supplementation that improves the rate of healing and reduces inflammatory tendencies. The need for such supplementation should be individually assessed by a specialist, taking into account your age, lifestyle and diet. Medical herbalists can advise you on both the appropriate herbal remedies and nutritional measures.

Must-have herbs

The herbs in this section are arranged in order of usefulness.

Arnica *Arnica montana*

For external use only. Do not apply arnica to open skin injuries.

Caution is needed in people who are allergic to plants belonging to the daisy family (the Asteraceae, formerly known as the Compositae).

Uses

This herb provides the best treatment for bruising and should be used only in cream, gel or ointment form. Any bumps, knocks or sprains, if treated immediately with arnica, will have minimal swelling and bruising and will heal much more quickly. This is an ideal treatment for children who have bumped their heads – a quick application of arnica cream to the injured spot (so long as the skin is not broken) will ease the pain within minutes, and no blue bump will develop. I have used it on fingers trapped in doors, toes crushed by heavy stones, innumerable bumps on the head and swollen knees after skiing – always with amazing results.

HOW TO APPLY IT: Arnica is not suitable for internal use as it can be quite toxic unless it is in a homeopathic form. For the same reason you should not apply it to open wounds and cuts, as too much arnica can then be absorbed into the bloodstream. However, it is safe to apply the ointment well away from the cut – keep a 2–3cm gap between the margin of the cut and the cream application, and apply a thinner layer of arnica than you would use for unbroken skin, where it can be applied quite liberally. Applying arnica to injuries that are more than one day old is less effective – it is very much a first-aid item that must be applied *as soon as possible after the injury* to prevent local haemorrhage and swelling.

HOW OFTEN TO USE IT: Normally, one generous application is sufficient to prevent bruise formation, but some injuries (e.g. swollen knees due to excessive exercise) will benefit from two to three applications every two to three hours.

SUITABILITY: Arnica cream is suitable for all age groups, including young children, and for use during pregnancy, so long as it is applied to unbroken skin. Use small amounts on very young children.

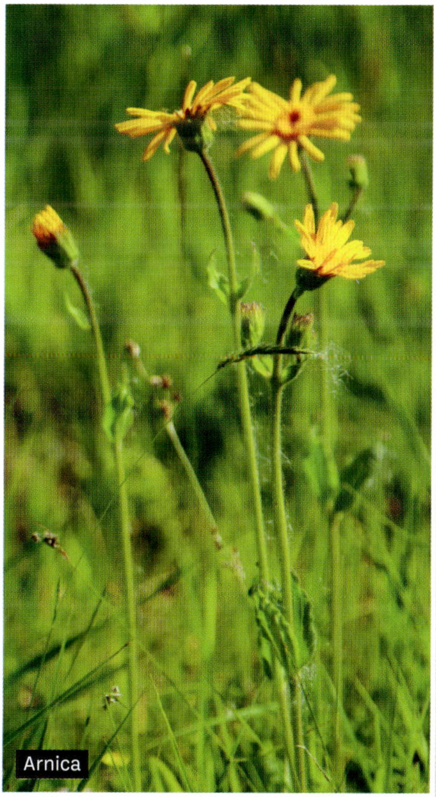

Arnica

Comfrey
Symphytum officinale

Use comfrey only for external treatment.

Uses

This is another herb that should be used only externally unless under the guidance of a medical herbalist. It is a great healer for fractures, sprains, a bad back and even broken bones! The old name for comfrey is 'knitbone', as it was traditionally used to aid the healing of broken bones. Comfrey ointment or a comfrey poultice can be applied to sprained ankles, to swollen knees, and to broken ribs, collarbone or fingers (as none of these can be put in plaster). Comfrey can be used to 'take over' from arnica to aid recovery from an injury, but you should avoid applying it directly to any injuries where the skin is broken. If you are using an ointment you can apply it around the cut but not directly to the open wound. Comfrey ointment or cream provides an excellent base for customising your remedy with the addition of different essential oils and tinctures.

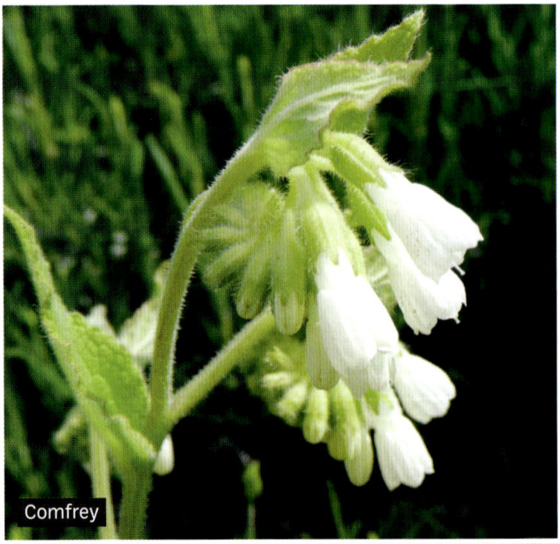
Comfrey

HOW TO APPLY IT: The type of external application of comfrey should be dictated by the type of injury. If there is a lot of recent swelling, choose a compress or poultice, but if it is a long-term treatment, use the cream or ointment.

HOW OFTEN TO USE IT: The frequency of application (irrespective of the type) depends on the injury. The more recent the injury, the more often you should apply the treatment (three to five times a day); for a long-term problem, apply the treatment once or twice a day.

SUITABILITY: Comfrey is considered safe for *external use* for all age groups, including small children, and for pregnant women.

Crampbark *Viburnum opulus*

Uses

Crampbark is a muscle relaxant, and is therefore suitable for problems caused by muscles going into spasm or becoming tense. It will help with muscular pain that is secondary to nerve pain – for instance, in sciatica – or when muscle tension leads to neck pain or tension headache. Crampbark is also useful for treating smooth muscle tension, and can be used for stomach cramps caused by IBS.

HOW TO USE IT: As a tincture, either added to ointments or taken internally.

HOW OFTEN TO USE IT: Ointments containing crampbark can be applied two to three times a day until the symptoms improve.

DOSAGE: **Adults:** 0.7–1.4ml diluted with some water, one to three times a day, tincture strength 1:2.

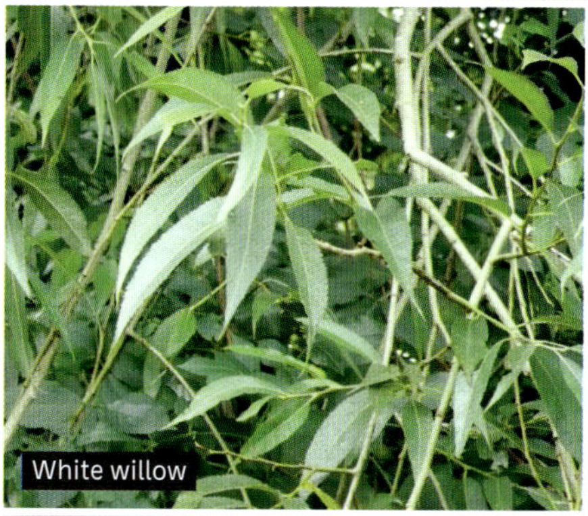
White willow

White willow and Purple willow bark *Salix alba* and *Salix purpurea*

Caution is needed in people who are allergic to salicylate compounds. Willow bark should also be avoided when breastfeeding or when taking high doses of blood-thinning medications.

Uses

Willow bark has been used to treat rheumatic complaints for centuries. The salicylate compounds in the willow bark extract are responsible for its anti-inflammatory and pain-killing properties, and the modern-day aspirin is derived from salicylic acid.

Willow bark extract can be used to treat any muscular or joint ailments of an inflammatory nature that are manifested as pain or swelling. It is the best treatment for back pain, whether this is of recent origin or a long-standing condition. Recommendations for using willow bark include any type of arthritis, joint inflammation, muscle ache (especially if secondary to joint ache), muscle tension and tension headache.

Purple willow (*Salix purpurea*) products are widely regarded as superior to those from white willow (*Salix alba*), but are more difficult to source.

COMBINATIONS: Willow bark combines well with other anti-rheumatic and anti-inflammatory remedies, such as wild yam and liquorice.

HOW TO USE IT: The tincture can be either added directly to the anti-inflammatory ointments (5ml per 20g of cream) or taken internally. In my experience the tincture dosage needed to obtain the anti-inflammatory and analgesic effect when taken internally is quite high and may prove difficult to achieve (willow bark extract has a strong unpleasant taste). Therefore I would recommend the tablets made from the freeze-dried extract.

DOSAGE: **Adults**: 1–4 tablets a day (each tablet should provide the equivalent of 8g of dried herb), or 1.2–2.4ml diluted with some water, one to three times a day, tincture strength 1:2 (if you are brave enough to put up with the taste!).

Rosemary *Salvia rosmarinus* (syn. *Rosmarinus officinalis*)

Do not use rosemary essential oil for external applications in pregnancy or for children under three years old without consulting a specialist.

If using it as a tincture, take it two hours before or after mineral supplements.

Uses

This herb is useful for all kinds of muscular pain. It helps to relax and soothe aching muscles after heavy exercise or when suffering from a cold. It also warms the muscles by stimulating the circulation to them, and it reduces muscular tension.

HOW TO USE IT: As rosemary essential oil. Add it to a bath, or to creams or ointments.

DOSAGE: **Adults**: 5 drops of essential oil in a bath, once a day, or 10 drops of essential oil mixed with 50g of comfrey cream and applied one to three times a day.

Optional herbs

Celery seed
Apium graveolens

Celery seed may lower the blood level of thyroxine in people who are taking that medication, so inform your doctor that you are taking the herb, and always take it a few hours before or after the thyroxine.

Caution is needed in people with kidney disorders and in women who are breastfeeding.

Uses

Celery seed can be used to treat a wide range of muscular and skeletal conditions, including gout, osteoarthritis, rheumatoid arthritis, rheumatic pains and muscular aches. It is one of the herbal detoxifiers, mainly through its diuretic action, which helps to remove metabolic waste products from the blood, including those that can exacerbate joint inflammation.

COMBINATIONS: Celery seed combines well with liquorice, wild yam and willow bark.

HOW TO TAKE IT: As a tincture.

DOSAGE: **Adults**: 1.4–2.8ml diluted with some water, one to three times a day, tincture strength 1:2. Remember to drink plenty of water to compensate for the diuretic action of the herb.

Chilli (cayenne pepper)
Capsicum annuum

Do not apply chillies to broken skin. Avoid contact with the eyes. Do not use chillies to treat acute inflammation such as an attack of gout. For internal use, chillies are best taken in the form of food rather than as a tincture.

Uses

Cayenne pepper is useful for rheumatic

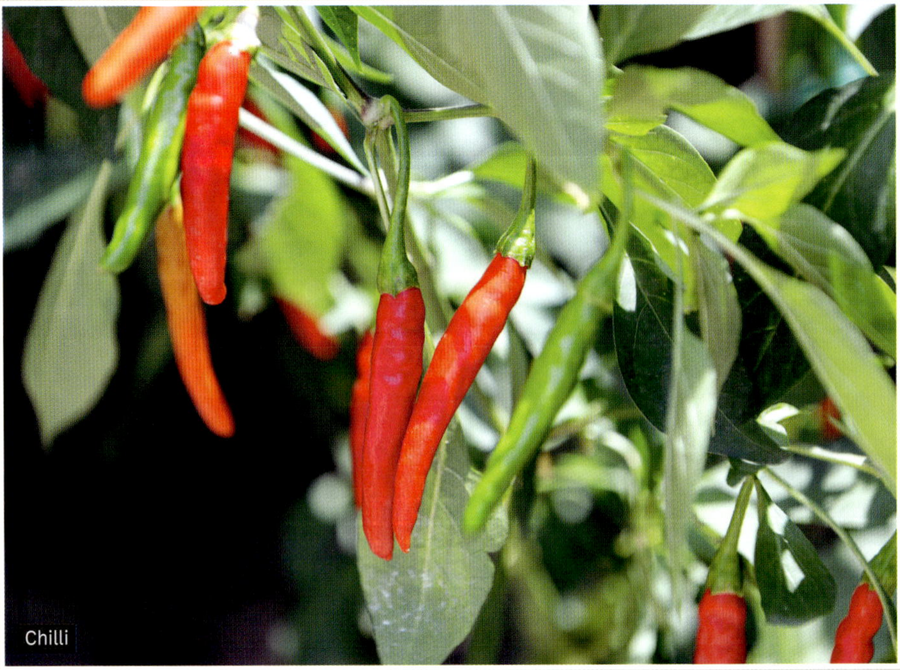

Chilli

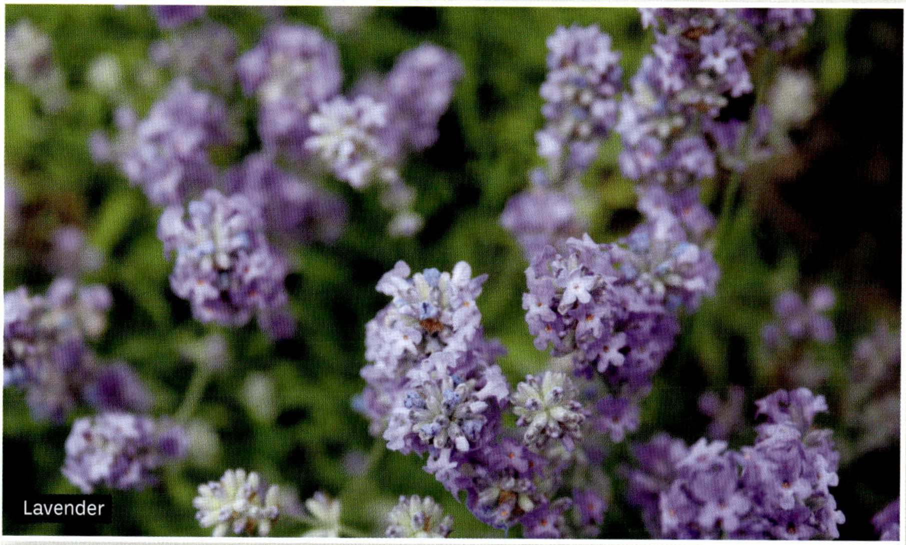

Lavender

complaints mainly because of its analgesic action (numbing the local nerves) and its ability to increase the local blood supply. The latter action helps to flush from a specific area the accumulated waste products or allergenic substances that often cause joint problems. The addition of chilli tincture to a healing cream will speed up recovery after an injury involving extensive bruising. Make sure that you wash your hands thoroughly after applying the cream. Chillies will not cause any harm, despite the burning sensation. If you experience any stinging, wash the affected area with plenty of cool water.

HOW TO USE IT: As a tincture added to comfrey cream or another cream or ointment base.

DOSAGE: **Adults**: add no more than 10 drops of the chilli tincture (strength 1:2) to 50g of the cream or ointment base (if the cream stings after application you have added too much).

Do not use this cream for children, as there is a risk that they will accidentally transfer it to their eyes.

Lavender *Lavandula angustifolia* (syn. *Lavandula officinalis*)

Do not use lavender essential oil for external applications in pregnancy or for children under three years of age without consulting a specialist.

Uses

Lavender is useful for treating pain resulting from a variety of rheumatic and post-traumatic causes (e.g. after a fall). It has a gently relaxing effect on the muscles and will therefore help to relieve any muscle tension or spasm caused by the inflammation or injury. It is also anti-inflammatory and anti-rheumatic.

I recommend adding it to the healing creams that are used to treat extensive bruising or non-specific rheumatic pains.

HOW TO USE IT: As lavender essential oil added to comfrey cream or another cream base.

DOSAGE: **Adults and children:** 5 drops of lavender essential oil mixed with 50g of the comfrey cream or other cream base.

Meadowsweet *Filipendula ulmaria*

Caution is needed in people who are allergic to salicylates.
If you are pregnant or breastfeeding, seek professional advice before using meadowsweet.

Uses

Meadowsweet has gentle anti-inflammatory properties due to its salicylate compounds. As it is also a digestive agent, it is most suitable for people who are sensitive to the effects of conventional anti-inflammatory medication on the stomach.

HOW TO TAKE IT: As a tea as an additional treatment for any joint or muscle pain.
DOSAGE: **Adults:** 1–2 cups a day.

Peppermint *Mentha* × *piperita*

Peppermint essential oil should never be used internally.
Caution is needed if using peppermint tea or oil while breastfeeding.

Uses

Peppermint applied externally has cooling and muscle-relaxing properties. These are very helpful where there is pain due to inflammation and/or muscle spasm.

HOW TO USE IT: As peppermint essential oil added to any cream for treating a recent injury (e.g. bruising after a fall, back strain, sprains) or for providing a gentle analgesic action for ongoing arthritic pain.
DOSAGE: **Adults and children (over four years old):** mix 5 drops of the peppermint essential oil with 50g of a base cream.

Birch *Betula pendula* (syn. *Betula alba*)

Caution is needed in people who are allergic to salicylates.

Uses

Birch has anti-arthritic, anti-inflammatory and detoxifying properties. It is used to treat all types of arthritis, including gout, especially if substantial swelling is involved.

COMBINATIONS: Birch can be combined with any other anti-rheumatic herbal remedies.
HOW TO TAKE IT: As a tincture.
DOSAGE: **Adults:** 0.7–1.3ml diluted with some water, two to three times a day, tincture strength 1:2.

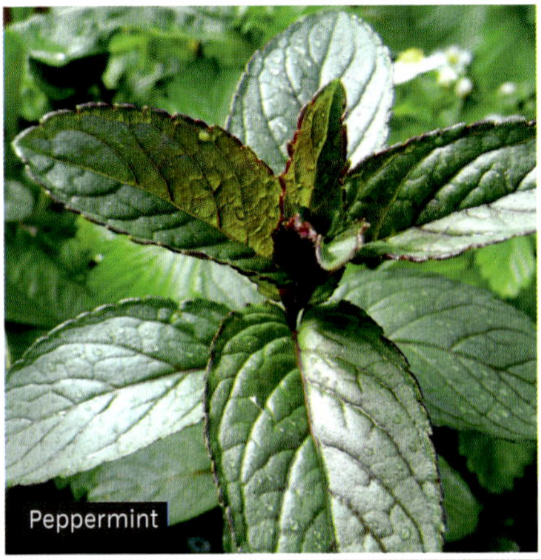
Peppermint

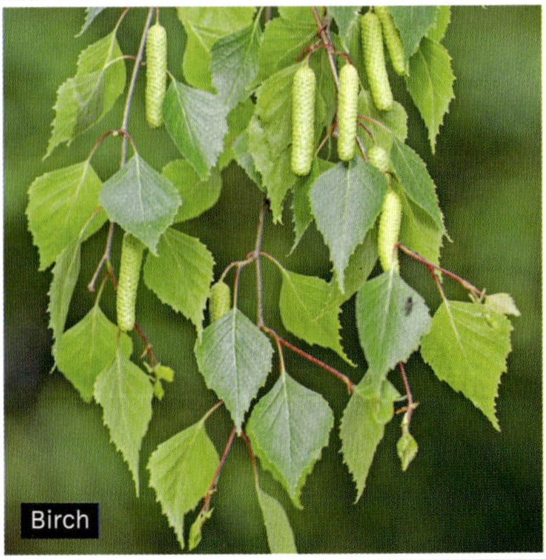
Birch

Turmeric *Curcuma longa*

Turmeric is contraindicated in people with gall-bladder problems, especially those caused by gallstones.

Caution is needed in people who are taking blood-thinning medications – doses of more than 15g/day should not be taken if they are on antiplatelet or anticoagulant medication. Turmeric may not be suitable for people with bleeding disorders, so it is important to consult a doctor first in such cases.

Uses

Turmeric – a well-known spice with a bright yellow colour – is one of the few herbs with general anti-inflammatory effects. It is used internally in cases of osteoarthritis, rheumatoid arthritis and back pain triggered by a variety of causes. It is often referred to as curcumin, which is the yellow pigment that gives the root its colour and is the main active constituent of turmeric.

COMBINATIONS: Turmeric combines well with wild yam and willow bark.
HOW TO TAKE IT: As a tincture or tablets.
DOSAGE: **Adults:** 1.7–5ml diluted with some water, two to three times a day, tincture strength 1:1, or 4–10g per day as tablets.

Wild yam *Dioscorea villosa*

Wild yam may cause or aggravate gastro-oesophageal reflux (heartburn).

Uses

Wild yam tincture has anti-rheumatic and anti-inflammatory properties. It is most useful for joint problems that often accompany the menopause, ranging from osteoarthritis or rheumatoid arthritis to non-specific general joint aches.

COMBINATIONS: Wild yam combines well with liquorice, celery seed and willow bark.
HOW TO TAKE IT: As a tincture.
DOSAGE: **Adults:** 1–2ml diluted with some water, one to three times a day, tincture strength 1:2.

Wintergreen *Gaultheria procumbens*

Do not use wintergreen essential oil for external applications in pregnancy or for children under three years old without consulting a specialist.

Caution is needed in people who are allergic to salicylate compounds.

Uses

This small evergreen bush yields an essential oil that has warming and anti-inflammatory effects when applied to the skin around a painful joint.

HOW TO USE IT: As wintergreen essential oil added to comfrey cream or another cream base.
DOSAGE: **Adults:** mix 10 drops of wintergreen essential oil with 50g of the comfrey cream or other cream base and apply to the affected areas two to three times a day.

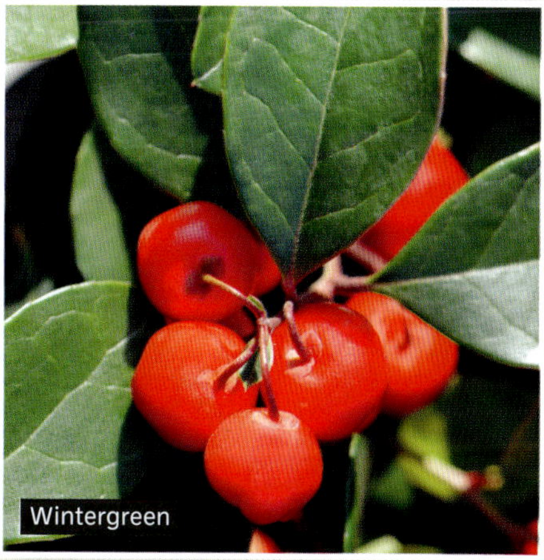
Wintergreen

Specific ailments affecting the muscular and skeletal systems, and herbs that can help

Back pain

All kinds of back pain can be eased with herbal remedies. I follow the approach of providing a warm treatment (a bath with essential oils or warming ointment) combined with anti-inflammatory remedies.

Treatment options

Please see pages 82–87 for herbal precautions.

- Apply arnica ointment – this should be your first line of treatment following an injury or strain to the back, and should be administered as soon as possible. **Adults and children:** apply once to the injured area, so long as the skin is unbroken. Repeat after a few hours if the injury was extensive.
- Apply comfrey ointment a couple of hours later after the arnica ointment, but do not apply it to the open injury. **Adults and children:** keep applying the comfrey ointment every few hours until there is an improvement.
- Take a hot bath with added essential oils of rosemary, lavender or wintergreen. **Adults:** 5–10 drops per bath.
- Take willow bark tablets. **Adults:** take the maximum dose for a day, according to the manufacturer's instructions, and then reduce to the average recommended dose until the pain eases.
- Apply the cream for muscular tension or spasm (see box below).

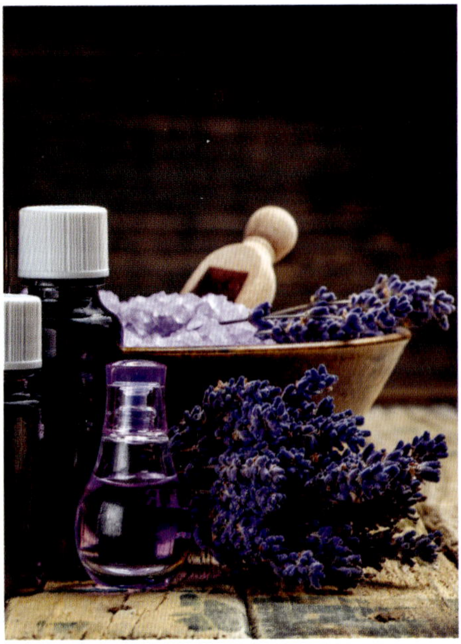

Cream for muscular tension or spasm

INGREDIENTS

- 5ml crampbark (tincture strength 1:2)
- 20g comfrey cream
- 5 drops of lavender essential oil
- 5 drops of rosemary essential oil

METHOD

1. Mix the ingredients well.
2. Transfer the mixture to a clean, dark glass jar, making sure that there are no air pockets left. Store for up to 12 months.

ADULTS: apply to the affected muscles two to three times a day.

Left Lavender essential oil and bath salts.

Bruising

Bruising results from varying degrees of bleeding under the skin following an injury. It can also follow any surgical procedure, and can be internal and not obvious on the surface of the skin. Spontaneous bruising that occurs without any injury is a circulatory disorder and should be investigated.

Treatment options

Please see pages 81–87 for herbal precautions. For more on bruising, see page 49.

- Arnica ointment or cream is the best treatment, and the more quickly it is applied the better the result. It is definitely an item to keep in your first-aid kit, both at home and on holiday. It is safe to use on small children, so long as the skin is not broken. You can use arnica around a surgical incision to reduce bruising, but make sure that you apply the ointment 2.5cm away from the edge of the wound. **Adults and children:** apply the ointment or cream once, as soon as possible, to the bruise site.
- If the skin is broken, comfrey cream or ointment is a better all-round remedy as it speeds up the healing of both bruises and cuts, but it still needs to be applied away from the cut – leave a margin of about 2cm around the broken skin. **Adults and children:** apply the cream or ointment one to three times a day, until the bruised area is no longer painful to touch.

Fractures

Fractured bones must be assessed by a doctor or the emergency services in a hospital. Most cases will end up in plaster, so you will not have much access to the actual site of the fracture. However, you can apply a herbal cream or ointment to the skin adjacent to the plaster, as enough will be absorbed in the area to speed up healing.

In some situations it is not possible to put bones in plaster – for instance, if you break a rib, upper arm, shoulder, finger or toe – in which case you can apply the external treatment directly to the skin over the injured part to speed up recovery.

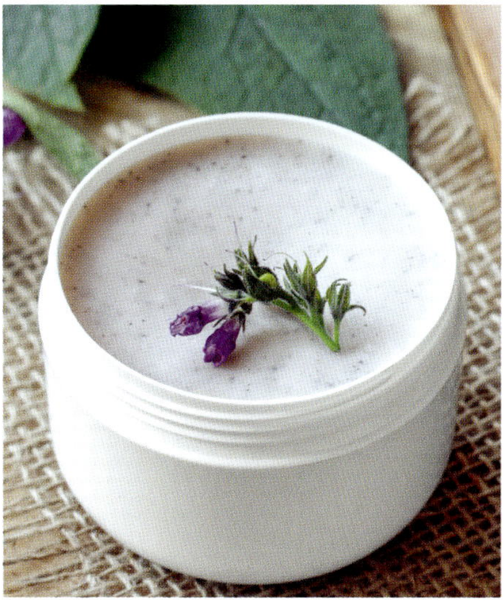

Above Comfrey ointment.

Treatment options

Please see pages 81–87 for herbal precautions.

- If the skin is intact, apply arnica ointment to the area over the broken bone before the plaster is put on. **Adults and children:** apply the ointment once, liberally.
- Apply a comfrey poultice or ointment to the area immediately adjacent to the plaster. **Adults and children:** apply once or twice a day for as long as you have to wear the plaster.
- Apply comfrey ointment directly but very gently to the skin over the fractured rib, toe, shoulder or finger. **Adults and children:** apply the ointment twice a day.

Gout

Practitioner treatment is recommended for this condition.

The symptoms of gout, which include swelling of the joint, shiny red skin around the joint and severe pain, can appear quite rapidly. The cause is the accumulation of uric acid crystals in the joint, which leads to sudden inflammation. The treatment options listed below will help to reduce the pain of acute attacks, but to treat recurrent gout you should consult a medical herbalist. Do not put any warming herbs on gout, as they can make the inflammation worse.

Treatment options

- For immediate relief of gout pain use a fresh cabbage leaf poultice. Bash a couple of leaves with a rolling pin until some juice appears on the surface, or mash the leaves in a food processor. Put the leaves or the mash on a bit of clingfilm and wrap it around the affected joint; secure it in position with an elastic bandage. **Adults:** apply a poultice as many times as necessary to achieve pain relief, keeping it in place for 30–60 minutes each time.
- Drinking celery seed and burdock root tea can help to prevent frequent attacks (see box below).

Tea to reduce the frequency of recurrence of gout

Please see page 84 for herbal precautions.

INGREDIENTS

- 50g dried celery seeds
- 50g dried burdock root

METHOD

1. Mix the herbs thoroughly.
2. Infuse 2 teaspoonsful of the mixture in a cup of freshly boiled water for 10 minutes.
3. Strain and drink warm. You can add honey to this tea.

ADULT DOSE ONLY: 1 cup a day for 6–12 months

Below Making fresh cabbage leaf poultice.

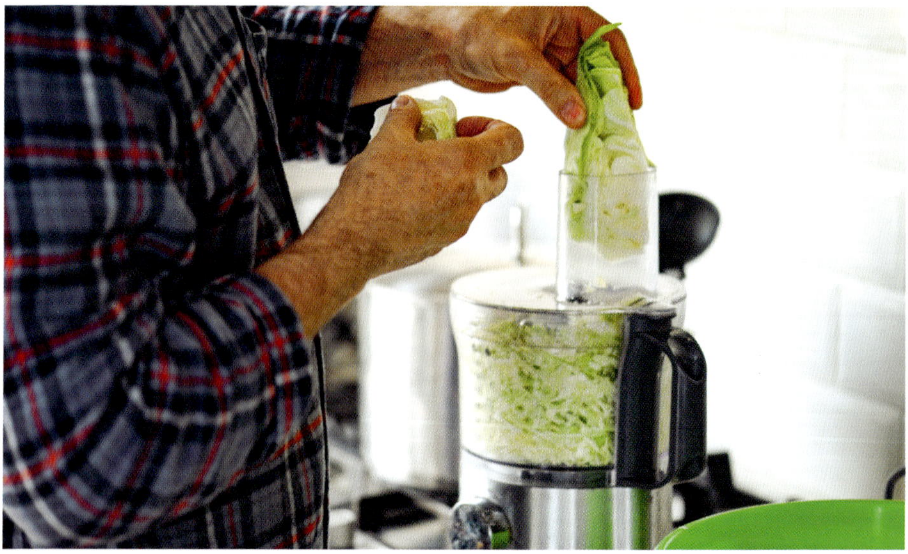

Joint pain

Joint pain can have many different causes, so it is best to see a health professional to get an accurate diagnosis. However, there are many anti-inflammatory herbs that can be safely tried at home for a variety of joint pains.

Treatment options

Please see pages 82 and 84 for herbal precautions.

- Apply comfrey ointment externally. **Adults and children:** two to three times a day.
- Apply a warming chilli cream – add no more than 10 drops of chilli tincture (strength 1:3) to 50g of the cream or ointment base. Do not use this cream in small children, as there is a risk that they will accidentally transfer it to their eyes. **Adults, and children over 10 years old:** apply two to three times a day to a painful joint.
- A general anti-rheumatic mix can be tried (see box, below left).
- Use the cream for painful joints described below.

Anti-rheumatic mix

Please see pages 83, 84, 99 and 164 for herbal precautions.

INGREDIENTS

- 40ml wild yam (tincture strength 1:2)
- 20ml liquorice (tincture strength 1:1)
- 20ml celery seed (tincture strength 1:2)
- 20ml willow bark (tincture strength 1:2)

METHOD

1. Mix the ingredients together.
2. Pour the mixture into a clean, dark glass bottle.
3. Label the bottle with the contents and the date.
4. Store at room temperature for up to a year.

ADULTS: 5ml diluted with some water, two to three times a day.

Cream for painful joints

Please see pages 81–87 for herbal precautions.

INGREDIENTS

- 50g comfrey cream
- 5 drops wintergreen essential oil
- 5 drops lavender essential oil
- 5 drops peppermint essential oil

METHOD

1. Mix the ingredients well.
2. Transfer the mixture to a clean, dark glass jar, making sure that there are no air pockets left.
3. Store for up to 12 months.

ADULTS: apply to the affected areas two to three times a day.

Muscle cramps

Muscle cramps can result from a magnesium deficiency, so supplementing with magnesium for a month or two may bring about a quick improvement. Alternatively, muscle-relaxing herbs can be used. Make sure you are well hydrated, as dehydration can also cause cramps.

Treatment options

Please see pages 81–87 for herbal precautions.

- Take crampbark tincture, especially if the muscle cramps are related to intensive exercise. **Adults:** 0.7–1.4ml diluted with some water, one to three times a day, tincture strength 1:2.
- Add muscle-relaxing essential oils, such as lavender or rosemary, to the bath. **Adults:** 5 drops per bath.

Muscular pain

Muscles can ache after intensive use or if you are suffering from flu or a cold. Sometimes muscle pain is caused by an underlying condition, such as fibromyalgia. In most cases, warming baths that stimulate the circulation are helpful. In addition, you can take a general anti-inflammatory herb and herbs that stimulate the circulation.

Treatment options

Please see pages 87 and 87 for herbal precautions.

- Add rosemary and wintergreen essential oils to the bath. **Adults:** 5 drops of either oil, or 2 drops of each if using them together.
- Take a tincture of turmeric. **Adults:** 1.7–5ml diluted with some water, two to three times a day, tincture strength 1:1.
- Take herbs that improve the circulation, such as ginger, yarrow, hawthorn or ginkgo (see pages 43–47), either as a tea or as a tincture.

Below A warm bath with essential oils is ideal for muscular pain.

Sprains

With sprains, as with bruising, the sooner you apply the treatment, the better the results. Immediate treatment will diminish the pain and swelling, minimise the development of bruising and speed up the rate of healing. Even if you can't administer a treatment straight away, it is worth using the herbs to aid recovery. Continue to apply the herbal ointment or compress until the symptoms improve.

Treatment options

Please see pages 81–82 for herbal precautions.

- Apply arnica ointment. **Adults and children:** apply once immediately after the injury, and repeat a few hours later.
- Apply comfrey ointment. **Adults and children:** apply two to three times a day until the symptoms improve.
- Apply a warm comfrey poultice or compress made from diluted tincture or a strong infusion. **Adults and children:** apply two to three times a day until the symptoms improve.

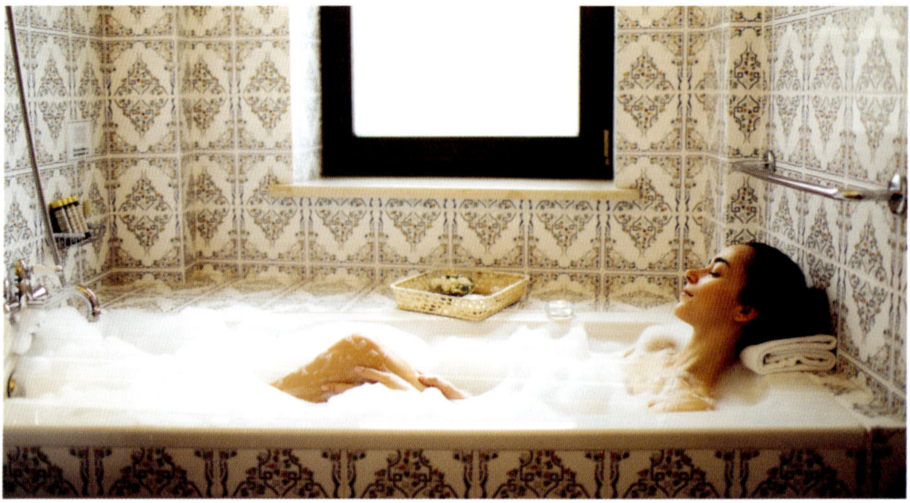

Conditions for which home treatment is not recommended

- Osteoarthritis: many cases of osteoarthritis respond very well to herbal treatment, but this condition does tend to need ongoing treatment, so it is best to have a prescription adjusted for long-term use.
- Rheumatoid arthritis: this is an autoimmune disorder that needs an individualised treatment and often requires a slow adjustment of conventional medication.
- Gout: this is often brought on by specific medication or the wrong diet, so it is important to look closely at the sufferer's general state of health.
- Restless leg syndrome: this can be related to stress, poor circulation and dietary deficiencies, and therefore requires a comprehensive treatment plan.
- Ankylosing spondylitis: this is another autoimmune disorder, which often improves dramatically in response to dietary adjustments combined with an individual prescription.
- Fibromyalgia: muscle pain is a prominent symptom of this complex disorder of the immune system, which requires a complex and long-term treatment.
- Juvenile arthritis: this is a type of rheumatoid arthritis that affects young children; excellent results have been achieved with individualised herbal treatment.

When to seek medical attention

- If you experience severe joint pain that is getting progressively worse.
- If you have a bad headache following injury to the head.
- If you experience severe back pain that is getting worse.
- If you have severe pain and swelling following a fall (as the possibility of a fracture needs to be assessed).
- If you have a widespread joint and/or muscle ache together with a feeling of general malaise that persists for a long time.

CHAPTER 10

The nervous system

The nervous system consists of the brain, the spinal cord and the network of nerve cells throughout the whole body. Disorders of the nervous system are often very complex. The nervous system is our 'control system', which means that the dysfunction of any body organ or tissue may be a result of nervous system dysfunction. Herbalists emphasise the importance of treating body and mind simultaneously, as the nervous system is intimately connected with every aspect of our body function.

Below Headaches, stress and tiredness are often caused by each other.

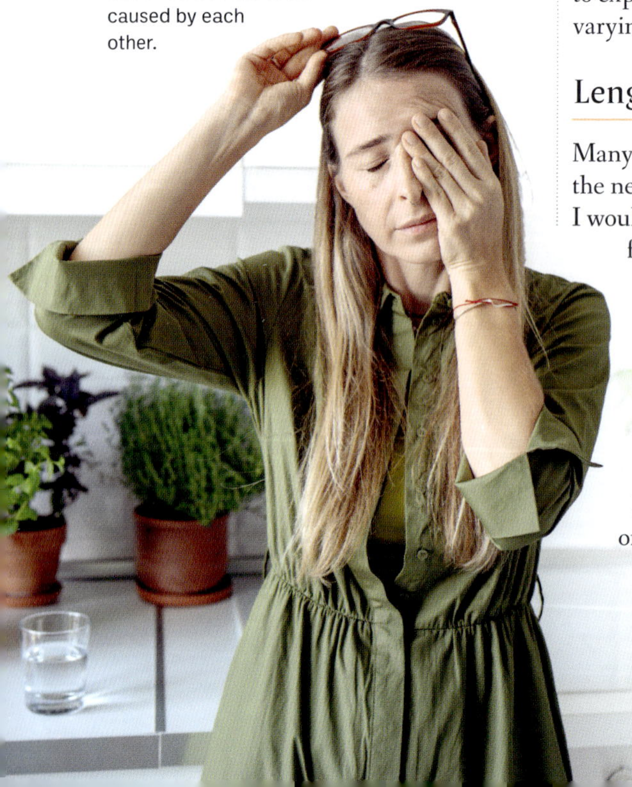

Symptoms and hormonal influences

Ailments that affect the nervous system can be manifested in many different ways – for instance, as physical pain or as an altered mood. Hormonal changes in the body may have a profound effect on the nervous system, and vice versa, so these two systems frequently need to be treated together. A familiar example of hormonal influence on the nervous system is premenstrual syndrome (PMS), which causes a significant proportion of women to experience emotional upheaval of varying severity.

Length of treatment

Many herbs have beneficial effects on the nervous system and nervous tissue. I would like to highlight the restorative function of herbs in relation to this system – some herbs have the capacity to aid the recovery of the nervous system from the effects of stress, illness or injury. Nervous tissue recovers slowly, so treatment of problems relating to the nervous system tends to be long term – a period of 6–12 months or even longer is not unusual.

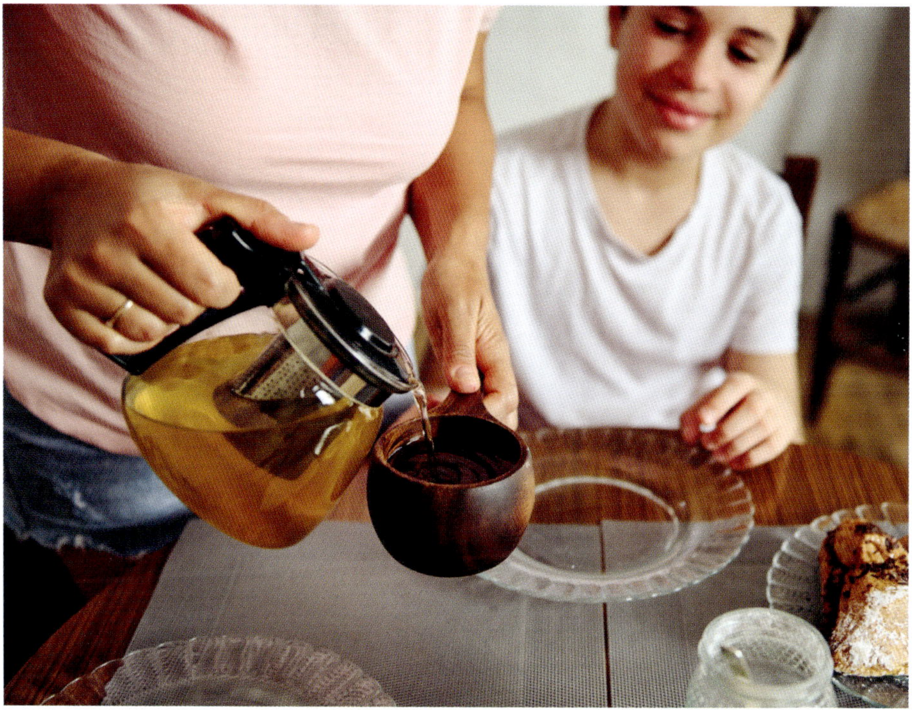

Above Drinking a medicinal herbal tea can be calming for the nervous system.

Non-addictive treatment

The biggest advantage of using herbs as opposed to conventional medicines in the case of the nervous system is that herbs are non-addictive. For example, many commonly prescribed types of medication for anxiety or sleep problems can lead to a dependency on the drug within a few weeks, and as a result it often takes a very long time to come off such medication. This is not a problem with medicinal herbs, because the mode of action is complex and involves many different constituents.

Variation in dosage

It is also worth pointing out that the nervous system tends to respond to herbal remedies in a very individual way. Some people may need 5 drops of a sleep mix, whereas others may need 2 teaspoonsful to achieve the same effect. Most people will feel more relaxed after taking valerian, but a tiny proportion will become anxious or over-animated after taking it. You may need to experiment a little to find which herbs and which dosage best suit your nervous system. In general it is best to start with a lower dosage, and gradually increase it if you do not see any improvement.

Mixing herbs and conventional medications

Many of the herbs described below can be taken alongside orthodox medication or used to help you to come off such medication, but I would strongly advise you to consult a herbal clinician in order to make the best choices.

Must-have herbs

Valerian *Valeriana officinalis*

Large doses of valerian can cause drowsiness or tiredness.

Uses

Valerian is a general relaxant for the nerves. It forms the basis of many over-the-counter remedies that help to improve sleep or relieve anxiety. It can be used in many situations – for example, when you have problems sleeping, when you are nervous before an exam or job interview, when you are upset by some bad news or when you feel stressed at work. It can be used for older children in some cases of hyperactivity, but the dosage should be adjusted by a herbalist (too much valerian can have a stimulating effect on such children). Valerian takes the edge off anxiety and works quite quickly – normally you should feel more relaxed within half an hour of taking a dose. It can also be used to relieve certain kinds of pain, namely tension headache, earache and period pain.

COMBINATIONS: Valerian works very well on its own, but also combines well with other anti-anxiety or sleep-inducing herbs.

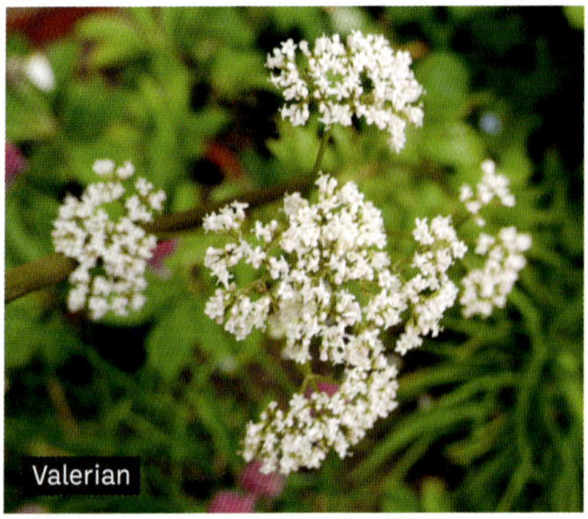

Valerian

HOW TO TAKE IT: This herb is best taken as a tincture. The dosage can vary a lot depending on how sensitive a particular individual is. My general advice is to try the minimum dose to begin with, but if you don't notice any effect after 30 minutes take another minimum dose. Next time you use valerian you can try the larger dose straight away. If you feel tired after a dose, you have taken too much (unless you are using it as a sleep remedy). I recommend that you use a concentrated tincture, at least strength 1:2.
DOSAGE: **Adults:** 0.7–2ml diluted with some water, one to three times a day, tincture strength 1:2. A larger dose can be taken as a one-off. I suggest specific amounts when particular ailments are discussed later in this chapter.

Lavender *Lavandula angustifolia* (syn. *Lavandula officinalis*)

Do not use lavender essential oil for external applications in pregnancy or for children under three years old without consulting a specialist.

Uses

Lavender works through the calming and relaxing effect of its lovely scent on the mind. It can induce deep sleep and can be safely used in children who become overexcited at bedtime.

HOW TO TAKE IT: Lavender is best used in the form of an essential oil, either in a bath, or directly applied to your pillow or in a vaporiser. You can also take a lavender tea.
DOSAGE: **Adults:** 5 drops in a bath, or 2–3 drops on a pillow, or 1–2 drops in a

vaporiser, or 1 cup of lavender tea (use 1 teaspoonful of herbs per cup of water). **Children (over four years old):** 1 drop in a bath or in a vaporiser.

Rosemary *Salvia rosmarinus* (syn. *Rosmarinus officinalis*)

Do not use rosemary essential oil for external applications in pregnancy or for children under three years old without consulting a specialist. If using it as a tincture, take it two hours before or after mineral supplements.

Uses

Rosemary is the opposite of valerian and lavender. It has an invigorating and stimulating effect on the nervous system, and it improves concentration and clarity of mind. It is a really useful aid when studying, as it improves both memory and mental performance. It can also be helpful for tension headaches.

HOW TO TAKE IT: Rosemary works through the effects of the sense of smell on the brain, so the essential oil is the best form in which to use it. If you need to revive your energy after a long day, or you need to be extra-switched-on in the morning, try adding a few drops of rosemary essential oil to your bath or shower tray. Sniffing a fresh twig of rosemary will also work – rub it with your fingers to release the scent. If you have a long drive ahead, put a few fresh twigs of rosemary in your car to help you to stay alert.

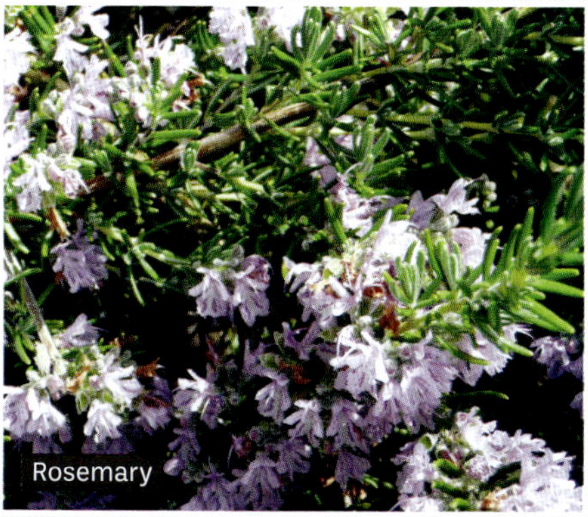
Rosemary

You can also take rosemary tincture, especially if you are looking for long-term effects on your concentration and memory.
DOSAGE: **Adults:** 5 drops of the essential oil in the bath or shower tray, or 1–2 drops in a vaporiser, or as a tincture, 0.7–1.4 ml diluted with some water, one to three times a day, tincture strength 1:2.

Chamomile (German) *Matricaria recutita* (syn. *Chamomilla recutita*)

Caution is needed in people who are allergic to plants belonging to the daisy family (the Asteraceae, formerly known as the Compositae).

Uses

Chamomile is an extremely versatile medicinal plant and has many applications in conditions related to the nervous system. If taken before going to bed, chamomile tea can have a relaxing effect and help you to fall asleep. Digestion issues caused by anxiety and stress can also be improved by chamomile. For children it is the best herb to use to induce peaceful sleep or treat tummy ache.

HOW TO TAKE IT: For adults, use a strong chamomile tea made with 2 tea bags or 2 heaped teaspoonful of loose herbs per cup of water. For children and babies, use a weak infusion made with 1 tea bag or 1 small teaspoonful of loose herbs per cup of water, infused for 1 minute. I suggest specific amounts for babies and young children with reference to specific conditions.
DOSAGE: **Adults:** 1 cup of tea as needed, up to a maximum of 4 cups a day.

Optional herbs

Lemon balm *Melissa officinalis*

Uses

Lemon balm is somewhat similar to lime tree flowers – it has a gentle relaxing effect and lifts the spirits, and its actions are readily observable within 30 minutes of taking it. This herb is also very effective for indigestion resulting from stress or anxiety. Drinking lemon balm tea before going to bed should ensure deep, uninterrupted sleep.

HOW TO TAKE IT: As a tea or tincture, ideally made from a fresh plant. Try to make the tea from fresh leaves, as the taste and action of these are superior to those of the dried herb.

DOSAGE: **Adults:** 1–3 cups of the infusion per day, or as a tincture, 1–2 ml diluted with some water, one to three times a day, tincture strength 1:2. **Children (over four years old):** lemon balm tea can be given to children, ranging from a few sips for young children to a cup for those over 12 years old.

Lime tree flowers *Tilia cordata, Tilia platyphyllos* and *Tilia × europaea*

Lime tree flowers should be avoided in people with a known allergy, and should be taken several hours before or after iron supplements.

Uses

The infusion made from lime tree flowers has a relaxing effect on an anxious, overactive mind. It is traditionally drunk in parts of France as an after-dinner drink, because it benefits the digestion as well as promoting sleep. The tea also lifts the spirits gently in situations where stress has become overwhelming. It is one of the most pleasant herbal teas to drink, as it has a lovely aroma and delicate flavour, which can be enhanced by adding a little honey. I regard this tea as the best remedy for the winter blues (and it will warm you up at the same time!) or for when you feel run down after having had a cold.

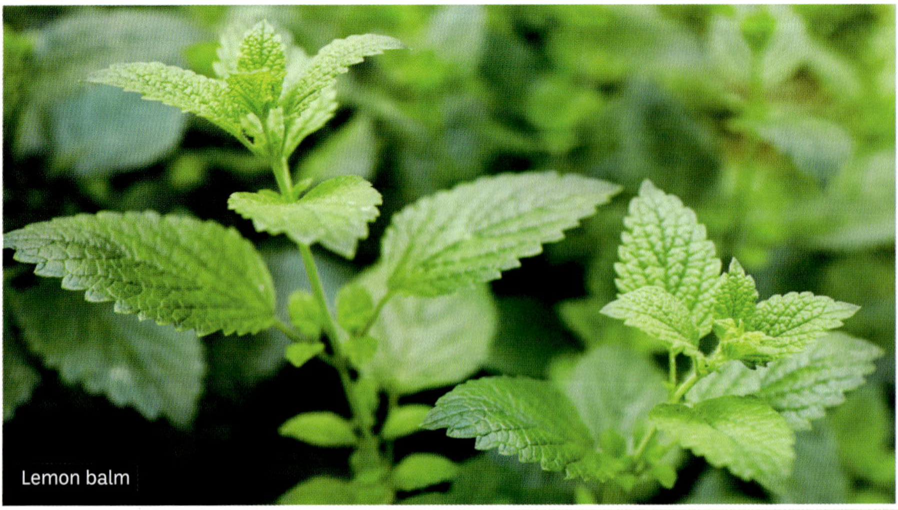

Lemon balm

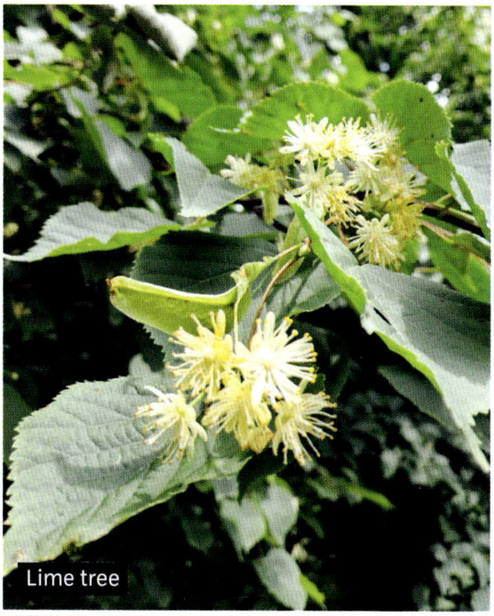

Lime tree

HOW TO TAKE IT: Dried flowers are normally used to make the tea. It is best drunk in the afternoon or evening to ensure sound sleep.
DOSAGE: **Adults**: 1–3 cups a day.

Liquorice *Glycyrrhiza glabra*

Liquorice should not be taken during pregnancy, or by the elderly.
Do not take liquorice for a prolonged period if you have high blood pressure, low potassium levels, problems with your heart, kidneys or liver, or water retention.

Uses

Liquorice affects the nervous system indirectly by supporting the functioning of the adrenal glands. These glands are responsible for the swift responses of the nervous system in stressful situations, and they can become exhausted if you are continually stressed. By gently supporting the adrenal glands, liquorice has a positive effect on mood and emotions. I recommend this herb for people who are experiencing prolonged stress, and for emotional fragility, mild depression and general nervous exhaustion.

HOW TO TAKE IT: For all of these uses a strong tincture is the best form to take. If you have a tendency towards water retention or high blood pressure, take only half of the recommended dose for a week at a time, and then have a week's break. You can repeat this 'on–off' procedure for two to three months, but make sure that you keep monitoring your blood pressure.
DOSAGE: **Adults**: 0.5–2ml diluted with some water, one to three times a day, tincture strength 1:1.

Oats (green oats) *Avena sativa*

Uses

Oats have a special place among the herbs used to treat the nervous system, as they are the restorative botanical for this system. For this purpose a green aerial part of the plant is used just when it starts to form the seeds, rather than the fully ripe grain that is used as food.

I recommend that you use green oats when you feel mentally or emotionally exhausted, when you have lost your motivation and drive, or when you have generally been under a lot of stress for a prolonged period. Oats support the nervous system and heal it after it has been under continual strain, and they will also help with anxiety and insomnia.

COMBINATIONS: Green oats can be mixed with any herbs that have relaxing, anti-anxiety or antidepressant effects.
HOW TO TAKE THEM: As a tincture, which should be made from fresh green oats (the aerial parts).
DOSAGE: **Adults**: 1–2ml diluted with some water, two to three times a day, tincture strength 1:2.

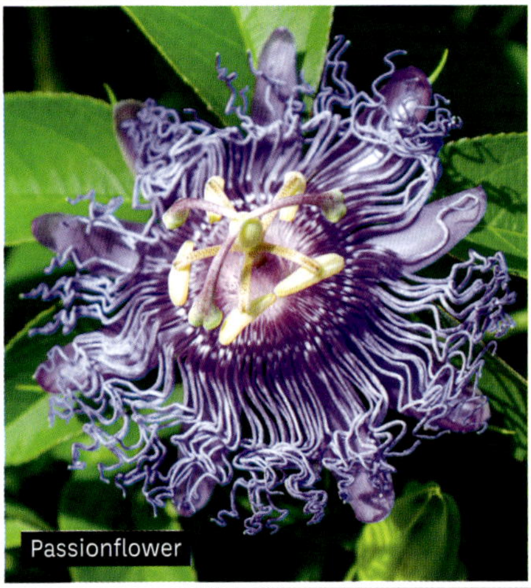
Passionflower

Passionflower
Passiflora incarnata

Uses

Passionflower is primarily a remedy for insomnia and anxiety. It is a good substitute for valerian as a treatment for sleep problems, but it is more suitable for long-term anxiety than for, say, exam nerves or stage fright.

COMBINATIONS: Passionflower combines well with green oats, lemon balm and valerian for the treatment of long-term anxiety.
DOSAGE: **Adults:** 1–2ml diluted with some water, one to three times a day, tincture strength 1:2.

Rose *Rosa × damascena, Rosa gallica* or *Rosa × centifolia*

Do not use rose essential oil for external applications in pregnancy without consulting a specialist.

Uses

Few people realise that rose has antidepressant properties. The medicinal part is the flower, mainly of the Damask rose (*Rosa × damascena*), and it is used in the Middle East as a remedy for shock and bereavement. Women seem to respond better to this herb than men, and I recommend using it for depressive moods related to hormone fluctuations, including those associated with the menopause, and also for people who are coping with any serious loss.

HOW TO USE IT: As a tincture, made from fresh rose petals. Good-quality rose tincture is not easy to source, so you may have to make your own. You need to use red or pink roses with a strong fragrance, preferably *Rosa × damascena, Rosa gallica* or *Rosa × centifolia*. You can also use rose essential oil (referred to as 'attar' or 'otto') in a vaporiser or in your bath, to lift the spirits.
COMBINATIONS: Rose combines well with lemon balm, St John's wort and vervain.
DOSAGE: **Adults:** 1–2ml diluted with some water, two to three times a day, tincture strength 1:2.
If using the rose essential oil add 2–5 drops to a bath, or 2–3 drops to a vaporiser.

St John's wort
Hypericum perforatum

Check that St John's wort is not contraindicated when you are on regular medication, as it can alter the metabolism of many drugs.

Avoid excessive exposure to sun and UV light when taking this medicinal herb

Uses

St John's wort is familiar to many people as a natural antidepressant. It works well for mild to moderate depression, and can be used in any circumstances where low mood is a symptom, but it is especially helpful for menopausal mood swings and post-viral depression. St John's wort is non-addictive and it has mild anti-anxiety properties. It is also a restorative herb, which means that it aids recovery from illnesses of the nervous tissue (e.g. neuralgia) or injury to this tissue.

The quality of the preparation is the key to this herb's effectiveness, so it is worth investing in high-quality products (see the Useful resources chapter). In my experience, St John's wort works relatively quickly – within a week or two – but occasionally people need to persevere for longer before they feel the uplifting effect. If you don't experience a significant improvement within six weeks you should seek an alternative treatment.

COMBINATIONS: St John's wort combines well with rose, green oats, vervain and valerian. Combination with valerian is particularly suitable for situations where anxiety is a pronounced feature.
HOW TO TAKE IT: As a tincture (this is preferable to a tea).

To be on the safe side, when you are on prescribed medication I would advise you to see a trained herbal practitioner to set an appropriate dose that is compatible with your specific type of medication. I do not recommend tinctures that are standardised to a single constituent, as the effectiveness of this herb depends on a whole spectrum of different constituents.
DOSAGE: **Adults:** 0.7–2ml diluted with some water, two to three times a day, tincture strength 1:2.

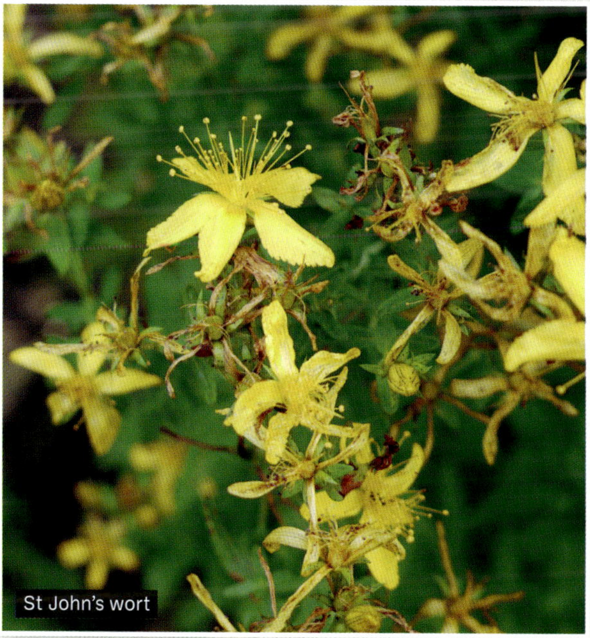
St John's wort

Vervain *Verbena officinalis*

Take vervain several hours before or after mineral supplements.

Uses

Vervain is a gentle relaxant and antidepressant. It also helps the body to cope with stress or to recover from the effects of stress, so it can be used in situations where prolonged stress begins to manifest as exhaustion, irritation or a low mood. It is also very useful for people who are recovering from illnesses that leave them feeling depressed and lacking energy, especially if they also have digestive problems. The low mood and emotional symptoms that can accompany menopausal changes also improve with vervain.

HOW TO TAKE IT: As a tincture or as a tea.
DOSAGE: **Adults:** 1–2ml diluted with some water, one to three times a day, tincture strength 1:2, or 1–3 cups of tea a day.

Specific ailments affecting the nervous system, and herbs that can help

Anxiety

Anxiety can be brought on by many circumstances, and you may need professional help to overcome anxiety that is persistent or severe. Occasional anxiety related to common life events such as a job interview, travelling, moving house or giving a presentation can be helped by taking relaxing herbs. All of these herbs work relatively quickly – within 30 minutes of taking them.

Treatment options

Please see pages 96–101 for herbal precautions.

- Take valerian tincture. **Adults (for regular use for up to a month):** 0.7–2ml diluted with some water, one to three times a day, tincture strength 1:2.

Below Freshly picked passionflowers.

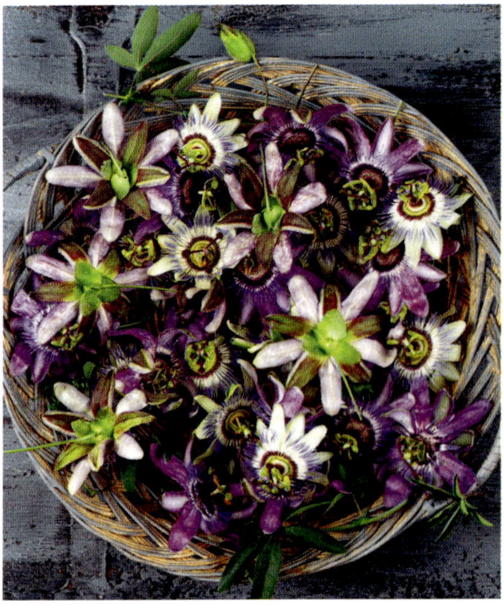

Adults (for one-off use): 5ml of tincture diluted with some water two hours before a stressful event, and a further 5ml diluted with some water 30 minutes before the event.
- Drink chamomile tea on a regular basis. **Adults**: 2–3 cups a day; use 2 teaspoonsful of loose herbs per cup, or two tea bags per cup.
- Take passionflower tincture if anxiety is disrupting your sleep. **Adults**: 1–2ml diluted with some water, one to three times a day, tincture strength 1:2.
- Drink lemon balm tea. Adults: 1–3 cups a day.
- Take the anti-anxiety mix below.

Anti-anxiety mix

Please see pages 96–101 for herbal precautions.

INGREDIENTS

- 20ml chamomile (tincture strength 1:2)
- 20ml lemon balm (tincture strength 1:2)
- 30ml valerian (tincture strength 1:2)
- 30ml passionflower (tincture strength 1:2)

METHOD

1. Mix the ingredients together.
2. Pour the mixture into a clean, dark glass bottle.
3. Label the bottle with the contents and the date.
4. Store at room temperature for up to a year.

Adult dose: 5ml diluted with some water, two to three times a day.

Concentration, problems with

Problems with concentration can be improved by a combination of diet, supplements, medicinal plants and lifestyle adjustments. Herbs will rarely provide the whole answer if there is a long-standing problem. The measures listed below are useful for situations in which you need to concentrate for prolonged periods of time – for instance, when studying for an exam or driving a long distance. Poor concentration often results from lack of sleep, so relaxing herbs taken before going to bed will improve your concentration the next day.

Treatment options

Please see pages 97 and 180 for herbal precautions.

- Take Siberian ginseng tincture. **Adults**: 1–4ml, once or twice a day, tincture strength 1:2.
- Use rosemary essential oil. **Adults**: add 5 drops to a bath, or use 2–3 drops in a vaporiser, or crush a twig of fresh rosemary with your fingers and inhale the fragrance for a few seconds, repeating this procedure whenever your concentration begins to flag again. You can also use the rosemary tincture.

Depression

Practitioner treatment is recommended for this condition.

A low mood can be lifted with many herbs, but severe depression needs treatment by a health professional. If you try the measures listed below, either singly or in combination, and you do not get results within six weeks, seek advice from a herbalist or your GP. Depression is a complex disorder, and often herbs other than antidepressant ones are required. For instance, if your depression is related to your menstrual cycle you may need herbs to balance your hormones, or if you feel down after having flu you will need herbs that boost your immune system.

Mix for mild depression with anxiety

Please see pages 96–101 for herbal precautions.

INGREDIENTS

- 20ml rosemary (tincture strength 1:2)
- 30ml vervain (tincture strength 1:2)
- 20ml valerian (tincture strength 1:2)
- 30ml St John's wort (tincture strength 1:2)

METHOD

1. Mix the ingredients together.
2. Pour the mixture into a clean, dark glass bottle.
3. Label the bottle with the contents and the date.
4. Store at room temperature for up to a year.

ADULT DOSE: 5ml diluted with some water, two to three times a day.

Treatment options

Please see pages 96–101 for herbal precautions.

- Take St John's wort tincture. **Adults**: 0.7–2ml diluted with some water, two to three times a day, tincture strength 1:2.
- Take rose tincture. **Adults**: 1–2ml diluted with some water, two to three times a day, tincture strength 1:2.
- Take vervain tincture or tea. **Adults**: 1–2ml diluted with some water, one to three times a day, tincture strength 1:2, or 1–3 cups of tea a day.

- Take green oats tincture. **Adults**: 1–2ml diluted with some water, two to three times a day, tincture strength 1:2.
- Use rosemary essential oil. **Adults**: 5 drops added to a bath, or 2–3 drops in a vaporiser.
- If anxiety is one of your symptoms, take the mix for mild depression with anxiety (see previous page).

Exam nerves and performance anxiety

Most people get nervous before big events such as sitting an exam, performing in front of an audience or speaking in public. Herbs can take the edge of such nervousness without impairing your performance. Depending on how nervous you get, you can opt for milder herbs, such as lemon balm, or stronger-acting ones, such as valerian or passionflower, and you can vary the dosage according to your requirements. All of the herbs listed below are suitable for children who get nervous before taking exams.

Below Valerian tincture.

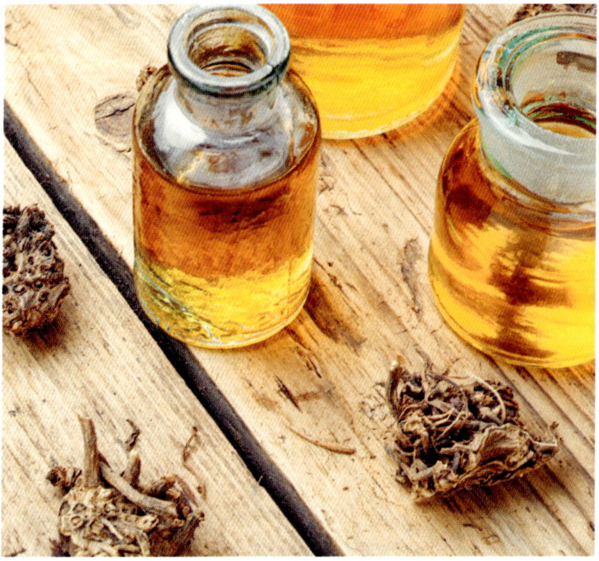

Treatment options

Please see pages 96–101 for herbal precautions.

- Take valerian tincture. **Adults**: take 5ml diluted with some water, tincture strength 1:2, a few hours before the event, and then a further 5ml diluted with some water 30 minutes before the event. If the event is in the evening you may need to take a dose in the morning, a dose at lunchtime and then a final dose 30 minutes before the event. Do not be tempted to take two doses at the same time, as this could send you to sleep!
- Take passionflower tincture. **Adults**: 1–2ml diluted with some water, one to three times a day, tincture strength 1:2.
- Drink lemon balm tea. **Adults**: 1–3 cups a day.

Headache, tension

Headaches can have many causes – for instance, dehydration, tension or eye strain. The most common type is the tension headache, which is related mainly to stress and sometimes to problems with the neck vertebrae. If you suffer from headaches regularly, you should see your doctor, optician and/or dentist to make sure that there is no serious underlying cause.

Treatment options

Please see pages 96–101 for herbal precautions.

- Take valerian tincture. **Adults**: if you already have a headache, take 5ml, once or twice a day, tincture strength 1:2; to prevent tension

Right Lavender bags are easy to make at home yourself.

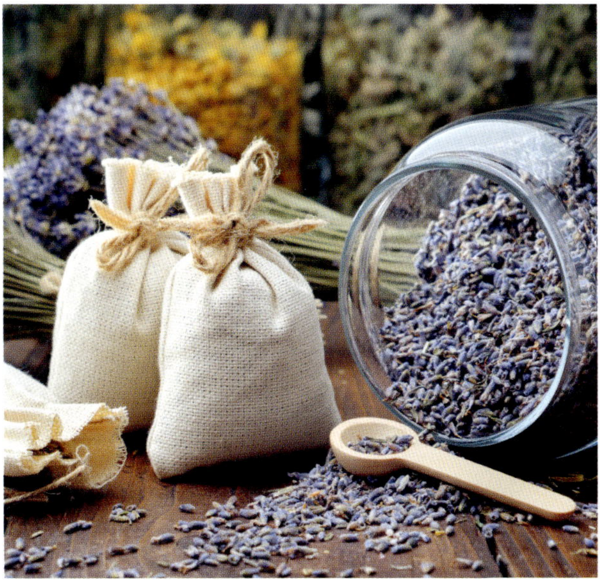

headaches if you get a lot of them, take 0.7–2ml, one to three times a day, tincture strength 1:2, for several weeks.

- Drink lavender tea. **Adults:** 1 cup as soon as you feel the headache coming on, using 1 teaspoonful of loose herbs per cup.
- Drink lemon balm tea. **Adults:** 1–2 cups when you feel the headache coming on.
- Drink chamomile tea. **Adults:** 1–2 cups when you feel the headache coming on.
- Drink the tea for tension headaches (see box).
- Drink lime tree flower tea. **Adults:** 1–2 cups when you feel the headache coming on.

Tea for tension headaches

Please see pages 96–101 for herbal precautions.

INGREDIENTS

- 25g dried lavender
- 25g dried lemon balm
- 25g dried chamomile
- 25g dried lime tree flowers

METHOD

1. Mix the herbs thoroughly.
2. Infuse 2 teaspoonsful of the mixture in a cup of freshly boiled water for 10 minutes. strain and drink warm. You can add honey to this tea.

ADULT DOSE: 1–2 cups when you feel the headache coming on.

Insomnia

Practitioner treatment is recommended for this condition.

Insomnia can be successfully treated with sleep-inducing herbs and there is no risk of becoming addicted to such herbs. Often, when you are under a lot of stress, you need both a daytime treatment to help you to relax and a night-time treatment to help you drop off to sleep and maintain your sleep through the night. The options listed below are primarily intended for one-off situations when you find it difficult to fall asleep or expect to have difficulty falling asleep.

Treatment options

Please see pages 96–101 for herbal precautions.

- Take valerian tincture – it is very useful in situations in which your mind is still very active despite the late hour. **Adults:** 5ml diluted with some water, tincture strength 1:2, taken once, if you cannot fall asleep. If you find that you feel slightly groggy in the morning, reduce the dose next time to 2–3ml.

- Put lavender essential oil in a bath or directly on the pillow you will sleep on. **Adults:** 5 drops in a bath, or 2–3 drops on a pillow.
- If you have had sleep problems for a long time, prepare a mix for insomnia (see box) and take it regularly for a month.
- Place a lavender pillow next to your head in bed so that you can smell and inhale the fragrance. You can make your own by buying about 100–200g of loose lavender and stuffing a small muslin bag with the herbs. Small lavender pillows are suitable for children.
- For children, taking chamomile tea before bedtime is usually sufficient to induce sleep. **Children:** four years old, a quarter of a cup; five to eight years old, half a cup; eight to twelve years old, a full cup.

Mix for insomnia

Please see pages 96–101 for herbal precautions.

INGREDIENTS

- 40ml valerian (tincture strength 1:2)
- 30ml lemon balm (tincture strength 1:2)
- 30ml passionflower (tincture strength 1:2)

METHOD

1. Mix the ingredients together.
2. Pour the mixture into a clean, dark glass bottle.
3. Label the bottle with the contents and the date.
4. Store at room temperature for up to a year.

ADULT DOSE: 5ml diluted with some water 30 minutes before sleep.

Nervous indigestion

Indigestion is often caused by anxiety or worry. At such times the two measures listed below can be used singly or in combination, depending on how severe the symptoms are. All of the measures can be used long term (for 6–12 months) if necessary.

Treatment options

Please see pages 96–101 for herbal precautions.

- Drink chamomile tea. **Adults:** 3–4 cups a day; if you suffer from heartburn, limit this to 1 cup a day.
- Take valerian tincture. **Adults:** 0.7–2ml diluted with some water, once or twice a day, tincture strength 1:2. Take marshmallow root powder if you get heartburn due to stress (see page 74).

Neuralgia

Practitioner treatment is recommended for persistent neuralgia.

Neuralgia is pain caused by damage to or inflammation of the nervous tissue. The most common types are trigeminal neuralgia, neuralgia that can follow shingles or herpes, and neuralgia associated with sciatica. Irrespective of which type you have, you will benefit from both internal treatment and the external application of herbs that have anti-inflammatory and regenerative effects on the nervous tissue. The antiviral properties of St John's wort are useful for neuralgia that is associated with shingles or herpes; use it internally as a tincture and externally as an infused oil.

Treatment options

Please see pages 96–101 for herbal precautions.

- Take St John's wort tincture. **Adults:** 2ml diluted with some water, three times a day, tincture strength 1:2, until the pain subsides; then reduce the dose to 1ml diluted with some water, three times a day, tincture strength 1:2, until the pain disappears.
- Take passionflower tincture for its calming and painkilling properties. **Adults:** 1–2ml, three times a day, tincture strength 1:2.
- Apply St John's wort as an infused oil externally over the affected area. **Adults and children:** apply the oil two to four times a day.
- Apply marigold ointment (see page 135) to the skin blisters caused by shingles. **Adults and children over four years old:** apply two to three times a day.

Panic attacks

Practitioner treatment is recommended for this condition.

Occasional panic attacks can be overcome using the measures listed below. Breathing into a paper bag during an attack is an effective measure for bringing the breath rate back to normal. In general, however, panic attacks are indicative of extreme anxiety, in which case professional help should be sought, as herbalists can provide an individual prescription with strong sedative properties.

Treatment options

Please see pages 96–101 for herbal precautions.

- Take valerian tincture. **Adults:** 10ml, taken once, diluted with some water, tincture strength 1:2, during a panic attack, or 0.7–2ml, two to three times a day, tincture strength 1:2, as a preventative measure.
- Drink strong lemon balm tea. **Adults:** 2–3 cups a day as a preventative measure.

Shingles

Practitioner treatment is recommended for this condition.

Shingles on the face, especially near the eyes, is a medical emergency and you will be prescribed antiviral medication.

Shingles is caused by reactivation of the chickenpox virus, usually when the affected person's immune system is weakened. It causes inflammation of the nerves that supply a specific part of the skin, and can manifest as tingling, itching, stinging or even severe pain in that area. There is a rash over the affected part which may either form a band or be quite diffused – it can resemble clustered insect bites

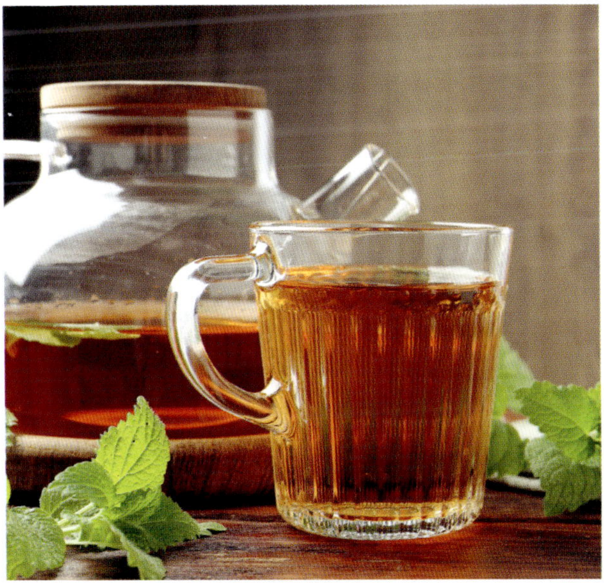

Right Lemon balm tea.

or eczema. The pain can occur early on or a few days after the rash appears. The internal and external treatment options listed below should bring relief within one or two weeks. I recommend that you use all three treatment options in combination. If you do not get satisfactory results, consult a herbal clinician, who can prescribe herbs with stronger immune support, analgesic and antiviral properties.

Treatment options

Please see pages 115 and 117 for herbal precautions.

- Take echinacea tincture. **Adults:** 1.2–3ml, three times a day, tincture strength 1:2.
- Take andrographis tincture. **Adults:** 1–2ml, three times a day, tincture strength 1:2.
- Apply the ointment for shingles (see box above right), which will ease the pain and speed up recovery.

Below Echinacea tincture.

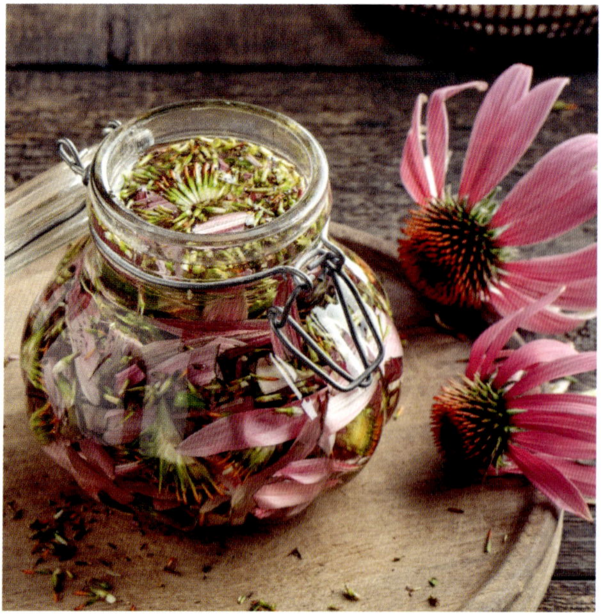

Ointment for shingles

Please see pages 96–101 for herbal precautions.

INGREDIENTS

- 50g marigold ointment or cream
- 5ml lemon balm tincture
- 5ml St John's wort infused oil

METHOD

1. Mix the ingredients well.
2. Transfer the mixture to a clean, dark glass jar, making sure that all air pockets are removed.
3. The ointment can be stored for up to 12 months.

ADULTS: apply to the affected area twice a day.

Stress

Coping with stress is not always easy, and our ability to manage it varies throughout our life and according to the nature of the stress. Siberian ginseng (see page 180) can increase your resistance to stress – it works as a general tonic for all of the body systems, including the nervous system, and it makes you more resilient to life's pressures. I recommend using Siberian ginseng in specific situations when you expect an unusual increase in stress – for instance, during exams or when you need to meet work deadlines. Korean ginseng works in a similar way, but it is much stronger and is not considered suitable for anyone under 40 years old according to the principles of traditional Chinese medicine.

The ability to cope with stress can also be related to your adrenal function, which can be improved by taking specific botanicals, so it may be worth consulting a medical herbalist about this (see also Chapter 15).

Treatment options

Please see pages 96, 99 and 180 for herbal precautions.

- Take Siberian ginseng tincture to increase your resistance to stress – this herb can be taken long term, for many months if necessary. **Adults**: 1–4ml diluted with some water, once or twice a day, tincture strength 1:2.
- Take valerian tincture if your reaction to stress manifests itself as anxiety or irritability. **Adults**: 0.7–2ml diluted with some water, one to three times a day, tincture strength 1:2.
- Take liquorice tincture if prolonged stress has left you feeling exhausted. **Adults**: 0.2–2ml diluted with some water, once or twice a day, tincture strength 1:1.
- Take green oats tincture if prolonged stress has left you feeling exhausted and depressed. **Adults**: 1–2ml diluted with some water, two to three times a day, tincture strength 1:2.

Conditions for which home treatment is not recommended

- Migraine: this condition has many causes, often related to dietary factors or hormonal imbalances.
- Depression that does not respond quickly to St John's wort: there are many herbs that can lift mood, but they need to be matched to the individual.
- Extreme anxiety: this condition requires careful adjustment of specific herbs and their dosage.
- Neuralgia: this ailment requires a careful balance of herbal painkillers with the herbs that restore the health of the nervous tissue.
- Multiple sclerosis: this disease of the nervous tissue can, in the early stages, be successfully put in remission by individualised herbal treatment. In cases of advanced disease herbs have much to offer in terms of supportive treatment.
- Shingles: this condition responds very well to herbal treatment, but may require specific immunostimulation.

When to seek medical attention

- If you have repeated, prolonged or very severe headaches.
- If you experience a sudden marked change in your vision or hearing.
- If you notice unusual sensations in your limbs (e.g. pins and needles, numbness) that will not go away or that are getting worse.
- If you suffer from extreme anxiety.
- If you have severe depression.

CHAPTER 11

The respiratory system

This chapter deals with problems associated with the respiratory system. The main parts of the respiratory system are the nose, throat and lungs. However, the ears and sinuses are closely associated with the respiratory system, and are therefore included here as well. The respiratory system tends to become diseased more often than other systems, as it is very easy to pick up all sorts of bugs just by breathing them in. Common infections of the respiratory system are usually viral but can occasionally be bacterial in origin. It is important to distinguish between viral and bacterial infections in order to choose the best treatment, whether herbal or conventional. The differences are pointed out in this chapter when discussing specific ailments in detail. However, sometimes it is not possible to tell whether you have been infected by a virus or bacteria unless you have a specialist investigation.

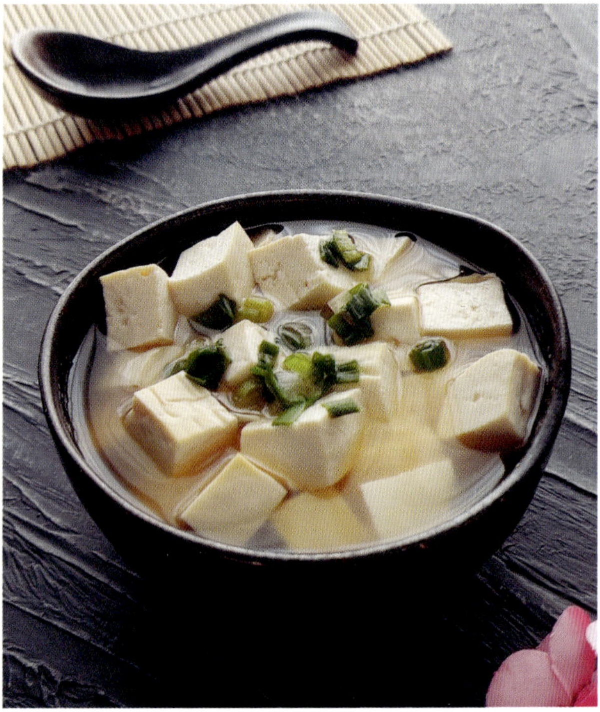

Right Miso soup is a delicious and healthy source of nutrients.

Temperature

An important point to remember with infections of the respiratory system is that there is a direct link between body temperature and the severity of the infection – the higher the temperature, the 'nastier' the bug. Children are more likely to develop a high fever very quickly, so it is really important to check the body temperature often and to keep it down by using appropriate measures (for further information on fever, see page 128).

Nutrition

Before moving on to herbal treatment I would like to recommend a couple of nutritional measures that are traditionally used when treating the common cold. The first measure is the traditional advice to drink lemon juice and honey with hot water. This makes good sense, as honey has mild antibiotic properties, soothes the lining of the throat, boosts your energy and warms you up, while lemon juice is a source of vitamin C, which reduces catarrh. You can use manuka honey for its stronger antibiotic properties – manuka honey is made by bees that collect pollen from the flowering tea tree plant. Use hot water, but let it cool slightly after boiling, as very hot water will destroy the vitamin C in lemon juice. I usually mix 2 teaspoonsful of honey with 1 teaspoonful of lemon juice per cup of water, but you can use your own proportions according to personal taste.

The second food that is traditionally used to relieve colds or flu-like symptoms is chicken broth. This is a common treatment in many European countries, as has been confirmed by a number of researchers.[12] A recipe that I use at home is shown in the box opposite. I recommend that you cook your own chicken broth, as it will contain more nutrients than a tinned or packet version.

The aim is to have clear broth, so do not blend the ingredients. I normally add some precooked noodles or rice to the broth, together with chunks of carrots and chicken meat. It is the most comforting, fortifying meal if you have a cold, but is also of benefit when convalescing from any serious illness. A good vegetarian and vegan equivalent would be a miso soup, which has a similar taste and mineral content to chicken broth. You could add lentils, chickpeas, mushrooms or tofu to provide additional protein, and carrots, parsnips and onion for additional minerals and vitamins.

Recipe for chicken broth

INGREDIENTS

- 4 drumsticks or 2 thighs – choose any parts of the chicken, preferably organic, with bones and skin
- 5 whole peeled carrots
- 2 peeled parsnips
- 1 whole peeled onion
- 1 litre of water

METHOD

1. Cover the chicken with water.
2. Boil for about 30 minutes.
3. Add the carrots, parsnips and onion.
4. Keep boiling on a low setting until the vegetables are tender.
5. Add salt and pepper to taste.

Rest

There has been a marked increase in the number of people suffering from post-viral fatigue over the last few years. This is largely a consequence of the fact that we are expected to push ourselves when we have a cold, instead of staying in bed and then recuperating at home until we have recovered. Two to five days at home will give your body enough time to recuperate properly, and will also prevent the spread of the infection to other people. Occasionally, a particularly virulent cold or flu variant emerges that requires a longer rest period. If you have had flu, glandular fever, bronchitis or a severe cold that you can't shake off, please refer to Chapter 20 on recovery from serious illness.

Must-have herbs

The herbs in this section are listed in order of usefulness.

Elderflower *Sambucus nigra*

This is my favourite herb for helping both to prevent the development of a cold or flu and to reduce the symptoms. In my experience, elderflower tea is one of the most effective treatments against viral infections.

Uses

Elderflower can be used both for nipping a cold in the bud and for treating the symptoms of a cold. If you start taking it straight away at the onset of symptoms, you may well not develop a cold at all, but if you do, it is still worth taking elderflower tea or tincture as it will help you to recover more quickly, and your symptoms will be milder. Apart from being antiviral, elderflower has anti-catarrhal properties, so it is especially worth taking this tea or tincture in situations when catarrh is a prominent symptom, and this applies to an ordinary runny nose as well as to allergic reactions and hay fever. As elderflower is a warming herb you can feel quite hot for a short while after taking it, especially after drinking a hot elderflower tea. This warming effect is useful for reducing a mildly raised temperature.

Elderflower tea is noticeably diuretic, so make sure that you drink plenty of water to compensate for this, and avoid drinking elderflower tea just before going to bed, if you want to avoid having to get up in the middle of the night.

While elderberries used as a tincture have similar properties, elderflower is more suitable for making an infusion.

Commercially produced elderflower cordials do not have any appreciable medicinal properties.

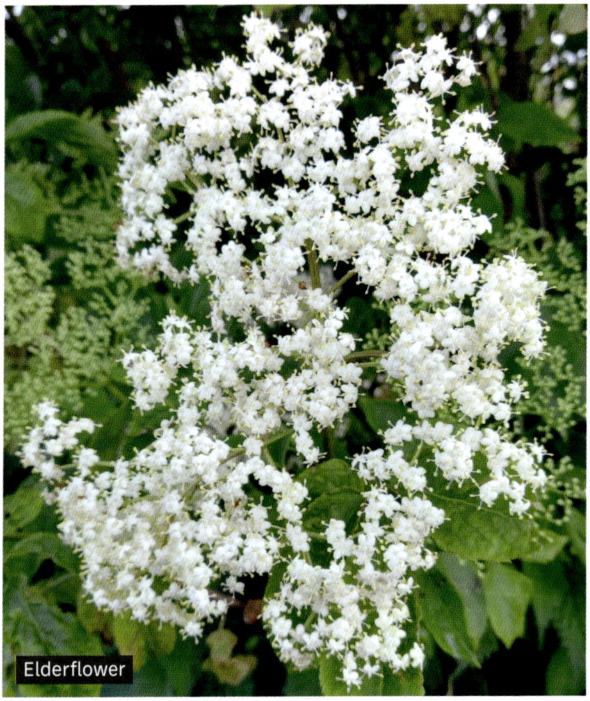

Elderflower

COMBINATIONS: Elderflower combines well with garlic or andrographis tablets or capsules.

HOW TO TAKE IT: Elderflower needs to be taken at the earliest possible stage of a cold or flu-like illness if you want to prevent it from developing.

You need 2–4 cups of infusion a day to prevent a cold from developing. It is best to drink 4 cups on the day you start feeling under the weather and 1–2 cups on the following day. Each cup should be brewed with 2 teaspoonsful of dried herbs or 2–4 tablespoonsful of fresh flowers. It is best to make a fresh brew of tea each time and drink it warm. You can add honey to the tea if you wish.

In my experience, warm, freshly brewed elderflower tea is the most effective of all the possible preparations that can be made from elderflower, but the tincture is also quite effective and may appeal to people who are travelling and who dislike the taste of elderflower tea.

DOSAGE: **Adults:** 1 cup of infusion one to four times a day; short-term dose for tincture, 5ml, two to three times a day, tincture strength 1:2, for two to three days; long-term dose for tincture, 0.7–2ml, three times a day, tincture strength 1:2.

Garlic *Allium sativum*

Do not take large doses of garlic for prolonged periods of time or when pregnant or breastfeeding. Discontinue garlic 10 days before undergoing surgery. This herb is not suitable for children under six years old.

Caution is needed in people who are taking blood-thinning (anticoagulant or antiplatelet) medications.

Uses

Garlic is an excellent anti-cold agent. You can take it in capsule form, eat it raw or drink garlic juice. Taking garlic regularly through the winter will prevent many milder colds, or you can take it in larger doses to treat a cold that has already developed. When garlic is cooked it loses most of its medicinal properties and is then safe to be consumed in all circumstances. It is important that you choose a good-quality preparation – look for freeze-

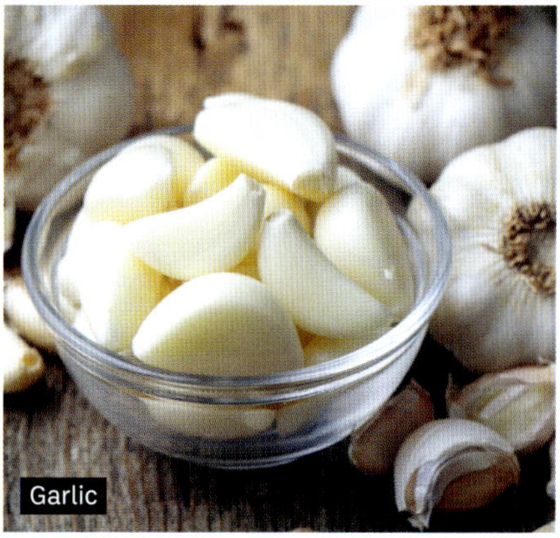

Garlic

dried garlic capsules or tablets that state the content of allicin or alliin (the most active ingredients of garlic, which are also responsible for its smell).

COMBINATIONS: Garlic combines well with elderflower and andrographis for the treatment of colds.

HOW TO TAKE IT: If you have a juicer you can make your own garlic juice, freeze it as small cubes (about 1 teaspoonful each) and then use it when you need it, mixing it with water or fruit juice in the same way as you would do with tinctures. Garlic juice mixed with fruit juice tastes much better than it sounds, especially if you use mango juice. Alternatively, you can stabilise the juice with alcohol for long-term storage (see box overleaf).

Based on my personal observations, confirmed by all of my patients who have used garlic juice, I have found that the juice does not give you garlicky breath! You will experience an aftertaste for a short time but it does not linger, and if you mix garlic juice with any fruit juice you will hardly notice it at all.

However, the simplest way to take garlic is to chop a single clove very finely, or crush it in a garlic press, mix it with a generous teaspoonful of honey and just swallow the lot. You can drink some water or juice to help it go down. The honey will mask the taste of garlic quite effectively, while preserving the garlic's curative, antimicrobial properties.

I do not recommend taking raw garlic for prolonged periods of time in large amounts (three cloves a day counts as a large dose), as such a habit may alter the bowel flora and lead to digestive problems; the same applies to garlic capsules and juice. Of course, cooked garlic is a completely different matter, and you can consume it regularly without any harmful effects.

DOSAGE: **Adults:** 1 teaspoonful of garlic juice, either freshly squeezed, defrosted or stabilised with alcohol, one to three times a day, or a crushed clove, one to three times a day, mixed with honey. If you opt for garlic capsules or tablets, follow the manufacturer's instructions.

Long-life garlic juice

INGREDIENTS

- 150ml freshly squeezed garlic juice produced with a juicer (for precautions, see page 113)
- 250ml of 40% pure vodka or brandy

METHOD

1. Mix the juice and alcohol together.
2. Pour the mixture into a clean, dark glass bottle.
3. Label the bottle with the contents and the date.
4. Store for up to two years in a cool, dark place.

Onion *Allium cepa*

Uses

Onion is milder than garlic but is particularly effective for chest infections and most types of cough. Fresh onion has an antimicrobial effect on the airways, as well as being soothing to an irritated

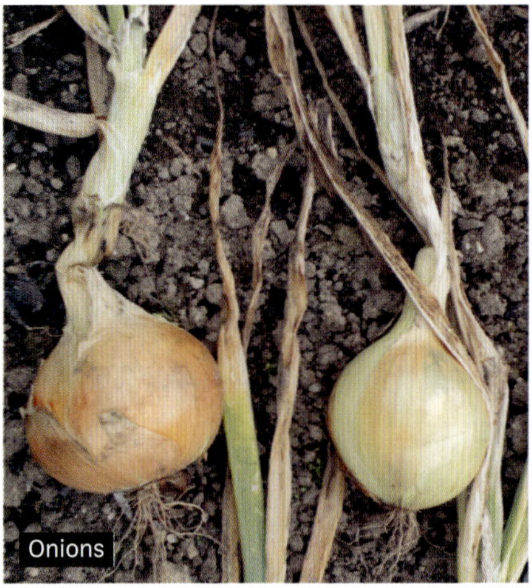

Onions

throat. Onion will reduce the intensity and frequency of coughing, and your cough should go away quite quickly. As a common food item that happens to have curative properties, onion is safe to use in all circumstances and for all age groups.

HOW TO TAKE IT: I recommend the use of freshly made onion syrup, which works best when taken as soon as you develop a cough. The recipe opposite was given to me by one of my teachers when I was training to be a herbalist, and from the very first time I used it I have been a firm supporter of this approach. Although the idea of onion syrup may not be very appealing, it tastes surprisingly nice despite the smell of raw onion. It is also easy to make when travelling (I once made it when trekking in the Himalayas). You can take onion syrup by itself or with any other herbal syrup.

DOSAGE: **Adults:** 1 teaspoonful, four to five times a day until the symptoms improve; for a slight cough take 1 teaspoonful once or twice a day, or for a severe cough take 1 teaspoonful seven to eight times a day. **Children (5–16 years):** 5–7 years, half a teaspoonful three times a day; 7–10 years, 1 teaspoonful three times a day; 11–16 years, 1 teaspoonful three to five times a day.

Recipe for onion syrup

INGREDIENTS

- 1 large onion
- 5–7 teaspoonsful of brown sugar or honey

METHOD

1. Peel and slice the onion into chunky slices about 5mm thick.
2. Put one slice in a cup and cover it with a teaspoonful of sugar or honey.
3. Follow this with alternate layers of onion slices and sugar or honey.
4. Leave the cup covered for a few hours.
5. The sugar will extract the juice from the onion, and you can collect the resulting syrup in a different cup (keep it covered for storage) or a small bottle.
6. Do not store onion syrup for more than two days.

Note: This syrup is only effective when freshly made, so you may have to make a fresh batch every two days if necessary. One onion produces on average a two-day supply of syrup.

Echinacea (purple coneflower) *Echinacea purpurea* and *Echinacea angustifolia*

Caution is needed in people who are allergic to plants belonging to the daisy family (the Asteraceae, formerly known as the Compositae).
Not suitable for transplant patients and children under 12.

Uses

The latest research on the use of *Echinacea* species to prevent colds favours its continuous use throughout the autumn and winter.[13] This prepares the immune system to respond more quickly to viral infections, and as a result you either do not develop any symptoms or, if you do catch a cold, the symptoms are much milder. Two distinct species are used medicinally – *Echinacea purpurea* (purple coneflower) and *Echinacea angustifolia* (narrow-leaved purple coneflower). A combination of the roots and aerial parts of these two species works best, and I would recommend that you source these from accredited herbalists to ensure good quality. *Echinacea angustifolia* is virtually extinct in the wild due to over-harvesting, so buy only from cultivated sources – it will be expensive because it is difficult to grow. However, *Echinacea purpurea* is easily cultivated in many parts of the world and, although slightly less effective, it is a more environmentally sustainable choice.

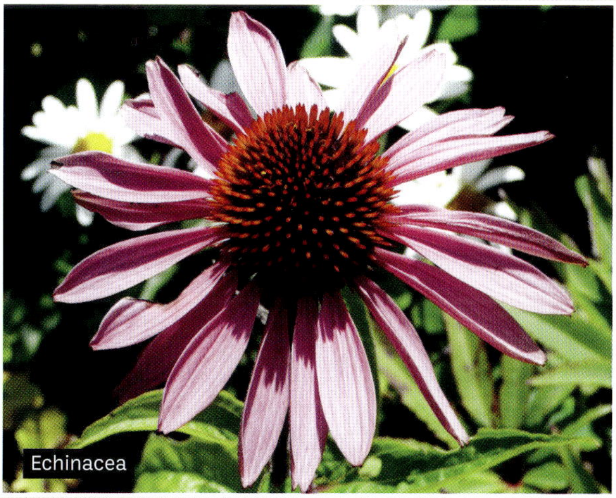

Echinacea

There is a simple test to assess the quality of echinacea tincture. If you put one or two drops of the neat tincture on your tongue you should feel a strong tingling sensation that is caused by alkylamides, the most relevant active constituents of the plant. If you feel no tingling sensation, the tincture is unlikely to have medicinal properties.

Traditionally, Native Americans used echinacea primarily as a wound-healing herb, both internally and externally. Scientific research has shown that stimulation of the immune system will improve all types of healing, as recovery from any disease depends on the immune system working efficiently.

HOW TO TAKE IT: I generally prescribe this herb in tincture form as a long-term treatment for people whose immune system is weakened (who tend to catch all of the bugs that are going round), or for those who take a long time to recover from a particular infection. As a general rule, I would avoid taking echinacea if you have severe symptoms, as it can occasionally make them worse.

I have found elderflower tea to be more effective than echinacea for nipping a cold in the bud, and it is certainly a cheaper option. However, I know plenty of people who use echinacea in larger doses at the onset of symptoms and get good results (a large dose is 5ml, three times a day, tincture strength 1:2, whereas a long-term adult dose is 1–2ml, three times a day, tincture strength 1:2). By careful experimenting you can find out what works best for you.

People who are prone to allergies should exercise caution with echinacea, as it is known to cause occasional allergic reaction, usually in the form of a skin rash. Start with very small doses if you have never taken it before, especially if you suffer from asthma, eczema or hay fever. Certain inflammatory disorders, such as rheumatoid arthritis, can occasionally be worsened by taking echinacea, but such reactions are not common.

DOSAGE: **Adults:** for long-term use take 1.2–3ml diluted with some water, one to three times a day, tincture strength 1:2; for short-term, intense treatment take 5ml diluted with some water, three times a day, tincture strength 1:2, for one to two days. **Teenagers (12–16 years):** Adjust the adult dose downwards, based on body weight (see Chapter 5).

Propolis

Propolis is not suitable for children under 12 years of age because of the risk of allergic reactions.

Caution is needed in people who have a history of various allergies.

Uses

Propolis is a resinous substance collected by bees from a range of different trees. The bees use propolis to protect the hive from infections, as it is a powerful natural antibiotic with a wide spectrum of activity against bacteria, viruses and fungi. Propolis can be used to treat a variety of respiratory conditions, including sore throat, tonsillitis, flu, chest infections, persistent coughs, severe colds and bronchitis.

Propolis has been shown to enhance the action of many antibiotics when taken at the same time as them.

COMBINATIONS: Propolis combines well with elderflower and echinacea.

HOW TO TAKE IT: You can use propolis spray (made from propolis tincture, strength 1:5) or propolis lozenges for sore throats, irrespective of whether the infection is viral or bacterial. By spraying the liquid directly towards the back of the throat you will be delivering a powerful local treatment, although the taste of propolis tincture is quite strong and you may experience some stinging. You should use the spray as soon as you develop a sore throat. Alternatively, you can take propolis internally, either as a tincture or as capsules. Always buy propolis from reputable suppliers, to ensure that it is of high enough quality for medicinal use.

DOSAGE: **Adults:** 0.5–2ml diluted with some water, one to three times a day, tincture strength 1:5, or 1g of powdered propolis in capsule or tablet form, one to three times a day, or 1–2 puffs from a spray bottle directed towards the back of the throat, two to four times a day, or propolis lozenges taken according to the manufacturer's instructions.

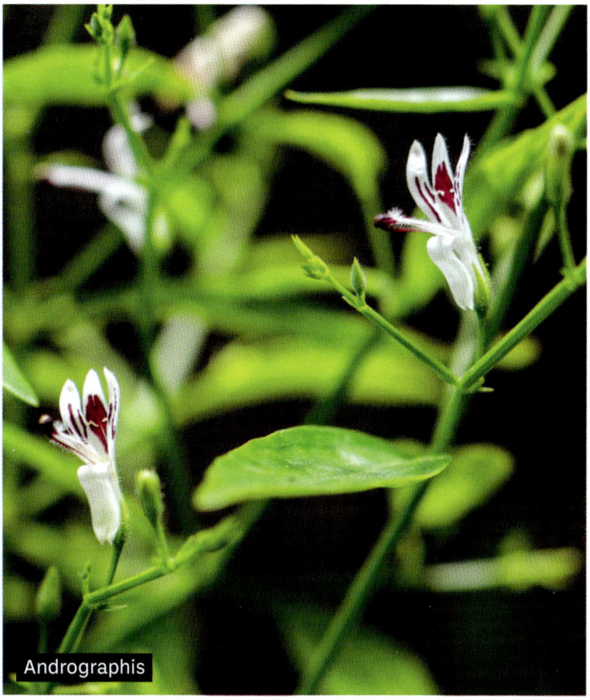

Andrographis

Andrographis
Andrographis paniculata

Andrographis should be avoided in the first trimester of pregnancy. Caution is advised in people who are taking immunosuppressive medication.

Uses

This herb is commonly referred to by its scientific genus name, but is sometimes also called 'king of bitters', as it is intensely bitter. Native to the Indian subcontinent, it has a long tradition of use to treat colds and fevers. It has immune-enhancing properties and is both antiviral and antibacterial. It can be used to prevent infections or to treat acute and chronic infections of the respiratory tract.

COMBINATIONS: Andrographis combines very well with echinacea and elderflower, especially at the onset of a cold, when such a combination can nip this in the bud.

HOW TO TAKE IT: I recommend a high dose (twice the normal dose) for adults if you suspect that you are coming down with a cold, at the stage when you only have vague symptoms, such as feeling unusually tired and achy. If you have already developed other symptoms of the cold take the standard dose. As the tincture is very bitter, for children you may need to disguise the taste with some juice (fresh mango juice works well for this). I do not recommend using increased doses for children.

DOSAGE: **Adults:** 1–2ml diluted with some water, three times a day, tincture strength 1:2; alternatively, for a short, intense treatment, 5ml diluted with some water, three times a day, tincture strength 1:2, for one to two days.

Optional herbs

There are many herbs that can lower the body temperature, ward off chills and soothe muscular aches and pains. You can customise your treatment according to your symptoms. For instance, if you have a cough, add one or two herbs that are specific for coughs. Some of these may be growing in your garden, in which case it makes sense to use what you already have.

Elecampane *Inula helenium*

Elecampane should be avoided by people who are allergic to plants belonging to the daisy family (the Asteraceae, formerly known as the Compositae).

Uses

Elecampane root is a traditional remedy for chest infections. It has a disinfecting action on the lung tissue as well as being an expectorant (i.e. it helps to remove excess mucus from the lungs). It can be used to treat any type of cough of recent origin, or to get rid of a lingering cough.

COMBINATIONS: Elecampane works well in combination with ground ivy, liquorice and thyme or elderflower (see the mix on page 126).
HOW TO TAKE IT: As a tincture.
DOSAGE: **Adults:** 1–2ml diluted with some water, two to three times a day, tincture strength 1:2.

Ground ivy *Glechoma hederacea*

Uses

Ground ivy belongs to the group of herbs that help to restore specific tissues to a healthy state. In particular it helps to heal the lining of the respiratory tract. It provides a supportive treatment for lingering coughs that cannot be shaken off.

COMBINATIONS: Ground ivy mixes well with tinctures of elecampane, thyme and marshmallow root or liquorice root to treat lingering chest infections (see page 126).
HOW TO TAKE IT: Ground ivy is best used as a tincture in combination with antimicrobial herbs.
DOSAGE: **Adults:** 1–2ml diluted with some water, two to three times a day, tincture strength 1:2.

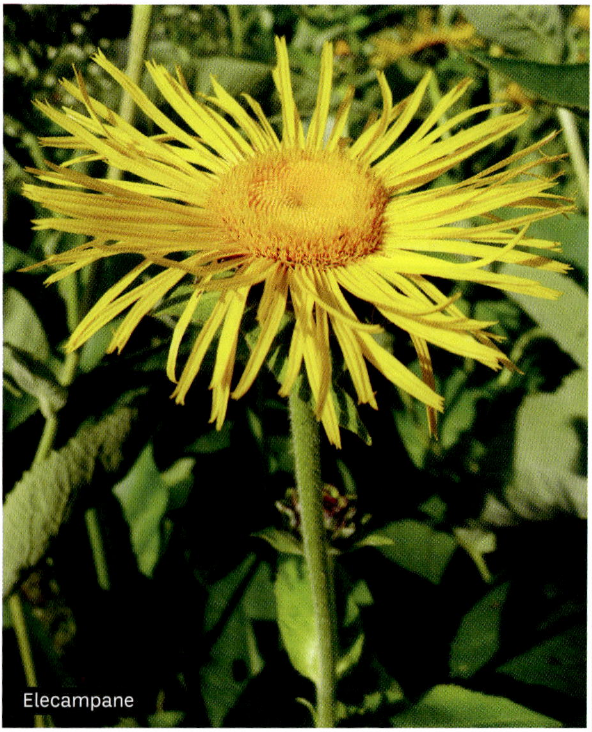

Elecampane

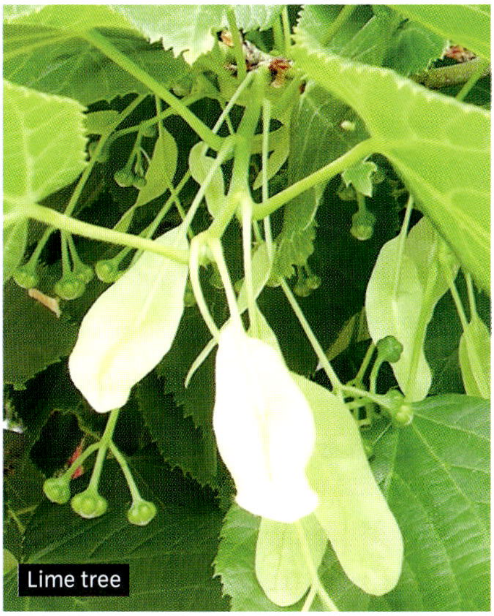

Lime tree flowers
Tilia cordata, Tilia × europaea and *Tilia platyphyllos*

Lime tree flowers should be avoided in people with a known allergy, and should be taken several hours before or after iron supplements.

Uses

Lime tree flowers are a traditional remedy used to reduce fever. This warming herb will induce slight perspiration if your body temperature is above normal. It will also improve disturbed sleep, which is often a problem for people who are unwell.

Use lime tree flowers for a moderately high temperature, between 37°C (98.6°F) and 38°C (100.4°F).

COMBINATIONS: Lime tree flowers can be combined with elderflower.
HOW TO TAKE THEM: Either as a tea made from dried flowers, or as a tincture.
DOSAGE: **Adults:** 0.5–1ml diluted with some water, one to three times a day, tincture strength 1:2, or 1 cup of warm infusion, one to three times a day.

Liquorice
Glycyrrhiza glabra

Liquorice should not be taken during pregnancy, or by the elderly.
Do not take liquorice for a prolonged period if you have high blood pressure, low potassium levels, problems with your heart, kidneys or liver, or water retention.

Uses

Liquorice is a demulcent (anti-irritant) and anti-inflammatory herb. It will reduce the irritation of the airways that is caused by infection and coughing. *People for whom long-term use of liquorice is not advised can safely use it for a few days to treat a cough.*

COMBINATIONS: Liquorice combines well with thyme, the latter having an antibacterial action and the former soothing the bronchi and throat.
HOW TO TAKE IT: Syrup made with liquorice and thyme is very effective for chest infections, and is my preferred preparation. You can take liquorice by itself as a tincture, or as a powder, which should be mixed with water until it has the consistency of runny custard.
DOSAGE: **Adults:** 0.5–2ml diluted with some water, one to three times a day, tincture strength 1:1, or 1g of liquorice powder, two to three times a day, mixed with water, or 1 teaspoonful of thyme and liquorice syrup, two to five times a day.

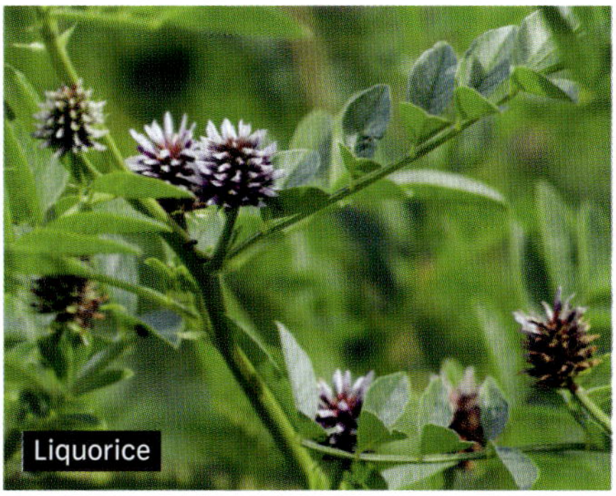

Marshmallow root *Althaea officinalis*

Marshmallow root preparations can be taken alongside any conventional medication, so long as they are taken two hours before or after the latter.

Uses

Marshmallow root, used as marshmallow syrup, is specifically recommended for a dry cough as it soothes the irritated airways. It is also good for a tickly cough resulting from a dry throat, which often occurs when the nose is blocked with catarrh.

HOW TO TAKE IT: As an adult you can take this syrup freely (1 teaspoonful at a time) whenever you have a bout of coughing, or throughout the day to prevent your throat from drying. However, if you are on prescribed medication you should take the syrup two hours before or after the medication.

Alternatively, you can use marshmallow root tincture, although in my experience the syrup is more effective.

DOSAGE: **Adults**: 1 teaspoonful of syrup, three to eight times a day, or 1–2ml of tincture diluted with some water, one to three times a day, tincture strength 1:2. **Children (over five years old)**: 5–7 years, half a teaspoonful of syrup twice a day; 8–12 years, 1 teaspoonful twice a day; 13–16 years, 1 teaspoonful three to four times a day.

Sage *Salvia officinalis*

Do not take sage internally during pregnancy or when breastfeeding. Do not take this herb continually for long periods of time. Sage is not suitable for children as an internal treatment.

Uses

Sage tea makes a soothing gargle for an inflamed throat, as it is very astringent. The tea can also be drunk to combat bacterial infections of the throat or bronchi.

HOW TO TAKE IT: Because sage is an evergreen plant I use it straight from my garden to make the gargle tea (10–15 chopped leaves per cup of boiled water), but you can also use dried sage (1–2 teaspoonsful per cup). I do not recommend using the tincture as a gargle, as it will sting (and if you dilute it too much it will not have any effect). Children usually find this remedy too bitter, but if they are willing to try it, let them do just one gargle once or twice a day. *Sage can be used as a gargle during pregnancy*.

DOSAGE: **Adults**: one mouthful of gargle, three times in a row. Repeat the procedure three to four times a day. **Children (5–16 years)**: one mouthful of gargle, twice in a row. Repeat the procedure once or twice a day.

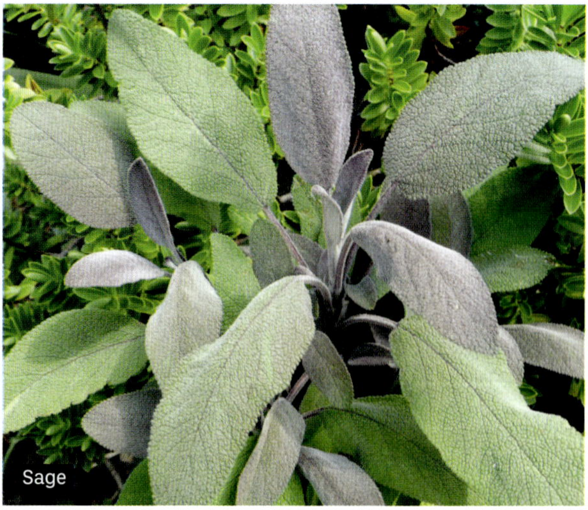

Sage

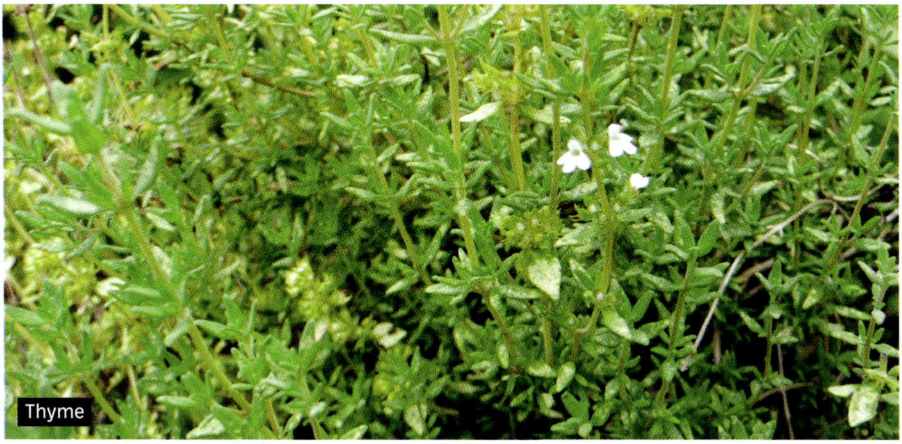
Thyme

St John's wort *Hypericum perforatum*

Check that St John's wort is not contraindicated when you are on regular medication, as it can alter the metabolism of many drugs.

Avoid excessive exposure to sun and UV light when taking this medicinal herb.

Uses

St John's wort has antiviral and antibacterial actions and can be added to any anti-cold treatment, either as a treatment during a cold or flu, or when experiencing post-viral fatigue.

The antiviral and anti-inflammatory properties of St John's wort are useful for external treatment of ear infections.

HOW TO USE IT: For its general antiviral and antibacterial actions, use as a tincture. **Adults**: 0.7–2ml diluted with water, three times a day, tincture strength 1:2.
For the treatment of earache, use St John's wort infused oil. You can either buy preparations from specialist retailers, or you can make your own (see Chapter 23). For directions on usage, see page 127. Precautions for the internal use of St John's wort do not apply to the infused oil.

Thyme *Thymus vulgaris*

Avoid the use of thyme in people with a known allergy to it.

Uses

Thyme is a powerful antiseptic for the lungs and is therefore useful for chesty colds with a bad cough, especially a dry one.

COMBINATIONS: Thyme combines well in tincture form with liquorice, elecampane and ground ivy for the treatment of chest infections, especially if the cough lingers for weeks.
HOW TO TAKE IT: Thyme is best taken either as a tincture or as a thyme and liquorice syrup (for precautions, see page 119).

You can purchase thyme and liquorice syrup directly from practising herbalists who run their own apothecaries, or you can make your own (see Chapter 23).
DOSAGE: **Adults**: 0.7–2ml diluted with some water, one to three times a day, tincture strength 1:2, or thyme and liquorice syrup, 1 teaspoonful two to five times a day.

Specific ailments that affect the respiratory system, and herbs that can help

Blocked nose, runny nose and catarrh

I am a great believer in allowing an ordinary runny nose to run, unpleasant though that may be. Trying to suppress this normal reaction of the lining of the nose just prolongs the problem and often shifts the infection to the sinuses, throat or chest. However, if your nose is so blocked that you can't breathe, the options listed below will ease the symptoms.

If your nostrils become sore as a result of constantly blowing your nose, apply a little marigold or comfrey ointment (see Chapter 12, pages 138 and 140).

Treatment options

Please see pages 58, 97, 113 and 121 for herbal precautions.

- Drink elderflower tea. It will reduce the secretions to a bearable level without suppressing them completely; this anti-catarrhal effect is often noticeable within minutes of drinking the tea. **Adults:** 2–4 cups a day.
- Inhale the steam from peppermint and thyme tea under a towel for 5–10 minutes (or for 2–3 minutes for children). **Adults:** steam inhalation once or twice a day.
- Add 2–3 drops each of rosemary and thyme essential oils to hot water, and inhale the steam under a towel for 5–10 minutes (or for 2–3 minutes for children). **Adults:** steam inhalation once or twice a day.
- Take fresh garlic. **Adults:** 1–3 cloves a day or 1–3 teaspoonsful of garlic juice a day.

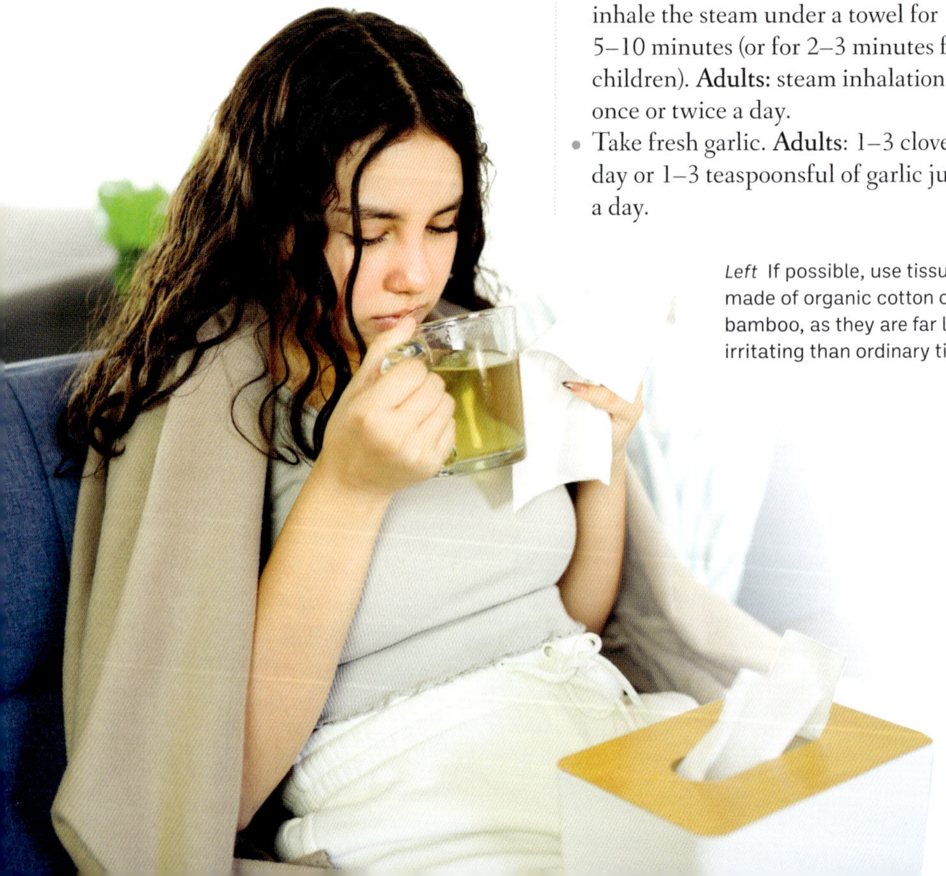

Left If possible, use tissues made of organic cotton or bamboo, as they are far less irritating than ordinary tissues.

Bronchitis

Practitioner treatment is recommended for this condition.

Bronchitis is inflammation of the lining of the bronchi, which are the large tubes that carry air to and from the lungs. The main symptoms are persistent cough (either dry or productive) and fever. Herbalists consider coughing to be a natural body defence mechanism that should not be suppressed. They use herbs to make coughing easier and less irritating, and to shorten the overall period of coughing. For a dry cough the aim is to make it productive, which means gently stimulating the production of mucus (herbs do not cause excessive mucus production). A productive cough is more effective in removing the infectious organism from the airways, and it is also less irritating to the bronchi. For a cough that is already productive, the aim is to change the consistency of the mucus so that it can be easily cleared from the lungs.

The best overall treatment is onion syrup, but you may need other syrups as well. Herbal syrups are very pure – they contain only herbs and sugar or honey – and they do not cause drowsiness. They work by reducing irritation in the airways as well as by having a mild disinfectant action. You may need to consult your local herbalist if you want to keep any of them in stock or make your own (see Chapter 23).

If there is any risk of bronchitis progressing to pneumonia or if it persists for a long time it may need to be treated with a professional prescription from a medical herbalist, or with antibiotics prescribed by your doctor.

Treatment options

Please see pages 116–121 for herbal precautions.

- Take onion syrup (see page 115), which is the best overall treatment for this condition. **Adults:** 1–8 teaspoonsful a day. **Children (5–16 years):** 5–7 years, half a teaspoonful three times a day; 7–10 years, 1 teaspoonful three times a day; 11–16 years, 1 teaspoonful three to five times a day.
- Take marshmallow syrup for a dry cough. **Adults:** 3–8 teaspoonsful a day.
- Take thyme and liquorice syrup for a chesty cough. **Adults:** 1 teaspoonful two to five times a day.
- Drink elderflower tea to lower the body temperature and in cases where there is a lot of catarrh. **Adults:** 1–3 cups a day.
- Take propolis tincture. **Adults:** 0.5–2ml diluted with some water, one to three times a day, tincture strength 1:5, or 1–2g a day as capsules.

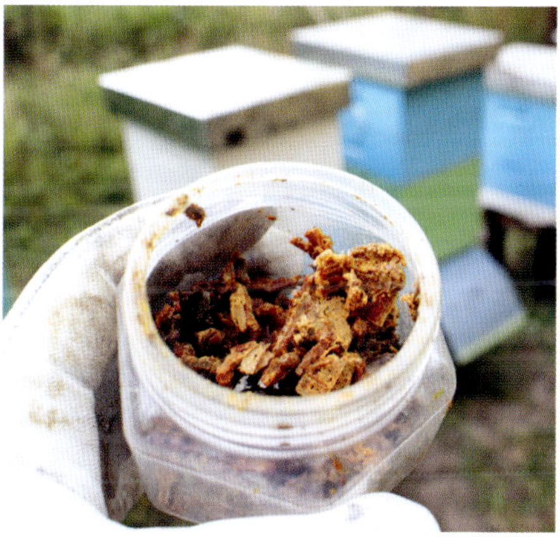

Above Fresh propolis.

Colds, frequent

If you catch more than two or three colds every winter, and if they linger for more than just a few days, your immune system may not be functioning as well as it should. There can be a number of reasons for this – for instance, your diet may be lacking in vital vitamins or minerals, or you may be under a lot of stress.

Treatment options

Please see pages 112–121 for herbal precautions.

- Take echinacea tincture for a few months. **Adults**: 1.2–3ml diluted with some water, three times a day, tincture strength 1:2.
- Take andrographis tincture or tablets. **Adults**: 1–2ml diluted with some water, three times a day, tincture strength 1:2.
- Drink elderflower tea during the winter months. **Adults**: 1 cup a day.
- Include raw garlic in your diet or take garlic capsules, according to the manufacturer's instructions. Garlic is not suitable for children under six years old. **Adults**: 1 fresh clove a day. **Children**: 7–12 years old ⅓ of fresh clove a day, 13–16 years old ½ fresh clove a day.

Colds, prevention of

Make sure that you eat a lot of fruit and vegetables and also plenty of garlic. There is no need to supplement your diet with vitamin C on a permanent basis, but it is worth using this vitamin supplement if you think that you have caught a cold. We are all more vulnerable to catching infections if our bodies are too hot or too cold (this is why Christmas shopping is an ideal situation for a cold virus to spread, as shoppers move constantly between overheated shops and excessively cold conditions outside), so dressing sensibly may ward off a lot of colds.

Supplement your diet with vitamin D in the winter months (from October to April), as this vitamin is essential for maintaining a strong immune system. The current guidance is that adults should take 400–1,000IU per day. This is equivalent to 10–22mcg (micrograms). As a lot of foods for children are now fortified with vitamin D, it is worth checking with a health professional what dose would be suitable for your child.

Avoiding crowded, air-conditioned areas is another simple way to minimise your risk of catching a cold, as is maintaining a distance from people who are already ill. Within a family, colds often spread through the use of the same cutlery or cups, so make sure that you put these on a hot wash cycle or wash them extra well by hand.

Treatment options

Please see pages 112–121 for herbal precautions.

- Drink 1 cup of elderflower tea every day throughout the winter season. **Adults**: 1 cup a day, or 2–4 cups a day if you develop any symptoms.
- Take good-quality echinacea tincture for 2–4 months. **Adults**: 1.2–3ml diluted with some water, three times a day, tincture strength 1:2. **Teenagers (12–16 years):** Adjust the adult dose downwards, based on the teenager's weight (see Chapter 5).

Below Orange juice is a good source of vitamin D.

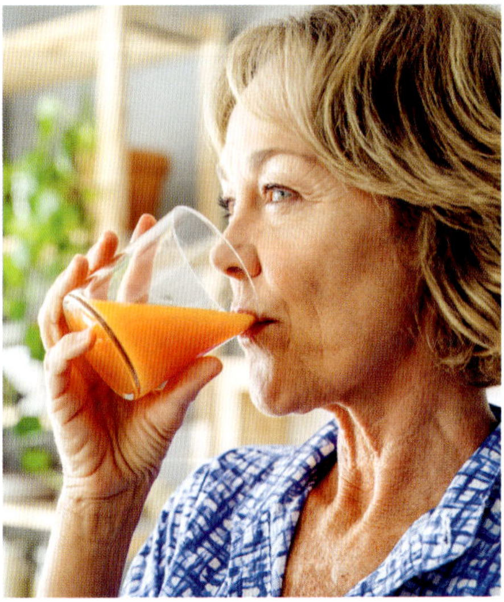

- Include raw garlic in your diet or take garlic tablets or capsules, according to the manufacturer's instructions. Garlic is not suitable for children under six years old. **Adults:** 1 fresh clove a day. **Children:** 7–12 years old ⅓ of fresh clove a day, 13–16 years old ½ fresh clove a day.

Colds, treatment of

If, despite adopting all of the preventative measures described earlier, you still develop a cold, you can minimise the symptoms with the help of herbs. Depending on the nature of the symptoms and their severity, you may need to use a combination of treatments. For more treatment options, look up the specific symptoms (e.g. cough, sore throat, runny nose) in this section of the chapter.

Treatment options

Please see pages 112–121 for herbal precautions.

- Drink elderflower tea. **Adults:** 2–4 cups a day.
- Drink warming teas (e.g. lime tree flowers or ginger, see page 63) if you are shivering. **Adults:** 1–3 cups a day.
- Reduce fever if it is above 38°C (100.4°F) (see Fever entry on page 128).
- Take fresh garlic with honey or garlic juice until the symptoms improve. *Garlic is not suitable for children under six years old.* **Adults:** 2–3 cloves a day or 1–3 teaspoonsful of garlic juice a day. **Children:** 7–12 years old ⅓ of fresh clove a day, 13–16 years old ½ fresh clove a day.
- Take the anti-cold mix (see box opposite).
- Take the mix for throat and chest infections (see box opposite) if your cold is really severe, and you have either a sore throat or a cough, or both.

Anti-cold mix

Please see pages 112–121 for herbal precautions.

INGREDIENTS
- 30ml elderflower (tincture strength 1:2)
- 20ml andrographis (tincture strength 1:2)
- 50ml stabilised garlic juice

METHOD
1. Mix the ingredients together.
2. Pour the mixture into a clean, dark glass bottle.
3. Label the bottle with the contents and the date.
4. Store at room temperature for up to a year.

ADULT DOSE: 5ml diluted with some water, one to three times a day.

Mix for throat and chest infections

INGREDIENTS
- 20 ml liquorice (tincture strength 1:1)
- 20ml thyme (tincture strength 1:2)
- 20ml elecampane (tincture strength 1:2)
- 40ml marshmallow root (tincture strength 1:5)

METHOD
1. Mix the ingredients together.
2. Pour the mixture into a clean, dark glass bottle.
3. Label the bottle with the contents and the date.
4. Store at room temperature for up to a year.

ADULT DOSE: 5ml diluted with some water, two to three times a day.

Cough, dry

A dry cough often results from a sore throat, but can also indicate a chest infection. The options listed below will reduce the frequency of coughing, especially at night. If the coughing wakes you up, take 1–2 teaspoonsful of marshmallow syrup, as this lubricates the dry throat almost immediately.

Treatment options

Please see pages 112–121 for herbal precautions.

- Take marshmallow syrup if your cough is caused by a dry or sore throat. **Adults**: up to 8 teaspoonsful a day.
- Take thyme and liquorice syrup if you think that the infection has spread to your chest. **Adults**: 1 teaspoonful two to five times a day.
- Use onion syrup (see page 115) to reduce the frequency of coughing, especially if you cough a lot at night. **Adults**: 4–5 teaspoonsful a day. **Children (5–16 years)**: 5–7 years, half a teaspoonful three times a day; 7–10 years, 1 teaspoonful three times a day; 11–16 years, 1 teaspoonful three to five times a day.
- Take echinacea tincture if your cough has persisted for more than 10 days, but do not take it at the onset of the cough. **Adults**: 1.2–3ml diluted with some water, three times a day, tincture strength 1:2.
- Take the tincture mix for a persistent cough (see box opposite).

Mix for a persistent cough

Please see pages 118–121 for herbal precautions.

INGREDIENTS

- 20ml thyme (tincture strength 1:2)
- 20ml liquorice (tincture strength 1:1)
- 20ml elecampane (tincture strength 1:2)
- 40ml ground ivy (tincture strength 1:2)

METHOD

1. Mix the ingredients together.
2. Pour the mixture into a clean, dark glass bottle.
3. Label the bottle with the contents and the date.
4. Store at room temperature for up to a year.

ADULT DOSE: 5ml diluted with some water, two to three times a day.

Cough, productive

Practitioner treatment is recommended for this condition.

A productive cough generally indicates that the airways are producing mucus in response to the infection – coughing is a mechanism for removing the excess mucus. Therefore it is best not to suppress this mechanism, but rather to aid it with syrups that unclog and disinfect the lungs. Yellow or green phlegm is a sign of bacterial infection, and you may need professional help for this from a medical herbalist, or antibiotics prescribed by your doctor.

Treatment options

Please see pages 112–121 for herbal precautions.

- Take onion syrup (see page 115). **Adults**: 4–5 teaspoonsful a day. **Children (5–16 years)**: 5–7 years, half a teaspoonful three times a day; 7–10 years, 1 teaspoonful three times a day; 11–16 years, 1 teaspoonful three to five times a day.
- Take thyme and liquorice syrup. **Adults**: 1 teaspoonful two to five times a day.

- Drink elderflower tea. **Adults**: 1–2 cups a day.
- Take the tincture mix for a persistent cough (see left) if your cough has not cleared up within 10 days.

Earache

Practitioner treatment is recommended for this condition.

This problem is most common in children. It is usually a sign of middle-ear infection, but can be a result of a growing wisdom tooth, or of a foreign body in the ear canal. The options listed below apply to mild infections, and will be most effective if used at the very onset of the symptoms. Earache that does not improve within a day of treatment, that gets progressively worse despite the treatment or that is exceptionally severe will need professional attention.

Treatment options

Please see pages 112–121 for herbal precautions.

- Apply St John's wort infused oil. Soak one end of a piece of cotton wool in the oil, shake off the excess so that it doesn't drip, and insert it gently at the entrance of the ear canal (make sure that you don't push it in too far, so that you can easily remove it later). Leave the cotton wool in place for a few hours, or ideally overnight. Use a smaller piece for children, and check periodically whether it is still in place.
- Apply marigold ointment *behind* the ear two to three times a day (see page 135).
- Take valerian tincture to reduce the pain (see page 96). **Adults**: 5ml diluted with some water, once or twice a day, tincture strength 1:2. **Children (5–16 years):** 5–7 years, 12 drops twice a day; 7–10 years, 16 drops twice a day; 11–16 years, 2ml twice a day. Please remember to dilute each dose in some water or juice. If your child is either very small or quite big for its age, use the calculation on page 33 that adjusts the dose according to the child's weight.

Ear infections, recurrent

Practitioner treatment is recommended for this condition in children.

This problem mainly affects children and young adults. Children with recurrent ear problems often respond extremely well to the removal of cow's milk from their diet (use goat's milk instead, or consult a nutritionist about other milk substitutes). Ice cream is a common culprit, as is getting water in the ears at a swimming pool.

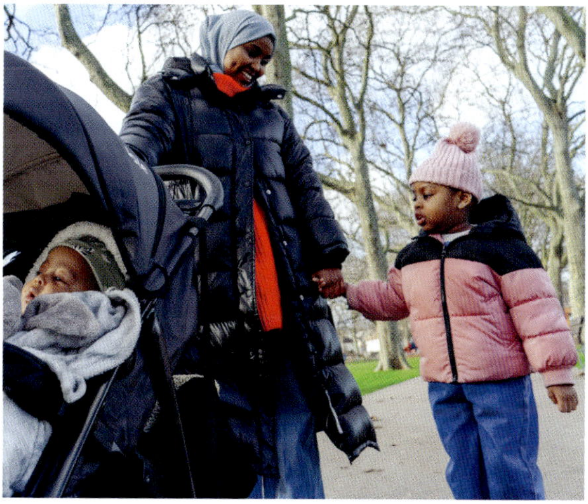

Right Having a cold head can make you vulnerable to infection, so wearing a warm hat in cold weather is the best preventative measure.

Treatment options

Please see pages 112–121 for herbal precautions.

- Take echinacea tincture for 1–3 months to improve the immune response. **Adults**: 1.2–3ml diluted with some water, two to three times a day, tincture strength 1:2.
- Drink elderflower tea to reduce the development of catarrh in the Eustachian tubes (the narrow passages that connect the inner ear to the throat). **Adults**: 1 cup a day.
- Apply marigold ointment *behind* the ear once or twice a day (see page 135).
- Use St John's wort infused oil at the very onset of the symptoms (see Earache entry on page 127).

External treatment is suitable for children over five years old.

Fever, reducing

Although fever is a natural defence mechanism that the body uses when fighting an infection, it can be very exhausting and can even cause fits in very young children, and loss of consciousness if allowed to run very high. In my view it makes sense to reduce fever if it is very high, so long as you do not immediately resume your normal activities. A lowered body temperature resulting from the use of either herbs or pharmaceuticals does not mean that the infection has gone away – your body will still be busy fighting it for a few more days, so you should give it a chance to do the job properly. This means staying in bed, or at least at home, for a day or two until your temperature no longer rises when you stop taking fever-reducing measures.

If your temperature creeps above 38°C (100.4°F) you may sometimes need to

Below Lime tree flowers tea.

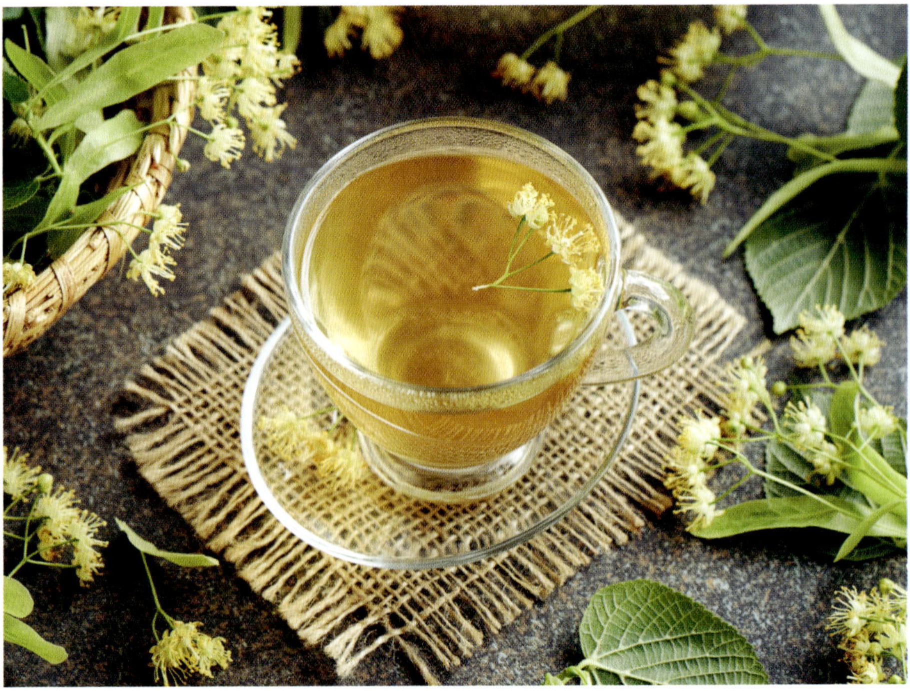

resort to aspirin or paracetamol (but be aware that the use of Calpol in children has been linked to an increased incidence of childhood asthma and hay fever).[14] A combination of elderflower tea and one of these conventional medicines is more effective than either on its own for reducing a fever, so by using both you will need less of the pharmaceuticals. It is not necessary to reduce the body temperature to the normal range – that is, 36.6–37°C (97.8–98.6°F). If your temperature is slightly raised, at somewhere between 37°C (98.6°F) and 38°C (100.4°F), this will help your body to fight the infection.

Children can develop a very high temperature very quickly, so you should monitor it with a thermometer every 2–3 hours and seek medical help if it goes above 39°C (102.2°F). Tepid sponging can be helpful. Strip the child to their underwear and, using a sponge or a flannel, gently moisten their limbs and trunk with lukewarm water. Do not be tempted to use cold water – lukewarm water evaporates more quickly and cools the body more effectively.

Tea for reducing fever

Please see pages 112 and 119 for herbal precautions.

INGREDIENTS

- 50g dry elderflower
- 25g dry lime tree flowers

METHOD

1. Mix the herbs thoroughly.
2. Infuse 2 teaspoonful of the mixture in a cup of freshly boiled water for 10 minutes, strain and drink warm. You can add honey to this tea.

ADULT DOSE: 1–3 cups a day.

Treatment options

Please see pages 112 and 119 for herbal precautions.

- Drink elderflower tea. **Adults**: 2–4 cups a day.
- Drink lime tree flowers tea. **Adults**: 1–3 cups a day.
- Drink a tea for reducing fever (see box left).

Flu

Practitioner treatment is recommended for this condition.

The difference between an ordinary cold and flu lies in the severity of the symptoms. Flu is caused by specific influenza viruses, some strains of which can be quite virulent. People with flu usually experience high fever, severe coughing, muscle ache, headache and nausea. They often feel very weak, and virtually unable to drag themselves out of bed. Flu usually lasts longer than a cold and can leave you feeling exhausted and depressed for weeks afterwards. It can be a serious disease and requires vigorous treatment.

The use of echinacea once the flu has already started is controversial, according to current research,[15] and I would not recommend using it while you are experiencing severe symptoms, such as a very high fever.

Treatment options

- If coughing is a prominent feature, use remedies that have an antiseptic action on the lungs (see Bronchitis entry on page 123, and Cough entry on page 126).
- Monitor the body temperature with a thermometer, and if necessary bring it down by using the measures described in the Fever entry on page 128.

- Take the antiviral mix, which combines four herbs that have antiviral properties (see box below).

Antiviral mix

Please see pages 112–121 for herbal precautions.

INGREDIENTS

- 25ml elderflower (tincture strength 1:2)
- 25ml garlic juice
- 25ml andrographis (tincture strength 1:2)
- 25ml St John's wort (tincture strength 1:2)

METHOD

1. Mix the ingredients together.
2. Pour the mixture into a clean, dark glass bottle.
3. Label the bottle with the contents and the date.
4. Store at room temperature for up to a year.

ADULT DOSE: 5ml diluted with some water, two to three times a day.

Hay fever

Practitioner treatment is recommended for this condition.

This condition is difficult to treat successfully at home, but many people seem to be able to decrease their sensitivity to pollen by eating local honey every day and well in advance of the pollen season. It is still worth using the measures listed below to reduce the symptoms.

Treatment options

- Drink elderflower tea, starting one month before and continuing throughout the pollen season. **Adults**: 1–2 cups a day.
- Drink eyebright tea before and during the pollen season. **Adults**: 1–2 cups a day.

Sinusitis

Practitioner treatment is recommended for this condition.

Sinusitis usually follows a bad cold with a runny nose and a lot of catarrh. The symptoms include a blocked nose, green or yellow discharge from the nose, dull pain above the eyebrows or below the eye sockets on either or both sides of the nose, headache and possibly a slight fever. Sinusitis can be quite tricky to treat yourself, especially if it is chronic (long-lasting). If you do not respond to the measures listed below, consult a medical herbalist.

Treatment options

Please see pages 112–121 and 139 for herbal precautions.

- Eat plenty of fresh garlic or take garlic juice. Garlic is not suitable for children under six years old. **Adults**: 2–3 cloves a day, or 1 teaspoonful of garlic juice twice a day. **Children**: 7–12 years old

Below Honey on toast.

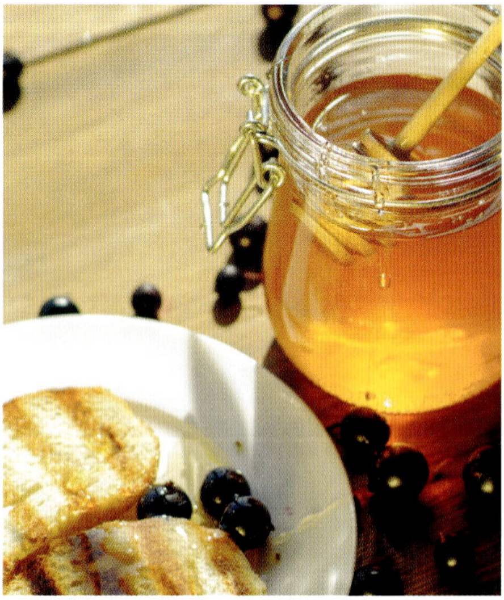

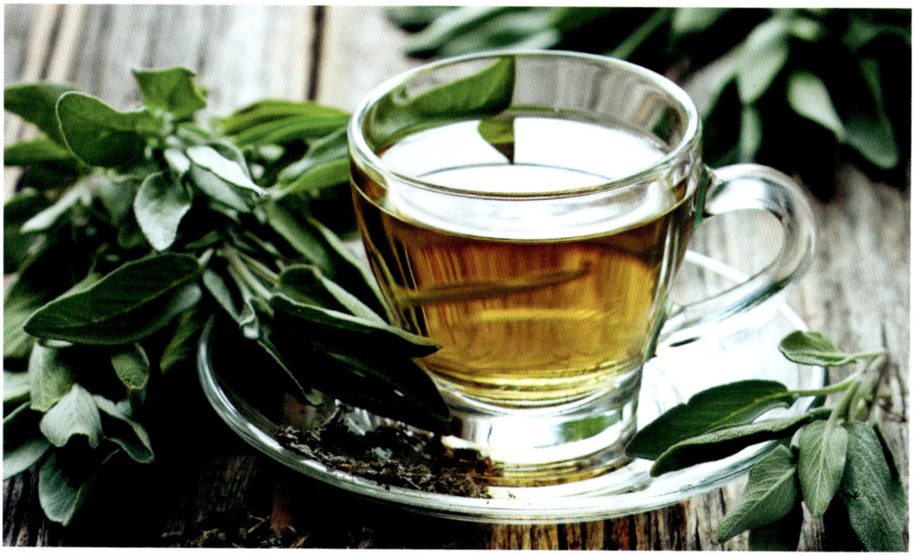

⅓ of fresh clove a day, 13–16 years old ½ fresh clove a day.

- Inhale the steam from tea tree essential oil and hot water under a towel for 5–10 minutes. **Adults**: add 5 drops of the essential oil to a large bowl of hot water.
- Massage tea tree essential oil into the painful areas over the eyebrows and on the cheeks. **Adults**: dilute 5 drops of the essential oil in 10ml of almond oil, and massage into the skin one to three times a day. Be careful to keep it away from the eyes.

Sore throat

If your throat is just red and swollen you are probably suffering from a viral infection, in which case use the normal measures applicable to any cold, but also use a gargle (see below). If your tonsils have white spots on them it is a bacterial infection, which may have to be treated with antibiotics. However, a natural antibiotic in the form of propolis spray or lozenges can combat many such infections.

Some texts recommend eating ice cream to relieve a sore throat. However, in my experience this only provides short-term relief from pain, after which the soreness returns with a vengeance!

Above Sage tea.

Treatment options

Please see pages 112–121 for herbal precautions.

- Drink elderflower tea. **Adults**: 2–4 cups a day.
- Gargle with warm sage tea. **Adults**: half a cup, two to four times a day.
- Gargle with one of the gargles listed on page 75.
- Apply propolis spray to the throat or take propolis lozenges. **Adults**: spray three to four times a day or take 1–4 lozenges a day. **Teenagers**: spray two to three times a day and use lozenges according to the manufacturer's instructions.
- Take fresh garlic with honey, or drink garlic juice. **Adults**: 1–2 cloves a day, or 1 teaspoonful of garlic juice once or twice a day.
- Take the antiviral mix described on page 130.

Tonsillitis

Tonsillitis can be distinguished from an ordinary sore throat both by white spots on the tonsils, which become very tender and swollen, and by a high temperature. See Sore throat entry on page 131.

Treatment options

Please see pages 112–121 for herbal precautions.

- Use propolis spray or take propolis lozenges. **Adults**: spray three to four times a day, or take 2–4 lozenges a day. **Teenagers**: spray two to three times a day and use lozenges according to the manufacturer's instructions.
- Prepare and take an antibacterial mix for tonsillitis (see box opposite).

Antibacterial mix for tonsillitis

Please see pages 112–121 for herbal precautions.

INGREDIENTS

- 20ml thyme (tincture strength 1:2)
- 20ml propolis (tincture strength 1:5)
- 30ml garlic juice
- 30ml andrographis (tincture strength 1:2)

METHOD

1. Mix the ingredients together.
2. Pour the mixture into a clean, dark glass bottle.
3. Label the bottle with the contents and the date.
4. Store at room temperature for up to a year.

ADULT DOSE: 5ml diluted with some water, three times a day until the symptoms improve, and then 2.5ml, three times a day for two days.

Below Checking for tonsillitis – see a doctor if your child shows symptoms.

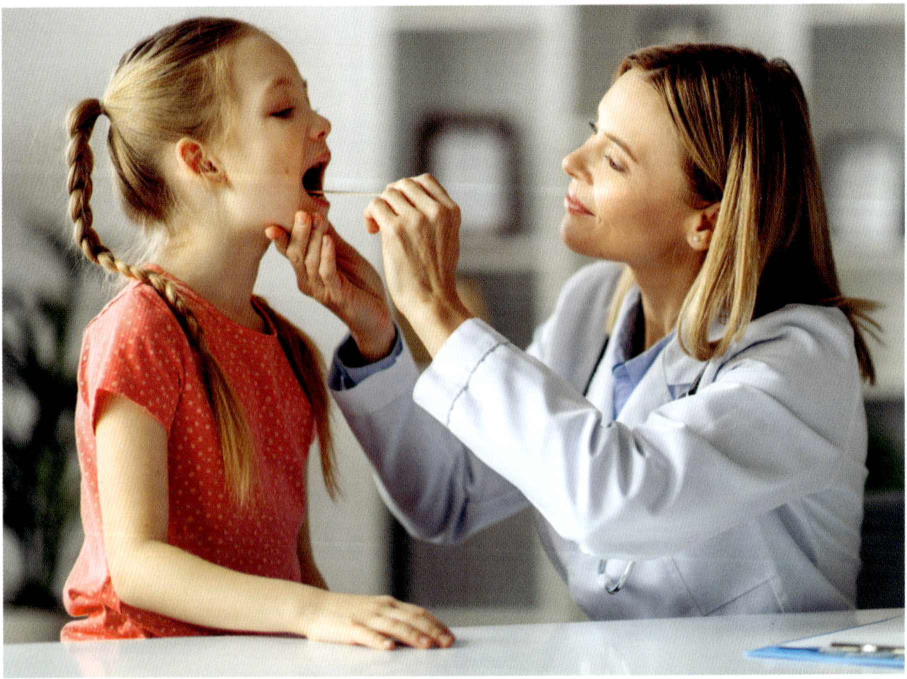

Conditions for which home treatment is not recommended

- Asthma: herbal treatment can greatly reduce the need for inhalers. The treatment will be highly individualised, depending on the type and severity of your asthma.
- Chronic bronchitis: this mostly affects older people, and needs an individual approach and the right combination of antibacterial, immune-modulating and anti-inflammatory herbs.
- Chronic fatigue syndrome (also called myalgic encephalomyelitis or ME): this condition causes profound tiredness, often following a viral infection or glandular fever. It can be very successfully treated with individually prescribed herbs – the treatment will depend on your case history and constitution.
- Hay fever: like eczema and asthma, this requires an individualised approach combined with adjustments to the diet and the patient's environment.
- Chronic sinusitis: this usually requires long-term treatment lasting for several months, depending on your health history.

When to seek medical attention

- If you experience a lot of chest pain when coughing.
- If you develop a high temperature – above 39°C (102°F) – and a dry/productive cough.
- If you have difficulty in breathing.
- If you have painful enlargement of the glands around the neck.
- If you have flu-like symptoms combined with a stiff neck and constant, severe headache.
- If you have a persistent cough, especially if this is accompanied by night sweats.

CHAPTER 12

The skin

Our skin is our interface with the outside world. It is the largest organ of the body, and is intimately connected with the vascular, immune and nervous systems.

Internal treatment

Although superficial skin problems can be dealt with most effectively by external treatment, many chronic skin problems involve the deeper layers of the skin and hence respond better to internal treatment.

Skin diseases often result from very complex interactions between our immune system, our hormonal system, our diet and the state of our nerves. Therefore it follows that a complex approach and a complex prescription are needed for complicated problems such as eczema, psoriasis, acne or acne rosacea. Careful observation is also often needed to identify the triggers for certain problems.

External applications

Most of the common, everyday skin problems, such as cuts, burns and stings, can be effectively treated with specific herbal preparations for external use that greatly increase the rate at which skin heals.

For external treatment, there is no distinction between adults and children when the area of affected skin is small. However, if a large area of the body is affected in a child, please consult a medical herbalist before applying large amounts of cream containing essential oils. Essential oils from the cream are partially absorbed into the bloodstream, and therefore caution is needed when using such preparations in young children.

I would also recommend that you do a small patch test first, especially when treating young children. Test a small amount of the cream or ointment and check the test area after 24 hours. If no reaction has occurred (redness, rash and/or itching) you can apply the preparation to a larger area.

Some of the ailments of eyes, scalp and hair can be easily tackled at home, but ***extra caution should be exercised when considering the treatment of eyes.*** If you are not entirely confident that you are applying the right treatment to your eyes it is best to consult your GP.

Must-have herbs

Marigold
Calendula officinalis

Caution is needed in people who are allergic to plants belonging to the daisy family (the Asteraceae, formerly known as the Compositae).

Uses

Otherwise known as calendula, pot marigold or common marigold, this plant has a broad range of uses as a treatment for the skin. Its scientific name is *Calendula officinalis*, and it should not be confused with French marigold (*Tagetes patula*). The medicinal marigold has large orange daisy-like flowers and does not have a strong smell, whereas the French marigold has aromatic, deeply divided leaves and smaller flowerheads with velvety frilly petals in shades of yellow, orange, red or brown. If in doubt, double check the scientific name.

Marigold has antibacterial, antiviral and antifungal properties. It promotes division of skin cells and hence the healing of any skin injury. It is also anti-inflammatory. Marigold petal preparations can be used in any situation where the skin has been broken due to either injury or skin disorders. Its main uses include the treatment of cuts, grazes, sunburn, heat burns, insect stings, dry lips, various skin rashes and nappy rash. Unless you are allergic to marigold, you can try it for virtually any skin problem except bruising, for which arnica would be a better choice.

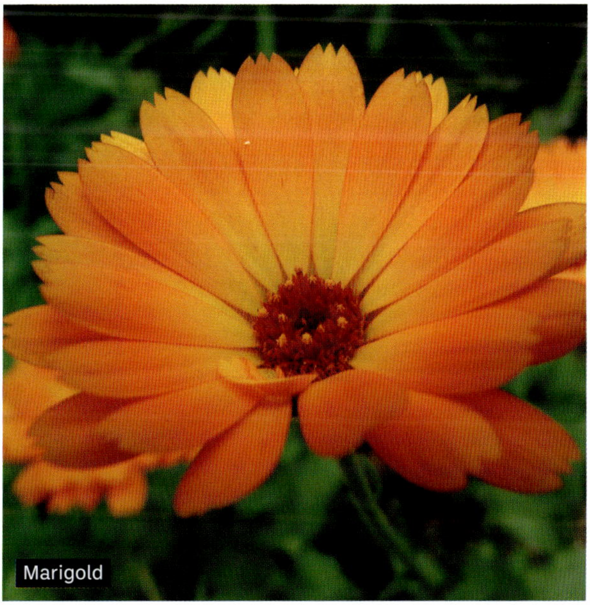

Marigold

Unfortunately, some people who suffer from multiple allergies may also be allergic to marigold. In my experience this precludes the possibility of using it internally in such cases, and eczema can sometimes be worsened by the application of marigold ointment to the affected areas.

HOW TO USE IT: You can use marigold as an ointment, cream, infused oil, poultice or compress, depending on the problem. It is easy to make your own marigold ointment, and I recommend that you do so (see Chapter 23), as home-made ointment will be far superior to anything that you can buy over the counter.

DOSAGE: This is specific to the problem (see the individual entries in the next section of this chapter).

Comfrey *Symphytum officinale*

Comfrey should only be used for external treatment.

Uses

Comfrey is very similar in its action to marigold, as it promotes division of skin cells and the healing of skin injuries. It is generally less allergenic and is therefore suitable for people who cannot tolerate marigold or chamomile. It is most useful in cases of 'mixed' injuries, where there is some bruising combined with an open wound.

HOW TO USE IT: You can apply this herb in the form of a cream, ointment, infused oil, poultice or compress.
DOSAGE: This is specific to the problem (see the individual entries in the next section of this chapter).

Chamomile (German) *Matricaria recutita* (syn. *Chamomilla recutita*)

Caution is needed in people who are allergic to plants belonging to the daisy family (the Asteraceae, formerly known as the Compositae).

Uses

This herb can be used as an internal or external remedy for many skin complaints. A very small proportion of people are allergic to chamomile, especially when it is applied to the skin. If you have never used it before, try it first on a small patch of skin for a few days before applying it to a larger area. Chamomile has an anti-inflammatory action and can therefore be used for any skin conditions where inflammation is a feature, including acne, swellings of various origins, dry eczema, insect bites and sore eyes.

HOW TO USE IT: You can apply chamomile as a cream, poultice, compress or use it internally as tincture.
DOSAGE: **External application:** this is specific to the problem (see the individual entries in the next section of this chapter).
Internal dose for adults: 0.5–1.4ml, one to three times a day, tincture strength 1:2.
Internal dose for children: specific dosages are indicated in the descriptions of specific health problems that affect children.

Thyme *Thymus vulgaris*

Do not use thyme essential oil for external applications in pregnancy or for children under three years old without consulting a specialist.
All other thyme preparations (tincture, tea and ointment) are safe for small children and in pregnancy if used *externally*.

Uses

Thyme can be used externally to treat skin infections, sunburn or a range of itchy conditions – for instance, it is an excellent remedy for treating itchy conditions of the genital area. It is the ideal remedy to try on fungal infections, either by itself or mixed with other antifungal herbs. It also acts as a good skin disinfectant for small injuries.

HOW TO USE IT: You can use thyme externally as a tincture, infusion, compress or essential oil. Tinctures or infusions that are applied directly to the skin with cotton wool are called lotions. Tinctures should be diluted slightly to avoid stinging – dilute 10ml of tincture with at least 50ml of water. The essential oil should generally be diluted either in carrier oil or in a cream or ointment base.
DOSAGE: **External application:** this is specific to the problem (see the individual entries in the next section of this chapter).

Optional herbs

Echinacea (purple coneflower) *Echinacea purpurea* and *Echinacea augustifolia*

Caution is needed in people who are allergic to plants belonging to the daisy family (the Asteraceae, formerly known as the Compositae). Not suitable for transplant patients and children under 12.

Uses

Although it is best known as a general modulator of the immune system, echinacea can also be useful as an external application in some cases of skin disease. Traditionally, Native Americans used it primarily as a wound-healing herb.

HOW TO USE IT: You can use diluted echinacea tincture to disinfect cuts and grazes, or you can take it internally if you suffer from a chronic skin problem such as acne or eczema, but make sure that you use a minimal dose initially, to avoid any possible worsening of the condition.
DOSAGE: **Adults:** 1.2–3ml diluted with some water, one to three times a day, tincture strength 1:2.
Teenagers (12–16 years): Adjust the adult dose downwards according to body weight (see Chapter 5).

Eyebright *Euphrasia* species

Uses

The name of this herb reflects its use – eyebright is the herb for external eye problems. It can be used to treat eye irritation, tiredness, watering, mild conjunctivitis, puffiness and itching.
HOW TO USE IT: Eye irritation that is a symptom of hay fever responds best to internal treatment with eyebright tincture. Other conditions can be treated with an eye bath containing a tiny amount of eyebright infusion (see Conjunctivitis entry on page 146).
DOSAGE: **External application:** this is specific to the problem (see the individual entries in the next section of this chapter).
Internal dose for adults: 1–2ml diluted with some water, two to three times a day, tincture strength 1:2.

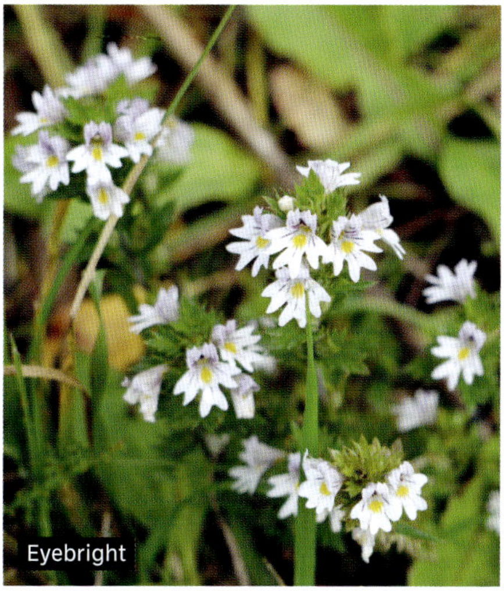
Eyebright

Lavender *Lavandula angustifolia* (syn. *Lavandula officinalis*)

Do not use lavender essential oil for external applications in pregnancy or for children under three years old without consulting a specialist.

Uses

Lavender is another herbal antiseptic, and though not as strong as tea tree (see page 139) it is less irritating to the skin. It is also mildly anti-inflammatory. Lavender is the only essential oil that I would add to eczema cream, as in my experience the others sooner or later cause skin irritation.

HOW TO USE IT: Lavender essential oil should be used for external applications mixed into a cream or carrier oil (see box below).

Antiseptic and healing cream (1)

INGREDIENTS

- 10–20 drops lavender essential oil
- 50g marigold or comfrey cream

METHOD

1. Mix the ingredients well.
2. Transfer the mixture to a clean, dark glass jar, making sure that all air pockets are removed.
3. Store for up to 12 months.

ADULTS, AND CHILDREN OVER THREE YEARS OLD: apply to the affected skin one to three times a day. Note: this cream may sting temporarily if the skin is broken.

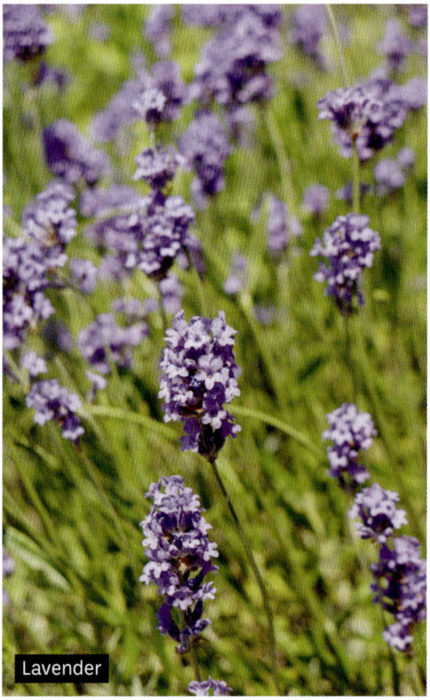

Lavender

Stinging nettle *Urtica dioica*

Caution is needed in people with a known allergy or histamine sensitivity.

Uses

Nettle leaves are an example of a medicinal herb that improves the detoxification of the body. Their action, when taken internally, is similar to that of antihistamines, so they are useful in skin conditions that are allergic in nature, such as eczema or urticaria (hives). You should only use well-dried leaves for a tea or a tincture. I do not recommend using fresh leaves for a tea, as the process of infusion may not neutralise all of the histamine present in the hairs of the plant.

HOW TO TAKE IT: Dried nettle leaves can be used as a tea or in a tincture.
DOSAGE: **Adults:** 1–2 cups of tea a day, or 0.7–2ml diluted with some water, one to three times a day, tincture strength 1:2.

Red clover *Trifolium pratense*

Caution is needed in people with oestrogen-sensitive conditions and those on blood-thinning medications.

Uses

Red clover can be used internally to treat most skin disorders. It is gently detoxifying and does not exacerbate any existing problems (whereas some stronger herbal detoxifiers can cause a temporary worsening of the skin condition). You can include it in any internal mix of tea or tincture for acne, eczema or psoriasis. If using a tincture, opt for the extracts based on 25% alcohol.

COMBINATIONS: Red clover combines well with yellow dock and chamomile.
HOW TO TAKE IT: As a tincture or as a tea.

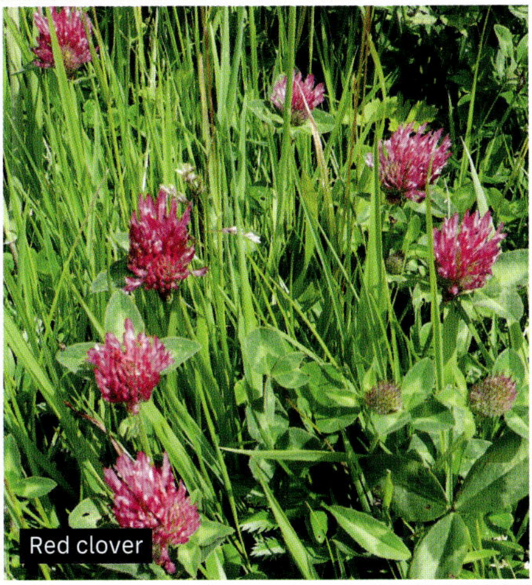
Red clover

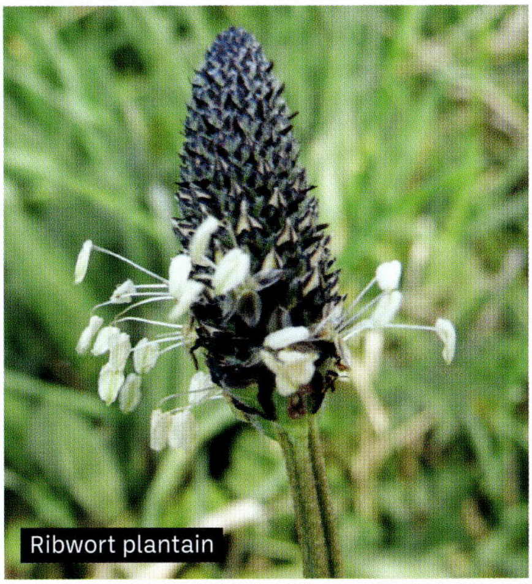
Ribwort plantain

DOSAGE: **Adults:** 1–2ml diluted with some water, one to three times a day, tincture strength 1:2, or 1–2 cups of tea a day.

Ribwort plantain
Plantago lanceolata

Uses

This herb has a generally soothing effect on skin conditions where inflammation is a feature, such as eczema. It also enhances the natural ability of the skin to heal. It is a very gentle herb that is suitable for people with multiple allergies. Ribwort plantain is a common plant with characteristic elongated leaves, and should not be confused with common plantain, which has rounded leaves and does not have the same medicinal properties.

HOW TO USE IT: Ribwort plantain can be taken on its own or combined with other skin remedies for internal treatment, either as a tea or as a tincture. It can also be applied externally as a compress or poultice to weeping and inflamed skin. For this purpose use a strong tea or freshly squeezed juice.

DOSAGE: **Adults:** 1–3 cups of tea a day, or 1–2ml diluted with some water, one to three times a day, tincture strength 1:2. **Children (4–16 years):** you can use it for external application once or twice a day until the inflammation improves. Alternatively take tincture (tincture strength 1:2): 5–7 years old, 12 drops twice a day; 7–10 years old, 16 drops twice a day; 11–16 years old, 2ml twice a day. Each dose diluted with some water/juice. If you want to use tea, the following dosage can be used: 5–7 years old, ¼ of a cup twice a day; 7–10 years old, ⅓ of a cup twice a day; 11–16 years old, ½ cup twice a day.

Tea tree
Melaleuca alternifolia

Do not use tea tree essential oil for external applications in pregnancy or for children under three years of age without consulting a specialist.

Uses

Tea tree is one of the strongest herbal antiseptics for external use. I recommend its use to treat fungal or bacterial infections of the skin.

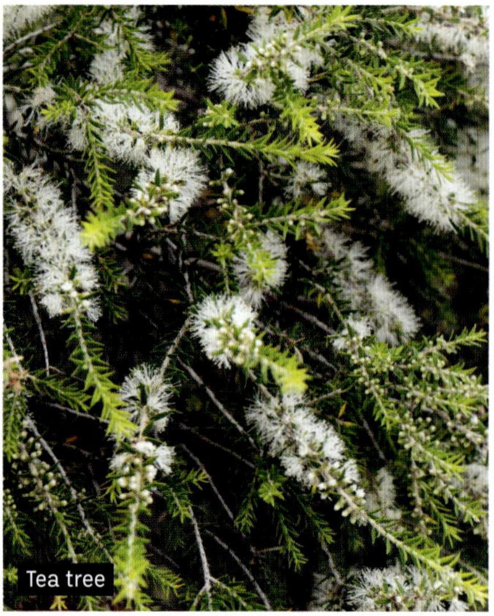

Tea tree

HOW TO USE IT: I do not advise using neat tea tree essential oil on the skin, as it can cause local skin irritation. However, it is very useful when applied in the form of a cream.

Antiseptic and healing cream (2)

INGREDIENTS

- 20 drops tea tree essential oil
- 50g marigold or comfrey cream

METHOD

1. Mix the ingredients well.
2. Transfer the mixture to a clean, dark glass jar, making sure that all air pockets are removed.
3. Store for up to 12 months.

ADULTS, AND CHILDREN OVER THREE YEARS OLD: apply to the affected skin one to three times a day. Note: this cream may sting temporarily if the skin is broken.

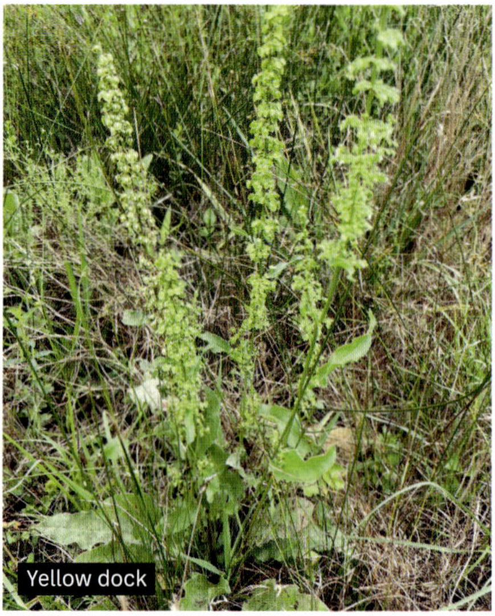

Yellow dock

Yellow dock *Rumex crispus*

Use only small doses of yellow dock in women who are breastfeeding.

Uses

Yellow dock is another general detoxifier (and a gentle laxative), and it is especially useful whenever skin problems are made worse by constipation. It can be used to treat eczema, acne and psoriasis.

COMBINATIONS: Yellow dock combines well with red clover, marigold and ribwort plantain.

HOW TO TAKE IT: Yellow dock is a fairly strong-acting herb, so it should be introduced gradually, at the lower end of the recommended dose range. If you mix it with other herbs, yellow dock should constitute no more than about 10–20% of the mix. It can be taken as a tea but has a rather strong taste, so it really needs to be mixed with other dry herbs, such as red clover and ribwort plantain (see pages 138–139).

DOSAGE: **Adults:** 1–2ml diluted with water, one to three times a day, tincture strength 1:2.

Specific ailments that affect the skin, and herbs that can help

Acne

Acne may require prolonged treatment, sometimes with herbs that can influence the hormones involved. The measures listed below can be tried singly or in combination, depending on the severity of the acne. The occasional single spot can simply be treated with external remedies. However, if there are quite a few spots, internal treatment is needed (again using either single or combined approaches) as well as external remedies. Internal treatment for acne often needs to be ongoing for months or even years to give sustained results. Supplementing with zinc will aid skin healing, though it may be necessary to improve the whole diet – in particular, chocolate (despite the conflicting scientific evidence), caffeinated drinks and alcohol should be avoided.

Below Around half of women in their 20s have acne.

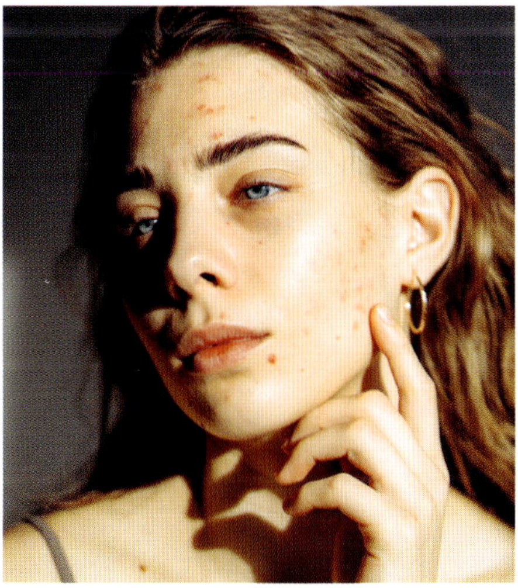

Treatment options

Please see pages 116 and 135–140 for herbal precautions.

- Drink chamomile tea on a daily basis. This is the simplest measure, but it is surprisingly effective – the key is to drink it every day! **Adults:** 1–2 cups a day, using 2 teaspoonsful of loose herbs or two tea bags per cup.
- Take propolis capsules daily if you get a lot of painful spots that resemble small boils. **Adults:** take the equivalent of 100–500mg of propolis a day, starting with 100mg and increasing the dose to 500mg if your symptoms are severe.
- Drink the tea for improving skin problems (see box overleaf).
- Take the tincture mix for skin disorders (see box overleaf).

Teenagers (11–16 years): use half the adult dose, or adjust the dose according to the body weight of the person being treated (see Chapter 5).

- Wipe the affected areas of the skin with witch hazel water after washing. Witch hazel water is a ready-made product available over the counter and can be applied undiluted to the skin with a piece of cotton wool. **Adults and teenagers:** do this once or twice a day, but if you find it too drying do it every other day.
- Dab the tea tree cream on the developing spots (for precautions, see pages 139–140). **Adults and teenagers:** do this twice a day.

- Apply undiluted marigold tincture directly to the spots with a cotton bud. If you start doing this as soon as you feel a spot beginning to develop, you should be able to prevent it from growing altogether (for precautions, see page 135). **Adults and teenagers**: apply two to five times a day.
- Large spots respond well to repeated application of marigold ointment. Gently rub on a small amount, preferably as soon as you develop a painful swelling, and keep reapplying it every couple of hours or so. **Adults and teenagers**: apply three to six times a day.

Mix for skin disorders

Please see pages 135–140 for herbal precautions.

INGREDIENTS

- 20ml yellow dock (tincture strength 1:2)
- 20ml red clover (tincture strength 1:2)
- 20ml marigold (tincture strength 1:2)
- 40ml ribwort plantain (tincture strength 1:2)

METHOD

1. Mix the ingredients together.
2. Pour the mixture into a clean, dark glass bottle.
3. Label the bottle with the contents and the date.
4. Store at room temperature for up to a year.

ADULT DOSE: 5ml diluted with some water, three times a day until the symptoms improve, and then 5ml a day for two to four months to maintain the improvement.
TEENAGERS (11-16 YEARS): use half the adult dose two to three times a day, or adjust the dose according to the body weight of the person being treated (see Chapter 5).

Tea for improving skin problems

Please see pages 135–140 for herbal precautions.

INGREDIENTS

- 10g dried yellow dock root
- 30g dried red clover flower
- 30g dried ribwort plantain
- 30g dried chamomile flowers

METHOD

1. Mix the herbs thoroughly.
2. Infuse 2 teaspoonsful of the mixture in a cup of freshly boiled water for 10 minutes, strain and drink warm. You can add honey to this tea.

ADULT DOSE: 1 cup a day until the symptoms improve, then half a cup a day for two to four months to maintain the improvement.
TEENAGERS (11-16 YEARS): use half the adult dose two to three times a day, or adjust the dose according to the body weight of the person being treated (see Chapter 5).

Below Dried chamomile flowers.

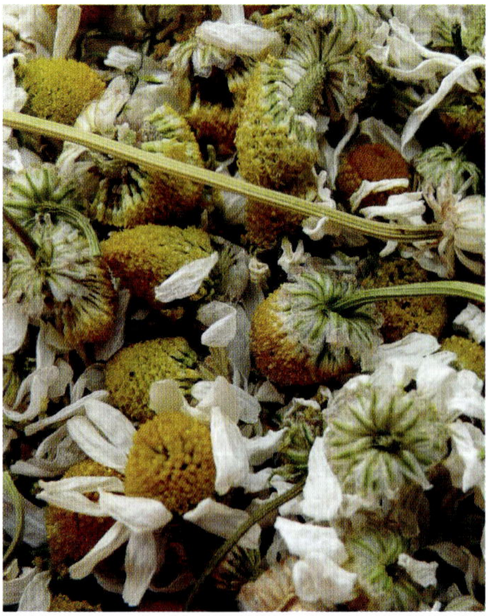

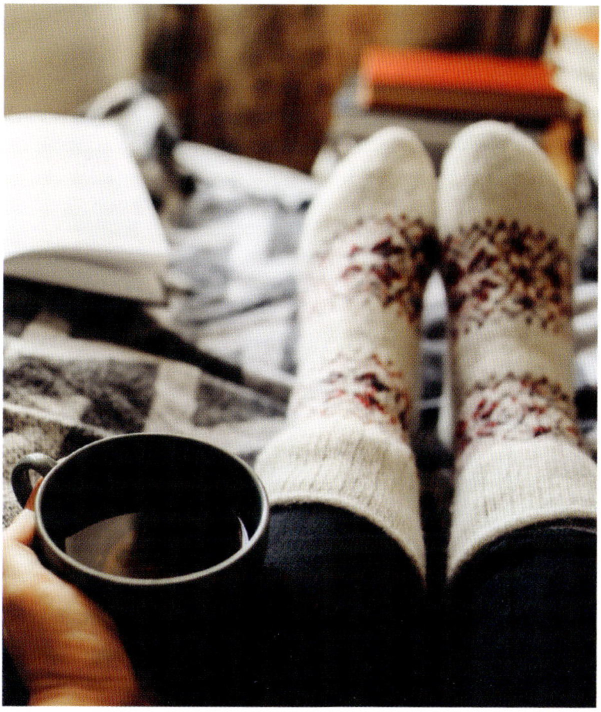

Right If you need to wear socks, opt for wool or cotton.

Athlete's foot

Athlete's foot is a fungal infection that usually 'sits' between the toes but can also infect other parts of the skin on the feet or spread to other parts of the body. Toenails can also be infected by a similar fungus. Fungal infections thrive in a warm, moist environment with little air circulation – wearing closed-toe shoes all day, especially in the summer, provides perfect conditions for this infection to develop. Whenever you can, let your feet 'breathe' to prevent this from happening. The measures listed below will help to heal the painful splitting of skin that athlete's foot often causes, and will reduce the itching. Unfortunately, it is very easy to get reinfected with the fungus, as the spores can persist in shoes, socks and towels. To minimise this risk, change your socks every day, do not share your towels with other members of the family, and try not to wear the same shoes every day (to prevent moisture build-up).

Treatment options

- Apply the antifungal ointment (see box on the right).
- Once the infection has cleared up, you can use the antifungal ointment as a preventative measure. **Adults, and children over four years old:** apply a small amount between the toes once a day for 6 to 12 months.

Antifungal ointment

Please see pages 135–140 for herbal precautions.

INGREDIENTS

- 50g marigold ointment or cream
- 10 drops tea tree essential oil
- 10 drops thyme essential oil

METHOD

1 Mix the ingredients well.
2 Transfer the mixture to a clean, dark glass jar, making sure that all air pockets are removed.
3 Store for up to 12 months.

ADULTS, AND CHILDREN OVER FOUR YEARS OLD: apply to the infected areas in the morning and evening, after a bath or shower.
Note: This cream may sting temporarily if the skin is split.

Boils

Practitioner treatment is recommended for this condition, especially when it occurs in children.

If you are not confident that the treatment is working, consult a doctor, as the bacteria from the boil can infect the blood and cause septicaemia (blood poisoning), which is a potentially life-threatening condition. Watch out for a red streak extending from the boil on the skin, as this can indicate that the infection is spreading.

This condition is quite rare today by comparison with earlier times, as people now live in much more hygienic conditions and have a more nourishing diet – both of these factors help to prevent skin infection. However, people with lowered immunity or nutritional deficiencies can still be prone to developing boils, so it is worth knowing how to treat them at home. The aim is to bring the boil to a head and then get rid of the accumulated pus by exerting gentle pressure. Healing usually occurs rapidly once the pus has been removed.

Treatment options

Please see pages 135–140 for herbal precautions.

- Make a warm poultice from 1–2 teaspoonful of slippery elm bark powder, and proceed as with the paste for drawing boils (see box on the right).
- Take propolis capsules or tincture. **Adults:** 0.5–2 ml, two to three times a day, tincture strength 1:5, or capsules equivalent to 100mg of propolis a day divided into three portions.
- Take echinacea tincture. **Adults:** 1.2–3ml two to three times a day, tincture strength 1:2.
- Apply the paste for drawing out boils (see box on the right).

Paste for drawing out boils

Please see pages 135–140 for herbal precautions.

INGREDIENTS

- 1–2 heaped teaspoonsful of slippery elm bark powder
- A little boiled water
- 5 drops tea tree essential oil
- 5 drops lavender or thyme essential oil
- 1–2g marigold ointment

METHOD

1. Mix all of the ingredients to a form a paste.
2. To apply the paste, put it on to a gauze dressing, press this gently against the boil and secure it in place with a large plaster or bandage.
3. Change the dressing every 24 hours until there is a definite white head at the centre of the boil. Apply gentle pressure around the boil until it bursts. You then need to continue gently squeezing until all the pus has gone.
4. Dress the area with some marigold ointment and a plaster.
5. Repeat the whole procedure if the boil starts to swell up again.

Burns

Ordinary burns usually happen at home while cooking, when using electrical appliances (especially irons) or while using fireplaces. If your burn is extensive, seek medical advice. Otherwise, place the injured area of skin under running cold water as soon as possible and keep it there until the pain subsides (sometimes it is easier to plunge a burned limb in a sink filled with cold water). Only then use the measures listed below.

Treatment options

Please see pages 135–140 for herbal precautions.

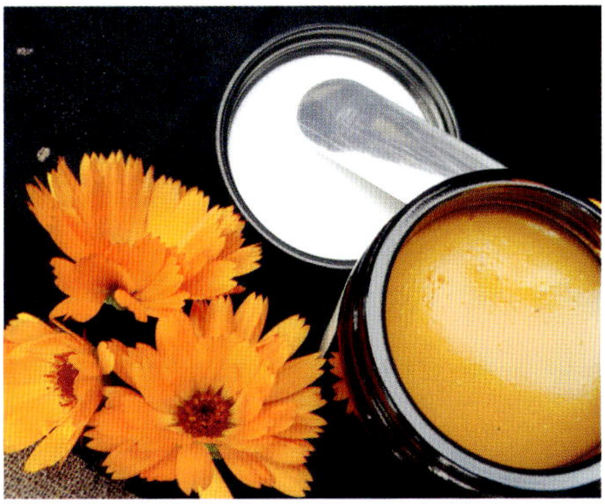

Above Marigold ointment.

- Apply a thin layer of marigold ointment. Do not cover the burn if the skin is unbroken.
- If the skin is broken you may need to cover the area once the pain has subsided. Put a thick layer of marigold cream on a plaster or gauze before covering the burn. This will prevent the dressing from sticking to the wound and will speed up the healing process.
- If you have no marigold cream, soak the burned area in a cold marigold infusion for 5–10 minutes, or apply a cold marigold infusion compress.

Cold sore

A cold sore is a viral infection that often accompanies a cold or flu. It is said that once you have a cold sore it will keep recurring, because the virus that causes it persists in the nerve cells. However, repeated treatment with marigold seems to reduce the frequency of eruptions. The ointment must be of the highest quality, or you can make your own (see Chapter 23).

Below Try not to touch your cold sore.

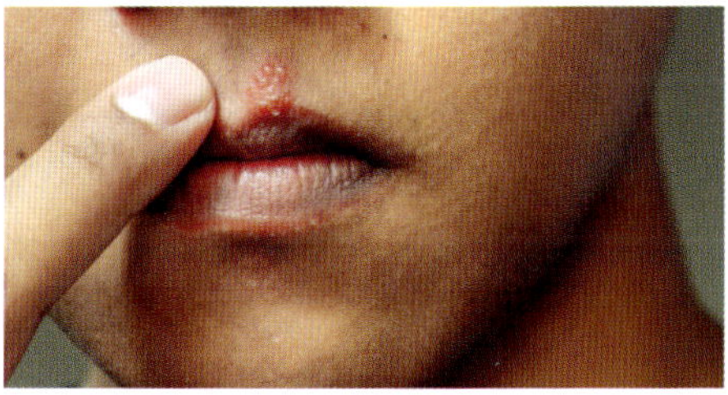

Treatment options

Please see pages 117, 135 and 136 for herbal precautions.

- Apply marigold ointment as soon as you feel the cold sore coming on to prevent it, and keep applying small amounts every hour or so.
- If the cold sore has already erupted, keep applying marigold ointment three to five times a day.
- Take elderflower tea for its antiviral properties. **Adults**: 2–3 cups a day.
- Take andrographis tincture for its antiviral and immunomodulating properties. **Adults:** 1–2ml of the tincture diluted with water, two to three times a day, tincture strength 1:2.
- Apply lemon balm cream for cold sores (see box below).

Lemon balm cream for cold sores

Please see pages 135–140 for herbal precautions.

INGREDIENTS

- 50g marigold or comfrey cream
- 10ml lemon balm tincture

METHOD

1. Mix the ingredients well.
2. Transfer the mixture to a clean, dark glass jar, making sure that all air pockets are removed.
3. Store for up to 12 months.

ADULTS, AND CHILDREN OVER FOUR YEARS OLD: apply thinly to the cold sore every 2–3 hours during the daytime until the sore has gone.
Note: this cream may sting temporarily.

Conjunctivitis

Practitioner treatment is recommended for this condition.

Conjunctivitis is best treated by a doctor, but mild eye irritation can be treated at home. The most successful treatment consists of an eye bath made with saline solution and a herbal infusion. You can get sterile saline from an optician or chemist, usually in the form used by contact lens wearers (make sure it is pure saline and does not contain any preservatives). I do not recommend using water for eye baths, as it does sting. If both eyes are affected, use a fresh eye bath for each eye. Always sterilise eye baths with boiling water before and after use, as eye infections can be very contagious. If the symptoms persist or worsen after you have tried the measures listed below, seek medical help.

Eyebright compress

INGREDIENTS

- 2 teaspoonsful of eyebright tincture mixed with 50ml freshly boiled water
- *or* half a cup of freshly infused eyebright tea

METHOD

1. Mix the tincture with the water or strain the tea, and make sure that the liquids are warm but not hot.
2. Soak two pieces of cotton wool in the liquid and squeeze out the excess liquid.
3. To apply the compress, place the cotton wool pieces on the eyelids. It is best to lie down for this treatment.

ADULTS: apply the compress for 5–10 minutes, then re-soak the cotton wool pieces and apply them again (the liquid should feel warm to the eyelids).

CHILDREN OVER FIVE YEARS OLD: use cool eyebright tea, not the tincture, and apply for only 1–3 minutes.

Treatment options

- Make an eye bath. Use 30ml of sterile saline plus half a teaspoonful of filtered eyebright tea. The tea should be brewed in the normal way and strained through a dense cloth or coffee filter.
- **Adults, and children over five years old:** bathe the affected eye for 10–20 seconds, one to three times a day.
- If the eyelids are sore and swollen, apply an eyebright compress (see box on the left).

Cradle cap

Although it is unsightly, this condition will eventually clear by itself. Sometimes it can still be present in older children, or even in teenagers. Cradle cap is not itchy and doesn't bother babies, so it is generally best left alone unless it is exceptionally thick and widespread. When trying the following treatment option, make sure that the olive oil doesn't get into the baby's eyes. You only need a small amount, and olive oil should be used rather than other oils, as it hardly ever causes an allergic reaction.

Below Cradle cap is considered to be a form of dermatitis, but it is unclear what causes it.

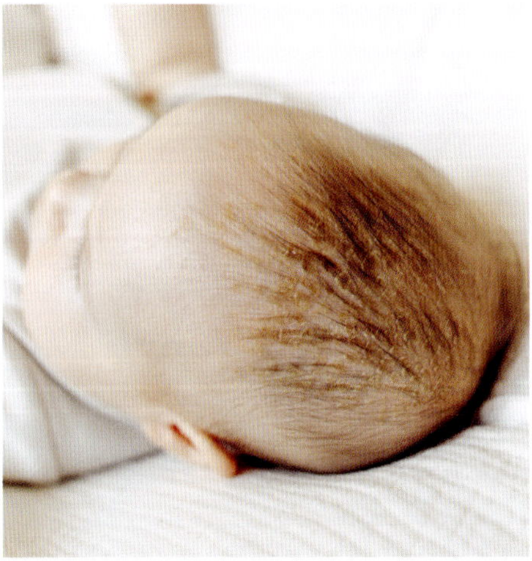

Treatment option

- Apply 1 teaspoonful of olive oil to the scalp in the evening, leave it there overnight and then gently wash it off with baby shampoo the next day. The dry skin scales should come off quite easily during washing or with gentle brushing afterwards. Don't pull off stubborn scales that seem to be stuck, but instead repeat the treatment a few days later.

Cuts, grazes and wounds

Make sure that you clean as much debris or dirt from the wound as possible before you apply any treatment. Run water from the tap over the cut if you can, or gently wipe the wound with cotton wool soaked in clean water, and then disinfect it as described below. If the cut is small, leave it exposed to the air, but if it is large or at risk of getting dirty or being knocked, cover it with a plaster. Always check the wound if any discomfort develops.

Treatment options

Please see pages 116, 135–137 and 161 for herbal precautions. All of the options listed below are suitable for children over three years old.

- After cleaning the wound you can disinfect it with any neat or slightly diluted herbal tincture (it is the alcohol that will do the most disinfecting, and it will sting!). Many herbs are antibacterial, and for a stronger disinfecting action you can choose from thyme, marigold or sage.
- If the cut is bleeding heavily, apply diluted yarrow tincture or yarrow juice (see page 49).
- Apply a small amount of marigold ointment around the cut if you intend to leave it exposed to the air.
- If you intend to cover the injury, apply marigold ointment liberally and leave the dressing in place for 24 hours. Repeat this process until the cut is healed.
- If the wound is difficult to clean and you are worried that it may become infected, you can use antiseptic and healing cream (2) (see page 140).

Dandruff and itchy scalp

Dandruff and itchy scalp often go together. The causes of dandruff are not always clear, but contributing factors include sensitivity to shampoos or other hair products, seborrhoeic eczema and mild fungal infection. If you have any spots or sores on your scalp you must consult a doctor for an accurate diagnosis.

For the treatment of common dandruff and/or itchiness I suggest that you make your own shampoo from a shampoo base that is free from sodium lauryl sulphate, and a combination of tinctures. Rinsing or rubbing the scalp with specific herbal teas can also help.

Below Homemade shampoos also reduce single-use plastic waste as you can reuse the containers.

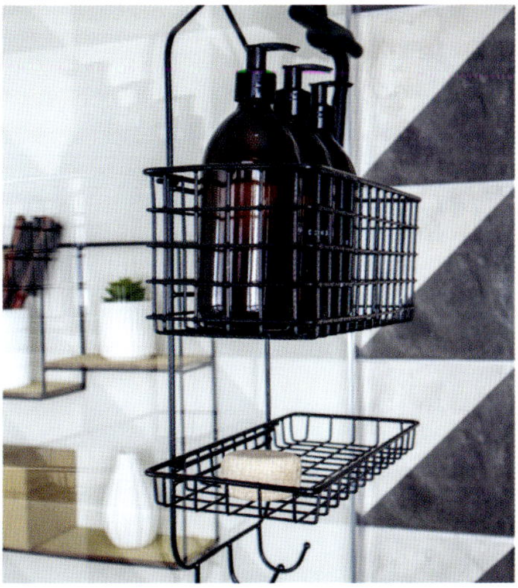

Treatment options

Please see pages 135–140 for herbal precautions. All of the options listed below are suitable for children over four years old.

- After washing your hair, add marigold tea to the final rinse (you will need to infuse a substantial amount – about 1 litre).
- Rub marigold or thyme tea directly on to the itchy scalp on a daily basis for a month or until the symptoms improve (use a small piece of cotton wool to apply the tea to the scalp).
- Use your own home-mixed herbal shampoo for a few months (see boxes).

Home-mixed herbal shampoo (1)

Please see pages 97 and 136 for herbal precautions.

INGREDIENTS

- 120ml mild shampoo base (available from many herbal retailers)
- 20ml chamomile tincture
- 20ml rosemary tincture
- 20ml thyme tincture

METHOD

1. Mix the ingredients together in a measuring jug.
2. Decant the herbal shampoo into a glass or plastic bottle. It will be quite runny.

ADULTS, AND CHILDREN OVER FOUR YEARS OLD: use like an ordinary shampoo, but lather your hair only once and then rinse it thoroughly; you can use this shampoo on a daily basis.
Note: this herbal shampoo can theoretically be made with strong infusions instead of tinctures, but unless you use the shampoo quickly it may go off.

Eczema

Practitioner treatment is recommended for this condition.

Eczema is very difficult to treat, as it is a condition caused by many contributing factors. Before trying a specific treatment you must look at any triggering factors and try to eliminate them as far as possible. Triggers for eczema include the following:

- Dietary causes: the most common ones are cow's milk and dairy products, chocolate, oranges, fizzy drinks, wheat and food additives; less common causes are bananas, strawberries, eggs, tomatoes and spicy food.

Home-mixed herbal shampoo (2)

Please see pages 46, 135, 138 and 139 for herbal precautions.

INGREDIENTS

- 120ml mild shampoo base (available from many herbal retailers)
- 20ml marigold tincture
- 20ml horsetail tincture
- 20ml horse chestnut tincture
- 20ml nettle leaf tincture
- 1–2 drops tea tree essential oil

METHOD

1. Mix the ingredients together in a measuring jug.
2. Decant the herbal shampoo into a glass or plastic bottle. It will be quite runny.

ADULTS, AND CHILDREN OVER FOUR YEARS OLD: use like an ordinary shampoo, but lather your hair only once and then rinse it thoroughly; you can use this shampoo on a daily basis.
Note: this herbal shampoo can theoretically be made with strong infusions instead of tinctures, but unless you use the shampoo quickly it may go off.

Mix for eczema (1)

Please see pages 119, 135 and 139 for herbal precautions.

INGREDIENTS

- 20ml liquorice (tincture strength 1:1)
- 30ml marigold (tincture strength 1:2)
- 50ml ribwort plantain (tincture strength 1:2)

METHOD

1. Mix the ingredients together.
2. Pour the mixture into a clean, dark glass bottle.
3. Label the bottle with the contents and the date.
4. Store at room temperature for up to 12 months.

ADULT DOSE: 5ml, diluted with some water, two to three times a day.
CHILDREN (4–16 YEARS): adjust the internal adult dose downwards, depending on the body weight of the child (see Chapter 5).

Mix for eczema (2)

Please see pages 135–140 for herbal precautions.

INGREDIENTS

- 30ml chamomile (tincture strength 1:2)
- 15ml yellow dock (tincture strength 1:2)
- 15ml red clover (tincture strength 1:2)
- 40ml ribwort plantain (tincture strength 1:2)

METHOD

1. Mix the ingredients together.
2. Pour the mixture into a clean, dark glass bottle.
3. Label the bottle with the contents and the date.
4. Store at room temperature for up to 12 months.

ADULT DOSE: 5ml, diluted with some water, two to three times a day.
CHILDREN (4–16 YEARS): adjust the internal adult dose downwards, depending on the body weight of the child (see Chapter 5).

- Environmental causes: biological washing powders, household chemicals (including artificial air fresheners), cosmetics, synthetic fabrics and dust mites.
- Stress.

Careful observation is needed to link particular triggers with eczema flare-ups. Often the selective exclusion of the most allergenic causes is enough to clear eczema completely. If this doesn't work you can try both internal and external treatment, but you must proceed very carefully, as some medicinal herbs have the potential to make eczema worse. Internal treatment usually consists of anti-inflammatory and detoxifying herbs, but sometimes an immune modulator and a relaxant for the nervous system are also required. In addition, it is worth optimising the microbiome by adding suitable probiotics. External treatment consists of a healing cream, but you must be very cautious and try each cream on a small area of skin to begin with. It is not uncommon to develop a reaction to a cream that worked very well to begin with, and sometimes you may need to use two or three different creams in rotation.

Treatment options

Please see pages 135–140 for herbal precautions.

- Apply marigold ointment or cream to the affected areas. **Adults, and children over three years old:** once or twice a day.

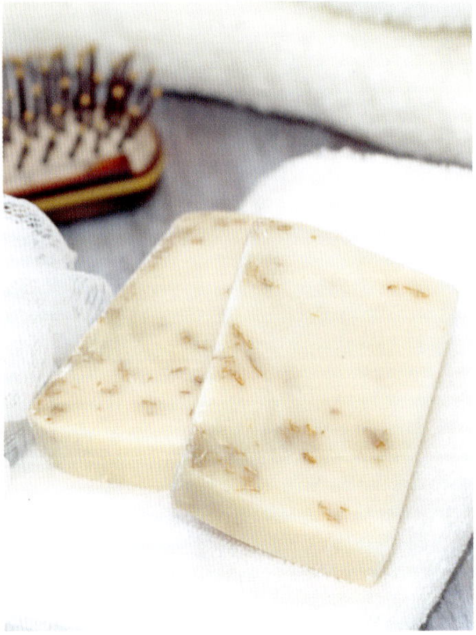

Above Oat soap bars can calm irritated skin.

- Apply either of the antiseptic and healing creams (see pages 138 and 140), especially if the eczema gets infected. **Adults, and children over three years old:** once or twice a day.
- A soothing treatment, especially for babies and small children, is an 'oat bath'. This is a little messy but very calming to the skin. You will need an old stocking or pair of tights, or a piece of muslin cloth, which you can fill with a couple of tablespoonsful of ordinary (preferably organic) porridge oats. Tie it tightly so that the oat grains can't escape, and then swish it in the bath water until the water acquires a milky appearance (or soak it for a few minutes until the oats release their milky contents). Adding a few drops of hemp seed oil to the bath will make it even more soothing. You can use this treatment every day or every other day.
- Try one of the mixes for eczema (internal use) (see boxes on previous page).

Itchy skin

Skin can itch as a result of many different conditions – some of these are visible, such as eczema, and others are less obvious, such as stress or liver dysfunction. Nutritional problems, such as an imbalance of essential fatty acids, are common among people who suffer from itchy skin. Often the cause can be found in the environment, such as washing powder or bubble bath. If the itching persists, consult a health professional.

Treatment options

Please see pages 135–140 for herbal precautions.

- Apply marigold ointment daily if your skin looks dry. **Adults, and children over three years old:** once or twice a day.
- Add marigold infused oil to your bath. **Adults, and children over three years old:** 10ml, once a day, until the skin improves.
- Add thyme or marigold to your bath, either as a tincture or as a strong tea. **Adults, and children over three years old:** add enough herbs to turn the bath water slightly yellow in colour (roughly 40ml of tincture or 500ml of infusion). Do this once a day for a week.

Nappy rash

Be careful if your baby suffers from eczema, as herbal preparations can occasionally make this worse.

Nappy rash occurs when the baby's skin becomes irritated. Keeping the nappy area well covered with a special protective cream will prevent the problem from occurring in the first place. Sometimes nappy rash is also caused by baby wipes or other baby skin products, which may contain ingredients that irritate the skin.

Treatment options

Please see page 135 for herbal precautions.

- Apply marigold cream to the nappy area and leave the baby without a nappy for 10–20 minutes after the application. **Dosage**: once or twice a day.
- Add some marigold tea to the baby's bath to promote healing. **Dosage**: 1 cup of infusion per bath, for two or three consecutive days.

Psoriasis

Practitioner treatment is recommended for this condition.

Psoriasis is a complex disease, and the treatments for it are exceptionally diverse and individual – there is no universal treatment. Dietary factors and lifestyle play a major role and often need to be modified. Looking at the microbiome and trying to improve the individual imbalance is often the key to successful treatment. The measures listed below will benefit some people, but most will need a unique treatment tailored to their own specific circumstances. The treatment for psoriasis is long term, lasting for at least 6–12 months.

Below Psoriasis patches are often found on elbows.

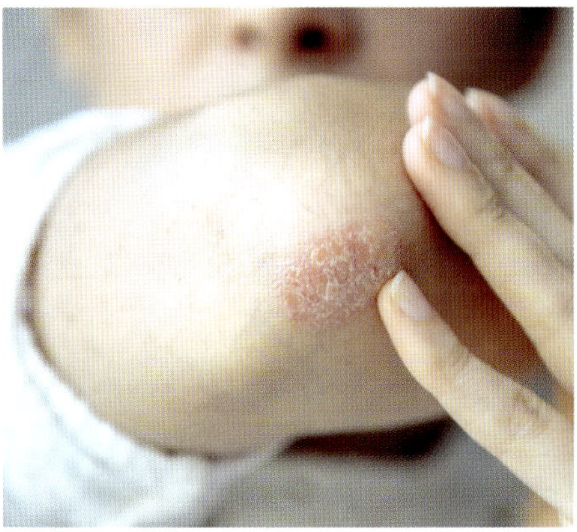

Treatment options

- Apply a cream for psoriasis that contains St John's wort infused oil (see box below).
- Take the mix for skin disorders (see box below).

Cream for psoriasis

Please see pages 116, 135 and 136 for herbal precautions.

INGREDIENTS
- 20g marigold or comfrey cream
- 5ml St John's wort infused oil

METHOD
1. Mix the ingredients well.
2. Transfer the mixture to a clean, dark glass jar, making sure that all air pockets are removed.
3. Store for up to 12 months.

ADULTS: apply to the affected areas twice a day.

Mix for skin disorders

Please see pages 119 and 138 for herbal precautions.

INGREDIENTS
- 20ml yellow dock (tincture strength 1:5)
- 20ml red clover (tincture strength 1:2)
- 20ml liquorice (tincture strength 1:1)
- 40ml ribwort plantain (tincture strength 1:2)

METHOD
1. Mix the ingredients well.
2. Pour the mixture into a clean, dark glass bottle.
3. Label the bottle with the contents and the date.
4. Store at room temperature for up to 12 months.

ADULT DOSE: 5ml diluted with some water, two to three times a day.

Puffy and/or tired eyes

Swollen eyelids or swollen areas underneath the eyes can be a sign of tiredness, allergy or water retention. If this happens regularly, you should consult a health professional to identify the underlying cause. However, if it is a one-off occurrence, the measures listed below will bring rapid improvement. The same measures can be used for tired eyes that feel uncomfortable due to lack of sleep or overwork. It is best to lie down for these treatments so that you can close your eyes and relax.

Treatment options

Please see pages 135–140 for herbal precautions. Both of the options listed below are suitable for children over three years old.

- Make a compress from ordinary, strong black tea, and apply it for 10 minutes. Use cotton wool pads soaked in freshly brewed warm tea, squeeze them gently to remove excess liquid and then apply as eye compresses (you don't want the compresses to dribble but you don't want to squeeze them too much either, otherwise they will be too dry to have an effect). You may need to re-soak the cotton wool pads, as the compress is most effective when warm. **Adults, and children over four years old**: apply for 10–15 minutes, once or twice a day. This treatment is surprisingly effective and is a good option for people who are allergic to marigold or chamomile.
- Make a compress from strong chamomile tea and apply it for 10 minutes, as described above. This option is only suitable for people who are not allergic to chamomile.

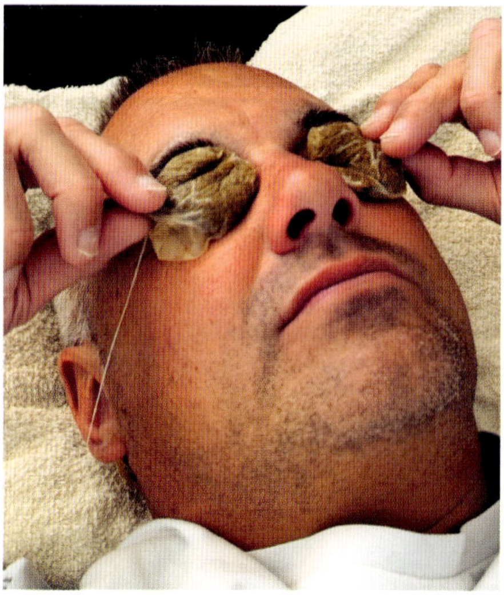

Above Chamomile teabags can be used to make an eyelid compress.

Skin rash

Skin rash can be a reaction to heat, contact with cosmetics and many other substances, or contact with certain plants. You should consult a health professional to obtain an accurate diagnosis. It is important to get the right diagnosis, as many skin problems can look the same to the untrained eye – for instance, some forms of eczema look like fungal infections or heat rash, and vice versa. Because the treatment will depend on the underlying cause, the measures listed below are of a rather general nature – they calm down the inflammation and stimulate the natural healing process.

Treatment options

Please see pages 135–140 for herbal precautions.

- Apply marigold ointment until the rash disappears (discontinue this treatment if the rash becomes worse). **Adults, and children over four years old**: apply once or twice a day.
- Apply a ribwort plantain poultice or compress (you can use fresh or dried

herbs). This is an extremely soothing treatment that can be applied even to a rash that is oozing fluid, such as weeping eczema (see page 30 for instructions on how to prepare and apply a poultice or compress). **Adults, and children over four years old:** apply for 15 minutes, once or twice a day.

Skin infection

Seek urgent medical help if you notice a red streak developing on the skin and extending away from the infected area, as this can indicate that the infection is spreading and there is a risk of septicaemia (blood poisoning), which is a potentially life-threatening condition.

Skin infections (including deeper skin infections, which are called cellulitis) usually follow some kind of injury, such as a cut, a scratch, a prick or a sting. Normally bacteria cannot penetrate the intact skin, and only when it is broken do they gain access to the deeper layers. The signs of infection are swelling around the point of entry, redness and tenderness. The swelling and redness have a sizeable diameter (5–15cm) and are quite diffuse, often with no clear boundary between the healthy and infected skin. Skin infection may be accompanied by a raised temperature. Most local skin infections can be treated with herbs, and I recommend use of a combination of an external and an internal antibacterial remedy. The measures listed below are applicable to small areas of infected skin (up to 5cm in diameter). If the area is much larger than this you need to see a health professional.

Treatment options

Please see pages 113 and 116 for herbal precautions.

- Eat raw garlic daily until the infection clears up. **Adults:** 1 crushed clove of garlic mixed with 1 teaspoonful of honey, two to three times a day.

Below Garlic contains a compound called allicin, which prevents fungi and bacteria from growing.

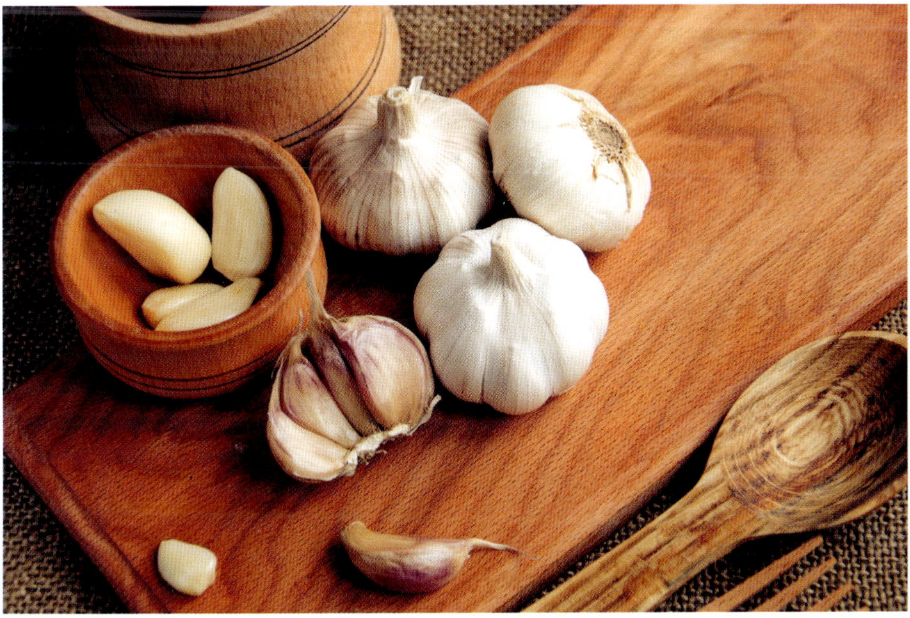

- You can secure a slice of garlic to the area with a plaster, but don't leave it in place for more than 2–3 hours or you may experience a local skin reaction that looks rather like a burn. For children you can rub the infected area with a sliced clove of garlic once or twice a day.
- Take propolis tincture. **Adults:** 0.5–2ml, two to three times a day, tincture strength 1:5, or propolis capsules that are equivalent to 100–500mg of propolis a day.
- Apply strongly antiseptic cream for skin infections (see box below).

Cream for skin infections

Please see pages 135–140 for herbal precautions.

INGREDIENTS

- 50g marigold cream
- 10ml echinacea tincture
- 10 drops thyme essential oil
- 10 drops tea tree essential oil

METHOD

1. Mix the ingredients well.
2. Transfer the mixture to a clean, dark glass jar, making sure that all air pockets are removed.
3. Store for up to 12 months.

ADULTS, AND CHILDREN OVER FIVE YEARS OLD: apply a thick layer to the infected area and cover it with non-absorbent dressing (as you want the ointment to be absorbed by the skin, not by the dressing). Change the dressing every 3–4 hours until the redness and swelling are visibly reduced and there is no tenderness.

Splinters

Small splinters that cannot be pulled out with tweezers can be drawn out with a paste made from herbal powder.

Treatment options

Both of the options listed below are suitable for children over three years old, and for use during pregnancy.

- Mix 1 teaspoonful of marshmallow root powder with a little warm water to form a thick paste. Apply the paste to the area where the splinter is, and cover it with a small square of plastic or clingfilm and then with sticking plaster. Keep the dressing on for an hour. When you remove the dressing there is usually no sign of the splinter, but the skin may have a puckered appearance for a while.
- If the area around the splinter is inflamed, add 1 drop of thyme or tea tree essential oil to the paste and proceed as described above.

Stye

Practitioner treatment is recommended for this condition.

A stye is a painful infection that affects the margins of the eyelid. It usually indicates poor immune function, exhaustion and nutritional deficiencies. The contributing factors need to be considered in addition to the external treatment.

Treatment options

Please see pages 135–140 for herbal precautions.

- Apply a small amount of marigold ointment directly to the stye until the symptoms disappear completely. Use a cotton bud for precise application, and

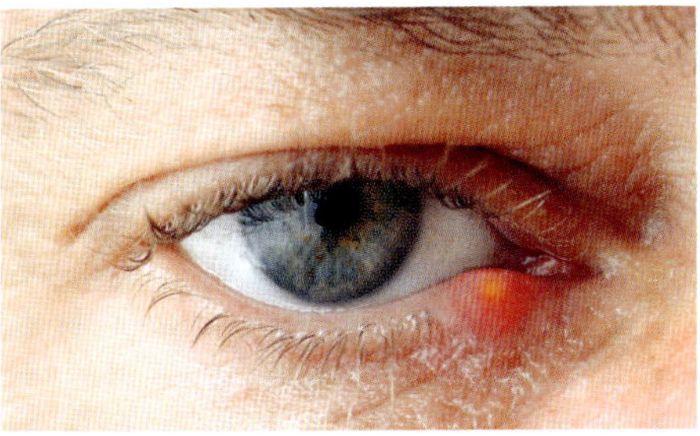

Above Styes can also form on the upper lid.

make sure that the ointment does not get into the eye. **Adults, and children over four years old:** apply three to five times a day.

- Apply a marigold compress twice a day to the affected eye (see page 30 for instructions on making a compress).
- Take eyebright tincture until the symptoms disappear completely. **Adults:** 1–2ml diluted with some water, twice a day, tincture strength 1:2.
- Apply a small amount of propolis cream directly to the stye until the symptoms disappear completely (see box below). This treatment is not suitable for children under 12 years old.

Propolis cream

Please see pages 116, 135 and 136 for herbal precautions.

INGREDIENTS

- 50g marigold or comfrey cream
- 5ml propolis (tincture strength 1:5)

METHOD

1 Mix the ingredients well.
2 Transfer the mixture to a clean, dark glass jar, making sure that all air pockets are removed.
3 Store for up to 12 months.

ADULTS, AND CHILDREN OVER 12 YEARS OLD: apply to the stye three to five times a day, making sure that the cream does not get into the eye.

Sunburn

Sunburn can range from a mild pinkness of the skin to a flaming red skin covered in blisters. If your sunburn is severe, do not use tinctures externally, as even a tiny amount of alcohol will sting. Marigold provides the best treatment I have ever come across – the marigold compress is immediately cooling and reduces the pain. Apply a cool but not ice-cold treatment.

Treatment options

Please see pages 135–136 for herbal precautions. All of the options listed below are suitable for children over three years old.

- Have a lukewarm bath to which marigold tincture or strong marigold tea has been added (enough tincture or tea to make the bath water yellowish in colour). Soak for 10–15 minutes.
- Apply cooled marigold tea directly to the skin with a sponge or cotton wool. Gently dab every hour until there is noticeable relief.

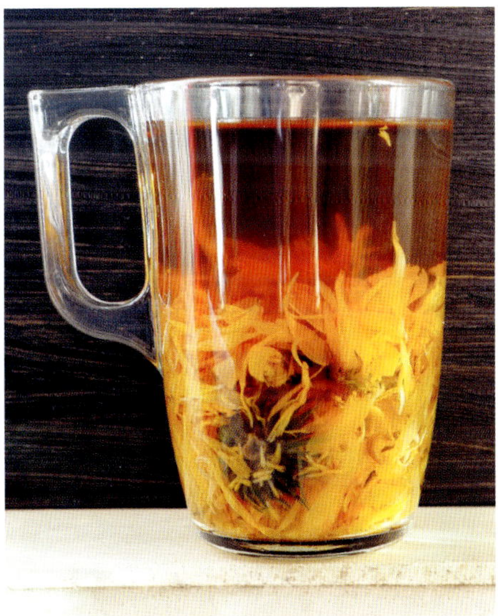

Above Use a strong marigold infusion to treat a burn.

- Apply a cool marigold tea compress (see page 30 for instructions on making a compress). **Dosage:** this can be applied repeatedly until relief is felt. Usually two or three applications are sufficient, but more may be necessary for severe sunburn.
- Apply marigold ointment or cream – this is best done after one of the above cooling treatments. The marigold ointment prevents the skin from peeling later on, and also provides a soothing effect. **Dosage:** one generous application is usually sufficient.
- Apply thyme tincture diluted with cold water as a gentle wipe. This treatment is suitable for minor sunburn. **Dosage:** 20ml of tincture (tincture strength 1:2) per cup of cool water; apply hourly two or three times.

Warts and verrucas

You need to be persistent when treating warts, as they often take a long time to disappear. Verrucas are a specific type of wart, usually found on the sole of the foot.

Widespread warts, and warts that don't disappear as a result of using the treatments described below, may require an internal treatment.

Treatment options

Please see pages 61 and 113 for herbal precautions.

- Apply a sliver of fresh garlic directly to the wart and hold it in place with a plaster for 2–3 hours (note that garlic may sting and cause a temporary skin rash around the wart). This is a one-off treatment, and I do not recommend it for children under six years old.
- Apply thuja tincture (tincture strength 1:2) to the wart for 5–6 weeks, or for up to 2–3 months if the wart is large. **Adults, and children over four years old:** apply one drop in the morning and one drop in the evening until the wart disappears.
- Apply fresh dandelion sap from the flower stalk directly to the wart for 6–12 weeks. **Adults, and children over four years old:** break a flowering stem and apply the fresh white juice to the wart two to four times a day.

Below Break the stem to get dandelion sap.

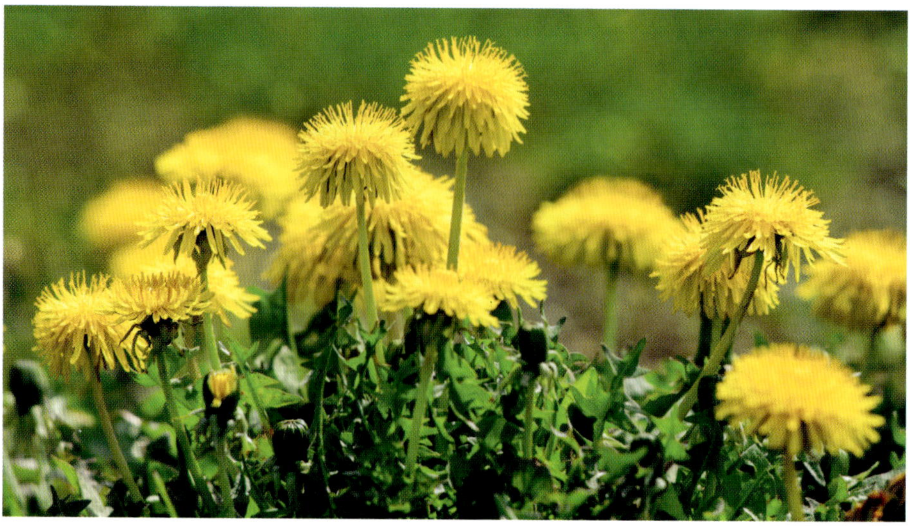

Conditions for which home treatment is not recommended

- Widespread eczema: this requires a comprehensive review of diet and lifestyle as well as individualised internal treatment.
- Psoriasis: the treatment varies enormously from one person to another, and may take up to a year.
- Acne rosacea: this is a complex condition that requires treatment of the circulatory system as well as the skin; it needs long-term medication with herbs.
- Molluscum contagiosum: although this viral infection will resolve by itself eventually, herbal treatment can significantly speed up recovery.
- Multiple warts: these usually require a combination of external and internal treatments.
- Fungal infection of the nails that cannot be eradicated: persistent fungal infection of the nails often requires an internal treatment as well as a combination of external remedies that can be rotated.
- Urticaria (hives): this condition is allergic in nature and therefore needs careful treatment; lifestyle and stress factors often also need to be addressed.
- Skin ulcer: a specialised treatment is required both internally and externally; you may need supervision on a daily or weekly basis to make sure that a particular treatment option is working.

When to seek medical attention

- If you have a severe eye infection (conjunctivitis).
- If you have an infected cut or wound that will not heal, especially if there is a lot of redness around the area and a red streak developing on the skin in the direction of blood circulation – this indicates the spread of the local infection, and there is a risk of septicaemia, which is a potentially life-threatening condition.
- If you experience sudden, patchy loss of hair.
- If you or your child have impetigo – a skin infection that produces yellow crusting and spreads quickly.
- If any skin lump develops that is tender, or does not go away, or becomes enlarged.
- If any mole undergoes a change in appearance and becomes enlarged or ulcerates.

CHAPTER 13

The urinary and reproductive systems

Although the urinary and reproductive systems are two independent physiological systems, they are closely connected due to their anatomical proximity and the influence of sex hormones.

The urinary system

The male and female urinary systems are essentially the same and consist of the kidneys, ureters, bladder and urethra. The urethra is much shorter in females than in males, which is the main reason for the higher prevalence of urinary tract infections in women. Infections of the urinary tract that are limited to its lower parts (the urethra and bladder) can be successfully treated at home, but if they are persistent you must consult your GP or a medical herbalist to make sure that the infection doesn't spread to the kidneys.

Reproductive system

Female

The female reproductive system consists of the vagina, cervix, uterus, Fallopian tubes and ovaries, and it is governed by a complicated interplay of sex hormones. Only mild hormonal disorders are suitable for self-treatment, but other common ailments of the female reproductive system are very amenable to home treatment. Some problems related to pregnancy (e.g. nausea, reflux) are discussed elsewhere.

Male

The male reproductive system consists of the penis, testicles and prostate gland. Disorders of the male reproductive system can be a result of impaired hormonal control, but they also often stem from lifestyle or psychological problems, or circulatory disease. Only a small proportion of such problems can be treated successfully at home.

Herb selection in this chapter

It is difficult to choose a small selection of herbs for the variety of medical problems that can affect the urinary and reproductive systems. The main reason for this is that such herbs often have a very narrow spectrum of action – for instance, saw palmetto is specifically used to treat prostate problems. It may not be practicable to store many of the herbs needed to effectively treat these systems unless you already use some of them to treat other problems. The selection provided here, which is larger than that for any other body system, will cover quite a few problems, but for many ailments of the urinary and reproductive systems you will need specific additional herbs.

Must-have herbs

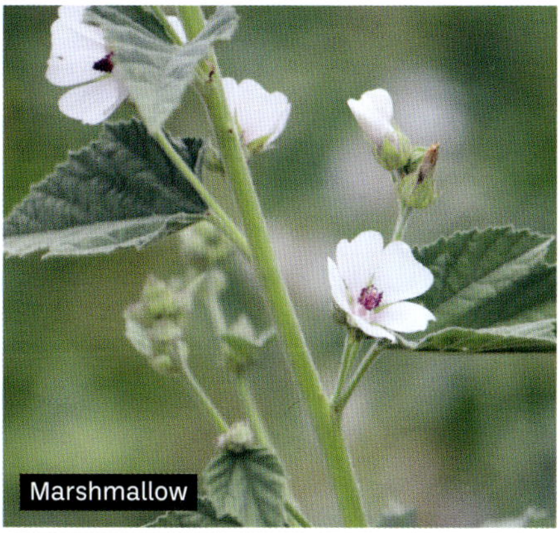

Marshmallow

Marshmallow root or leaves *Althaea officinalis*

Marshmallow preparations can be taken alongside prescribed medication, so long as they are taken at least two hours before or after the latter.

Uses

You can use marshmallow root or leaves to make a very soothing drink if you have cystitis or urethritis. Marshmallow infusion provides rapid relief from the pain and stinging sensation in the urethra.

HOW TO TAKE IT: As a tea. Start drinking it as soon as you develop symptoms of cystitis or urethritis. It is best to drink this tea warm, and to let it brew for a long time to allow the release of the mucilage (the anti-irritant constituent of the plant) from the leaves. You can infuse a large amount of the herb (5–10 teaspoonsful of dried root or dried leaves) in one go in a cafetière or a teapot and then drink three to five portions throughout the day, mixing each portion with a small amount of hot water.

DOSAGE: **Adults**: 3–5 large cups a day.

Crampbark *Viburnum opulus*

Uses

Also known as guelder rose, crampbark is a muscle relaxant, and is therefore suitable for relieving menstrual cramps.

HOW TO TAKE IT: As a tincture, as and when needed.

DOSAGE: **Adults**: if you experience period cramps, take 2ml diluted with some water three times a day, tincture strength 1:2, for one to two days.

Teenagers (11–16 years): 11–13 years, take half the adult dose; 14–16 years, take three-quarters of the adult dose. Alternatively, you can adjust the dose according to the body weight of the person being treated (see page 33).

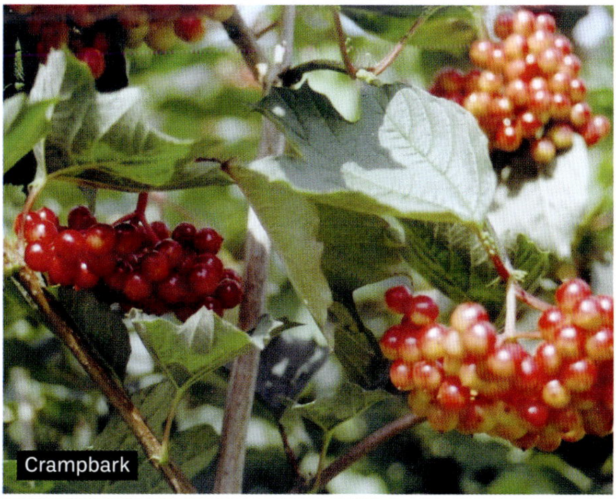

Crampbark

Couch grass *Elymus repens* (syn. *Agropyron repens*)

Uses

Couch grass is mildly diuretic and soothes irritation of the urinary tract. It is suitable for conditions in which passing urine causes pain or a burning sensation (e.g. cystitis, urethritis), and for conditions where there is general inflammation of particular parts of the urinary tract (e.g. prostatitis, kidney stones).

COMBINATIONS: Couch grass combines well with herbs that have antiseptic effects on the urinary tract, such as celery seed or thyme, and with other herbs that have anti-irritant properties, such as marshmallow leaf.
HOW TO TAKE IT: Couch grass can be taken as a tea or as a tincture.
DOSAGE: **Adults:** 1–2ml diluted with some water, three times a day, tincture strength 1:1, or 3–4 cups of tea a day.

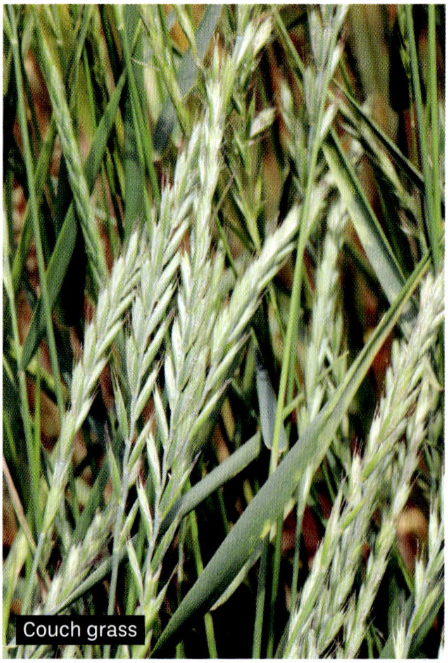

Couch grass

Echinacea (purple coneflower) *Echinacea purpurea* and *Echinacea angustifolia*

Caution is needed in people who are allergic to plants belonging to the daisy family (the Asteraceae, formerly known as the Compositae). Not suitable for transplant patients and children under 12.

Uses

As a general modulator of the immune system, echinacea can be taken to help with any infection, so it is a useful supplement if you experience repeated bouts of cystitis or thrush.

HOW TO TAKE IT: Take it for at least a month to boost your immune system after the worst of your infection is over.
DOSAGE: **Adults:** 1.2–3ml diluted with some water, two to three times a day, tincture strength 1:2.

Thyme *Thymus vulgaris*

Do not use thyme essential oil for external applications in pregnancy or for children under three years old without consulting a specialist. All other thyme preparations (tincture, tea and ointment) are safe for small children and in pregnancy if used *externally*.

Uses

Thyme works as an antiseptic for the urinary system, and can therefore be used to treat urinary tract infections. It is also useful for relieving the itchy symptoms of thrush.

HOW TO TAKE IT: To treat cystitis, take thyme as a tincture until the symptoms completely disappear. It is best to drink marshmallow leaf tea at the same time. To treat cystitis and thrush you can combine thyme tincture with

echinacea or andrographis tincture.
DOSAGE: **Adults**: 0.7–2ml diluted with some water, two to three times a day, tincture strength 1:2.

Yarrow *Achillea millefolium*

Do not take yarrow during pregnancy.

Caution is needed in people who are allergic to plants belonging to the daisy family (the Asteraceae, formerly known as the Compositae).

Uses

Yarrow can be used as a treatment for periods that are irregular or too heavy. It is also useful if you experience digestive symptoms around the time of your period.

COMBINATIONS: Yarrow combines well with herbs such as chamomile or crampbark to reduce period pain.
HOW TO TAKE IT: As a tea or as a tincture.
DOSAGE: **Adults**: 1–2 cups a day, or 0.7–2ml, one to three times a day, tincture strength 1:2.
Teenagers (11–16 years): 11–13 years, take half the adult dose; 14–16 years, take three-quarters of the adult dose. Alternatively, you can adjust the dose according to the body weight of the person being treated (see page 33).

Saw palmetto *Serenoa repens* (syn. *Serenoa serrulata*)

This herb is not suitable for children, or for women who are pregnant or breastfeeding. Prostate cancer should be excluded before commencing treatment with saw palmetto, as the herb may mask the symptoms of the disease.

There is a possibility of temporary digestive upset. Caution is needed in people who are taking warfarin.

Uses

Saw palmetto is specific for prostate problems, particularly benign prostatic enlargement (also known as benign prostatic hyperplasia or BPH), but it can also be used to treat other inflammatory disorders of the male genitourinary tract, such as urethritis or orchitis. It is worth noting that saw palmetto does not alter the levels of prostate-specific antigen (PSA), which is a marker used both to screen for prostate cancer and to monitor patients who have been diagnosed with the latter. Sometimes this herb can cause a stomach upset or diarrhoea, in which case it needs to be combined with herbs that have an anti-irritant effect on the digestive system (e.g. marshmallow root, see page 159). Alternatively, a smaller dose can be taken.

HOW TO TAKE IT: As a tincture, or as capsules or tablets.
DOSAGE: **Adults only**: 1–3ml, two to three times a day, tincture strength 1:2, or the equivalent of 2.2–3.2g of dried herb a day as tablets or capsules.

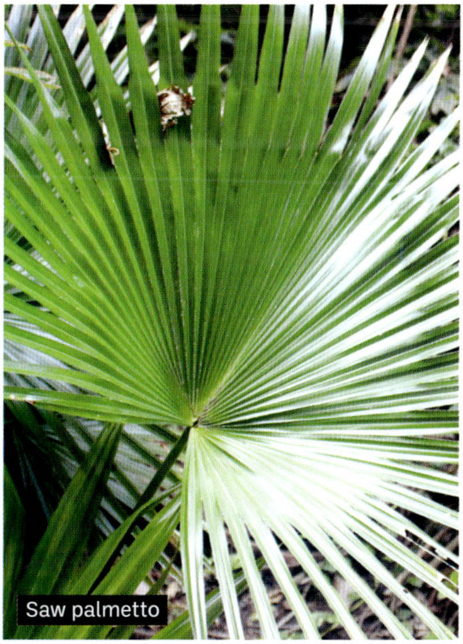
Saw palmetto

Optional herbs

Selection of diuretic teas

Many of the herbs discussed in previous chapters have diuretic properties, and can therefore be used whenever it is desirable to increase the volume of urine – for instance, during a bout of cystitis or urethritis. It is preferable to take diuretic herbs as a tea, although a tincture diluted with a cupful of warm water will work just as well. Suitable herbs include marshmallow leaf, celery seed, birch, shepherd's purse, dandelion leaf, lime tree flowers, meadowsweet and nettle leaf. Before using any of these plants, please check for any precautions in the detailed account of the plant in the relevant chapter of this book.

Celery seed *Apium graveolens*

Celery seed may lower the blood level of thyroxine in people who are taking that medication, so inform your doctor that you are taking the herb, and always take it a few hours before or after the thyroxine.

Caution is needed in people with kidney disorders and in women who are breastfeeding.

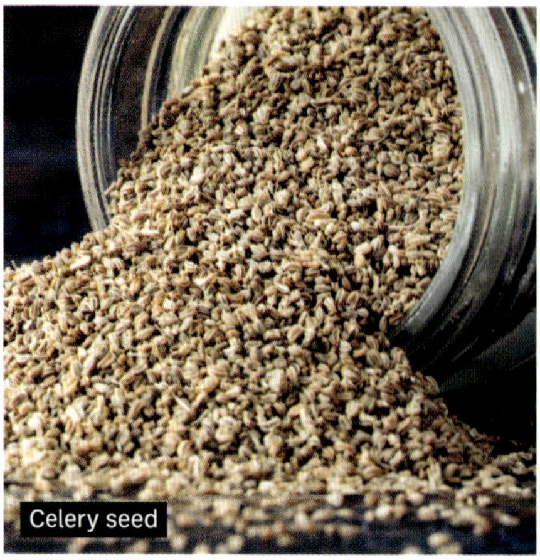

Celery seed

Uses

Celery seed is most useful for infections of the urinary tract, as it has an antiseptic effect on this part of the body.

COMBINATIONS: Celery seed combines well with couch grass (see page 160).
HOW TO TAKE IT: As a tincture.
DOSAGE: **Adults**: 1.4–2.8ml diluted with some water, one to three times a day, tincture strength 1:2.

Damiana *Turnera diffusa* (syn. *Turnera aphrodisiaca*)

Damiana is not suitable for children. It should be avoided during pregnancy and when breastfeeding.

Caution is needed in people who are prone to extreme anxiety.

Uses

Damiana is considered to be a tonic for both the male and female reproductive systems, and can therefore be used in a number of circumstances in which these are not functioning optimally. It seems to possess a mild aphrodisiac action as well as providing a general sense of improved well-being.

HOW TO TAKE IT: As a tincture.
DOSAGE: **Adults**: 1–2ml diluted with some water, one to three times a day, tincture strength 1:2.

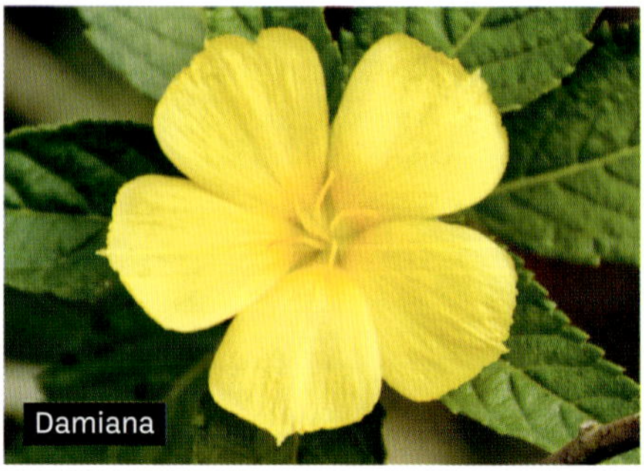

Damiana

Dandelion leaves *Taraxacum officinale*

Caution is needed in people who are allergic to plants belonging to the daisy family, and in those who have gall-bladder problems.

Uses

Dandelion leaves are used primarily as a diuretic (though they also mildly stimulate the liver and the release of bile), and this herb is useful in many cases of water retention and oedema, or whenever an increased flow of urine is indicated.

HOW TO TAKE IT: As a tea or as a tincture.
DOSAGE: **Adults:** 2–4ml, one to three times a day, tincture strength 1:2.

Sage *Salvia officinalis*

Do not take sage internally during pregnancy or when breastfeeding.
Do not take this herb continually for long periods of time.
Sage is not suitable for children as an internal treatment.

Uses

Sage preparations inhibit sweating and are therefore useful for hot flushes. It is best to combine sage with other herbs for menopausal symptoms, such as red clover or wild yam.

HOW TO TAKE IT: I recommend using sage as a tincture, but it can also be taken as an infusion. You should not take sage continually, so whichever form you use, have a two-week break every four weeks or so.
DOSAGE: **Adults only:** 0.7–1ml diluted with some water, two to three times a day, tincture strength 1:2, or 1–2 cups of infusion a day.

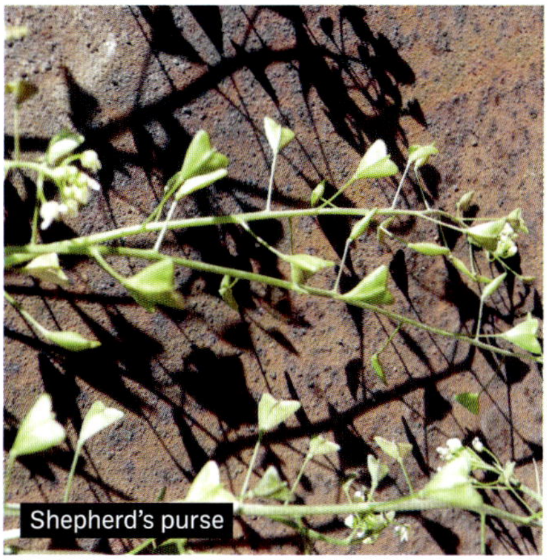
Shepherd's purse

Shepherd's purse *Capsella bursa-pastoris*

Caution is needed during pregnancy and when breastfeeding.

Uses

This herb can be used to decrease the amount of bleeding during a heavy period, but a large dose is needed to achieve this effect. Shepherd's purse can also improve the tone of the uterine muscle and can help to relieve symptoms of a partial uterine prolapse.

HOW TO TAKE IT: As a tincture or as a tea.
DOSAGE: **Adults (heavy periods):** 10ml diluted with some water, three to four times a day, tincture strength 1:2, for one or two days only.
Adults (uterine muscle tone): 2–3 cups of tea a day, or 1–2ml of tincture diluted with some water, three times a day, tincture strength 1:2, until symptoms improve.
Teenagers (11–16 years): 11–13 years, take half the adult dose; 14–16 years, take three-quarters of the adult dose. Alternatively, you can adjust the dose according to the body weight of the person being treated (see page 33).

White deadnettle
Lamium album

Uses

This herb is used specifically to treat excessive vaginal discharge. It provides a useful addition to the treatment of thrush or other infections of the female reproductive tract.

COMBINATIONS: White deadnettle combines well with thyme and marigold, either as a tincture or as a tea.

HOW TO TAKE IT: As a tincture or as a tea.

DOSAGE: **Adults:** 1–2 cups of tea a day, or 2ml diluted with some water, two to three times a day, tincture strength 1:2. **Teenagers (11–16 years):** 11–13 years, take half the adult dose; 14–16 years, take three-quarters of the adult dose. Alternatively, you can adjust the dose according to the body weight of the person being treated (see page 33).

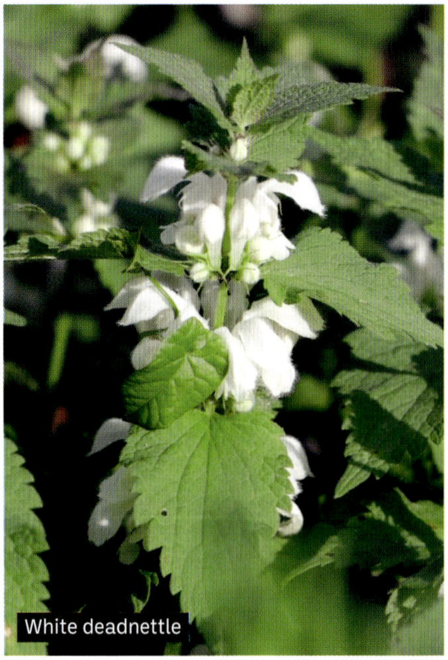
White deadnettle

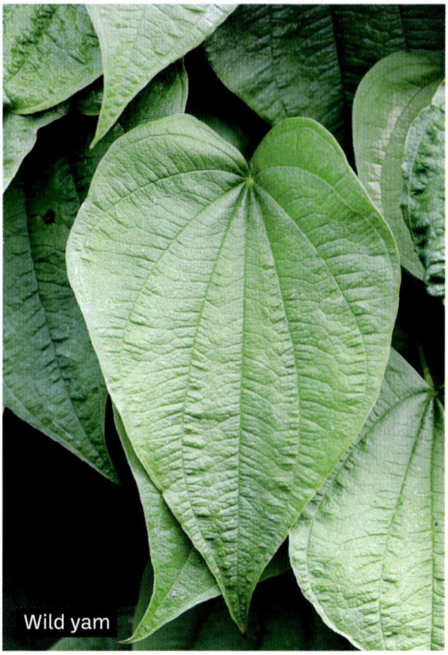
Wild yam

Wild yam
Dioscorea villosa

Wild yam may cause or aggravate gastro-oesophageal reflux (heartburn).

Uses

Wild yam is one of the main herbs used in the treatment of menopausal problems. It is especially useful if you also have joint pain and stiffness.

Combine it with other herbs depending on the particular combination of menopausal symptoms (see the Menopause entry on page 170).

HOW TO TAKE IT: As a tincture.

DOSAGE: **Adults:** 1–2ml diluted with some water, two to three times a day, tincture strength 1:2.

Specific ailments that affect the urinary and reproductive systems, and herbs that can help

Bedwetting (in children)

This problem normally resolves by itself as the child grows up, but gentle herbal support may help with the natural maturing of the brain–bladder alarm system. Sometimes emotional issues are involved, in which case you should seek professional help.

Treatment options

Please see page 159 for herbal precautions.

- Crampbark tincture. **Children (3–7 years):** 7 drops diluted in water or juice, twice a day, tincture strength 1:2.
- Marshmallow leaf tea. **Children (3–7 years):** a quarter of a cup, twice a day.

Benign prostatic enlargement (benign prostatic hyperplasia)

Practitioner treatment is recommended for this condition.

This condition must be diagnosed by a GP, as the symptoms are very similar to those of prostate cancer. Herbs can decrease the urge to pass urine frequently, especially at night. Men with prostatic enlargement are prone to cystitis and urinary retention, both of which can be successfully treated with herbs to reduce the need for antibiotics.

Treatment options

Please see pages 138, 159 and 164 for herbal precautions.

- Take saw palmetto tincture on a regular basis. **Adults only:** 1–3ml diluted with some water, two to three times a day, tincture strength 1:2.
- Drink marshmallow leaf, nettle leaf and nettle root tea (see box overleaf) on a daily basis to prevent cystitis.

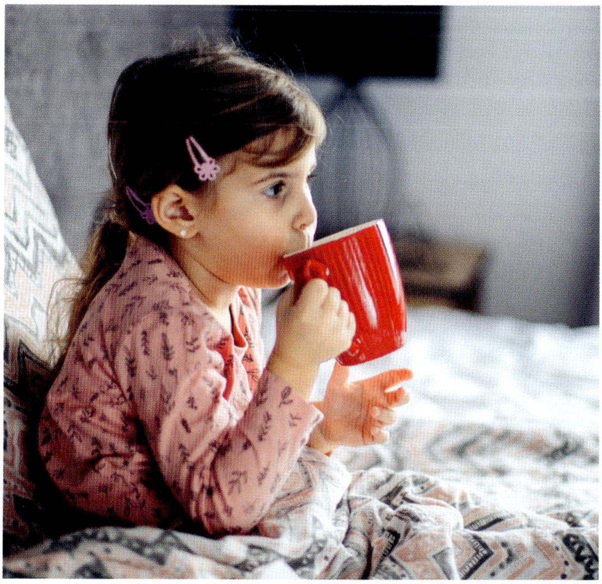

Left Marshmallow leaf tea soothes the lining of the bladder.

Cystitis and urethritis

Practitioner treatment is recommended for recurrent episodes of these conditions.

Cystitis is an infection of the bladder, and it is as common as urethritis, which is an infection of the urethra (the narrow passage connecting the bladder to the outside of the body). If your symptoms consist of a burning sensation on passing urine, an increased urge to pass water, and you need to urinate very often, you are most probably suffering from urethritis. If, in addition to these symptoms, you develop a pain above your pubic bone, you become feverish and your urine becomes cloudy and smelly, you are most probably suffering from cystitis. In addition to using the measures described below, it is important to drink 1–2 litres of water or herbal tea a day to dilute the urine, as this will reduce the stinging and flush out the bacteria. Another common measure is to take cranberry tablets or capsules, although this is only effective for some bacteria that can infect the urinary tract. I do not recommend cranberry juice, as it is normally sweetened and less effective than tablets or capsules. You can also speed up recovery by eating plenty of parsley and celery, avoiding hot spices and alcohol, and using a hot water bottle at bedtime.

Remember that if your infection does not clear up within a couple of days you must see a health professional, as there is a risk that the infection will spread to the kidneys. If you notice that there is a link between your cystitis and sexual activity, be fastidious about your own and your partner's hygiene, and empty your bladder both before and after sex.

Tea for preventing cystitis

Please see pages 138, 159 and 164 for herbal precautions.

INGREDIENTS

- 50g dried marshmallow leaf
- 25g dried nettle leaf
- 25g dried nettle root

METHOD

1. Mix the herbs thoroughly.
2. Infuse 2 teaspoonsful of the mixture in a cup of freshly boiled water for 10 minutes. Strain and drink warm.

ADULT DOSE: 1 cup a day for 3–12 months.

Mix for cystitis and urethritis

Please see pages 159–164 for herbal precautions.

INGREDIENTS

- 20ml thyme (tincture strength 1:2)
- 20ml celery seed (tincture strength 1:2)
- 20ml couch grass (tincture strength 1:2)
- 40ml marshmallow leaf (tincture strength 1:2)

METHOD

1. Mix the ingredients together.
2. Pour the mixture into a clean, dark glass bottle.
3. Label the bottle with the contents and the date.
4. Store at room temperature for up to 12 months.

ADULT DOSE: 10ml diluted with some water for the first dose, then 5ml diluted with some water twice more that day, and then three times a day until the symptoms have gone, and for one further day after the symptoms have gone.

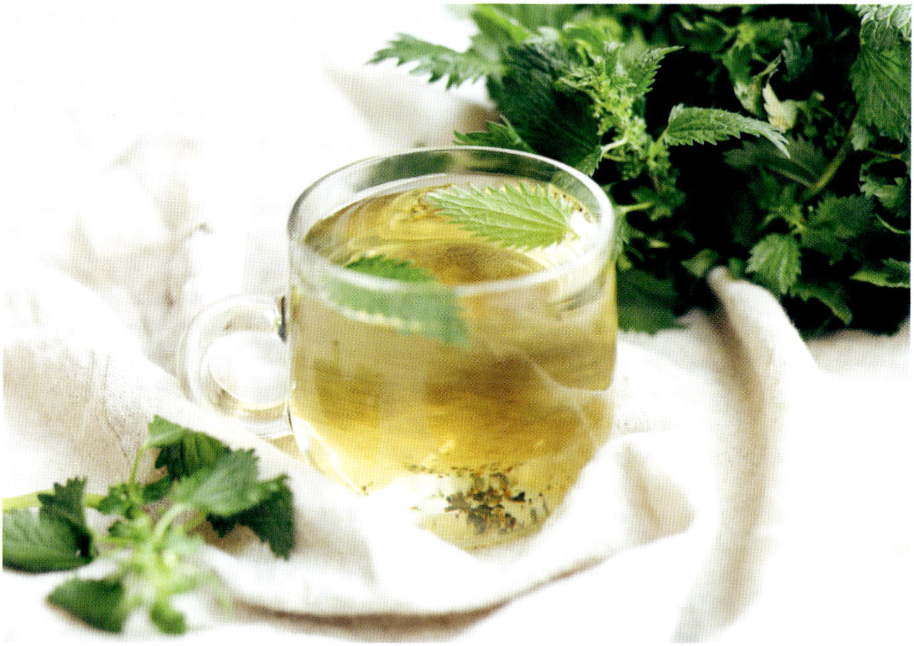

Above Nettle tea.

Treatment options

Please see pages 117, 159 and 160 for herbal precautions. The treatment is the same for cystitis and urethritis.

- Drink marshmallow leaf tea to soothe the pain and the irritation. **Adults:** 3–5 cups a day.
- Drink any of the diuretic teas listed in the optional herbs section. **Adults:** 1 cup a day if you are already drinking marshmallow tea, otherwise 3 cups a day.
- Take thyme tincture for its antiseptic properties (if you are not taking the mix for cystitis, see right). **Adults:** 0.7–2ml diluted with some water, one to three times a day, tincture strength 1:2.
- Take echinacea tincture if you are experiencing recurring episodes. **Adults:** 1.2–3ml diluted with some water, two to three times a day for a month, tincture strength 1:2.
- Take andrographis tincture for its antibacterial and immune-enhancing properties. **Adults:** 1–2ml diluted with some water, two to three times a day for three to five days, tincture strength 1:2.
- Take the mix for cystitis and urethritis (see box on page 166).

Erectile dysfunction

Erectile dysfunction can be a complex ailment and has a diverse range of causes – for example, having diabetes, taking a particular medication, drinking too much alcohol or having psychological problems. You need to address the causes, and the primary treatment is often long term. The measures listed below can provide supportive treatment only.

Treatment options

- Improve your circulation with hawthorn and blueberries (for more information, see pages 43 and 45).
- Take relaxing herbs if anxiety is a contributing factor (see Chapter 10).

Hot flushes

Practitioner treatment is recommended for this condition.

Hot flushes are usually experienced by women around the time of the menopause, most often after their periods have stopped. Many herbs and supplements can be useful, though the choice of herbs will depend on the stage of the menopause. For instance, if you are still having periods, chaste tree can be helpful, but if you have stopped having periods or have had a total hysterectomy, this herb would be of little benefit.

A healthy diet – for example, eating less meat and more soya products, and drinking less alcohol and coffee – can make a big difference. Vitamin E supplements (400–500IU a day) can be helpful for some women. If your hot flushes are really severe and disruptive you will need a complex prescription to restore the balance of female sex hormones as well as other hormones, especially thyroid hormones. If your hot flushes are caused by side effects of your medication you should consult a practitioner before taking any herbs.

Below Hawthorn flowers

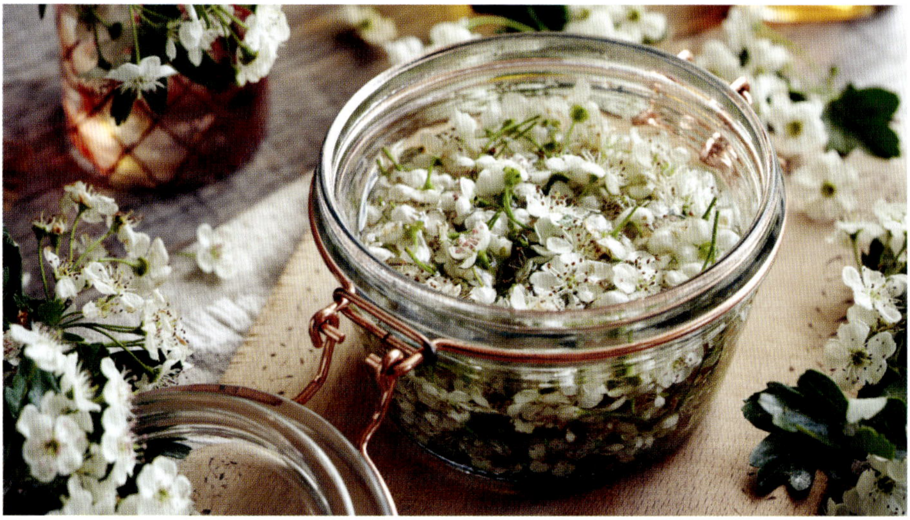

Mix for hot flushes

Please see pages 100, 163, 164 and 195 for herbal precautions.

INGREDIENTS

- 25ml sage (tincture strength 1:2)
- 35ml wild yam (tincture strength 1:2)
- 20ml hawthorn flowers (tincture strength 1:2)
- 20ml St John's wort (tincture strength 1:2)

METHOD

1. Mix the ingredients together.
2. Pour the mixture into a clean, dark glass bottle.
3. Label the bottle with the contents and the date.
4. Store at room temperature for up to 12 months.

ADULTS ONLY: 5ml diluted with some water, two to three times a day.

Treatment options

Please see pages 100, 163, 164 and 195 for herbal precautions.

- Take sage tincture, but have a two-week break from this herb every four weeks if you take a large dose. **Adults**: 0.7–1ml diluted with some water, two to three times a day, tincture strength 1:2.
- Take wild yam tincture. **Adults**: 1–2ml diluted with some water, two to three times a day, tincture strength 1:2.
- Take hawthorn flower tincture. **Adults**: 1–2ml diluted with some water, one to three times a day, tincture strength 1:2.
- Take St John's wort tincture if the menopausal symptoms make you feel depressed or if you have mood swings. **Adults**: 0.6–2ml diluted with some water, two to three times a day, tincture strength 1:2.
- Take one of the mixes for hot flushes (see box overleaf and page 168), but take it instead of – not as well as – the above herbs.

Incontinence

Practitioner treatment is recommended for this condition.

Involuntary passing of urine can affect both men and women, and can be a result of many different factors, including stress, infection, weakness of the pelvic floor muscles, urinary retention and post-surgery inflammation. As there is such a variety of causes the core treatment will vary from person to person, and should be prescribed by a herbal clinician. The measures listed below are therefore intended to provide only a supportive treatment to the main treatment prescribed by a professional.

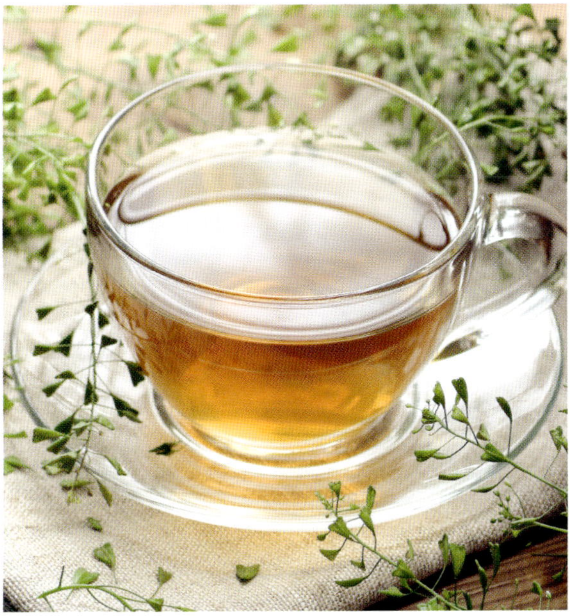

Right Shepherd's purse tea.

Treatment options

Please see pages 159–164 for herbal precautions.

- Drink marshmallow leaf tea daily to reduce any irritation that leads to an urgent need to pass urine. **Adults**: 1–2 cups a day.
- Drink shepherd's purse tea as a gentle diuretic that aids urinary retention. **Adults**: 2–3 cups a day.

Libido, low

This is a surprisingly common problem in both sexes. Its root causes normally include factors such as overwork, emotional problems and lifestyle issues, although a hormone imbalance is occasionally responsible. For more information on how to improve sex drive, see Chapter 16.

Treatment options

Please see pages 162 and 181 for herbal precautions.

- Take damiana tincture. **Adults**: 1–2ml diluted with some water, one to three times a day, tincture strength 1:2.
- Take Korean ginseng as a general tonic for the whole body, as this also improves the sex drive. Adults: 300–500mg a day in tablet form, or 0.5–2ml diluted with some water, once or twice a day, tincture strength 1:2.

Menopausal problems

Practitioner treatment is recommended for this condition.

The menopause can be associated with a whole array of health problems, such as hot flushes, mood swings, low libido, discomfort during sex and joint aches. Each woman will experience a different combination of symptoms that will also vary in severity. As a result, individual prescriptions are recommended, which may need to be adjusted as the symptoms

Mix for menopausal symptoms (especially hot flushes and lack of energy)

Please see pages 100, 101, 163, 164 and 195 for herbal precautions.

INGREDIENTS

- 20ml sage (tincture strength 1:2)
- 20ml hawthorn (tincture strength 1:2)
- 20ml wild yam (tincture strength 1:2)
- 20ml vervain (tincture strength 1:2)
- 20ml St John's wort (tincture strength 1:2)

METHOD

1. Mix the ingredients together.
2. Pour the mixture into a clean, dark glass bottle.
3. Label the bottle with the contents and the date.
4. Store at room temperature for up to 12 months.

ADULT DOSE: 5ml diluted with some water, two to three times a day.

Below Consider joining a menopause support group if you are struggling.

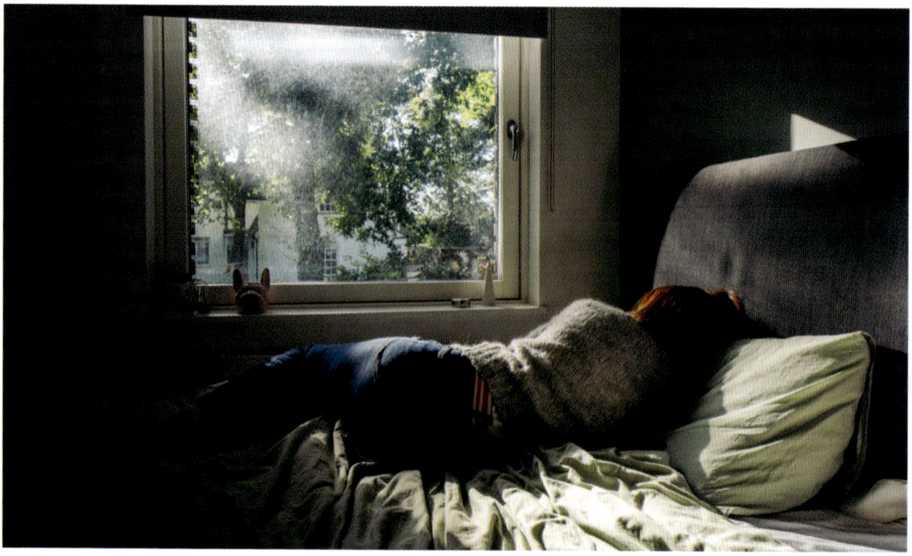

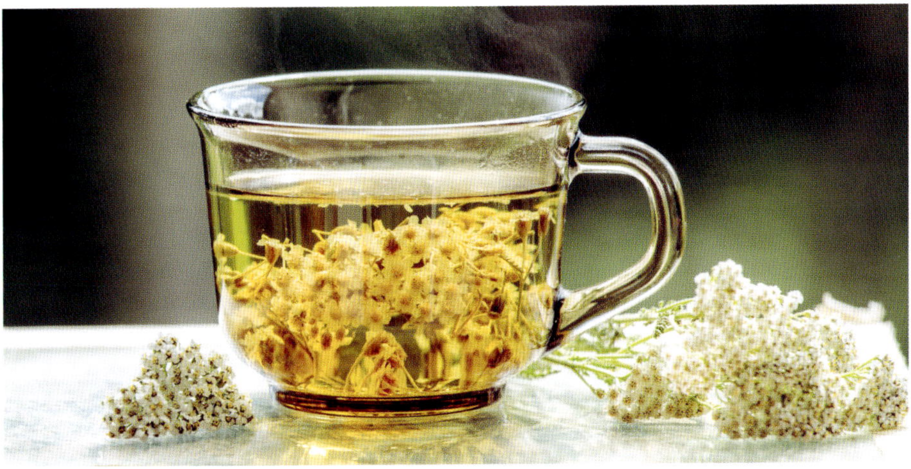

Above Yarrow tea.

improve. The two prescription mixes described here will not suit all women, and should be customised to treat your own unique set of symptoms.

Mix for menopausal symptoms (especially mood swings or feeling low)

Please see pages 100, 101 and 164 for herbal precautions.

INGREDIENTS

- 25ml rose (tincture strength 1:2)
- 25ml vervain (tincture strength 1:2)
- 25ml St John's wort (tincture strength 1:2)
- 25ml wild yam (tincture strength 1:2)

METHOD

1. Mix the ingredients together.
2. Pour the mixture into a clean, dark glass bottle.
3. Label the bottle with the contents and the date.
4. Store at room temperature for up 12 months.

ADULT DOSE: 5ml, diluted with some water, two to three times a day.

Periods, heavy

Heavy periods can be due to fibroids or endometriosis, so it is important to consult your doctor and have a proper check-up. If these diagnoses are excluded, you can use the measures listed below. You may need to take Floradix or another iron supplement if you are experiencing very heavy blood loss.

Treatment options

Please see pages 161 and 163 for herbal precautions.

- Take yarrow tincture or tea for a few months to achieve a sustained effect. **Adults**: 0.7–2ml diluted with some water, one to three times a day, tincture strength 1:2, or 1–2 cups of yarrow tea a day.
- Take a large dose of shepherd's purse tincture or tea on the first two days of your period only. **Adults**: 10ml diluted with some water, three to four times a day, tincture strength 1:2, or 3–4 cups of tea a day.

Teenagers (11–16 years): 11–13 years, take half the adult dose; 14–16 years, take three-quarters of the adult dose.

Periods, painful

Practitioner treatment is recommended for this condition.

Treatment of painful periods often requires a holistic approach that includes a herbal prescription, improvements to one's diet and changes to one's lifestyle. There may be a specific hormonal imbalance that is best corrected by a medical herbalist. The measures listed below can be used to ease the pain during a period – it is important to start taking the herbs on the day when the period pain starts. It is possible that the dosages stated will make you feel sleepy, in which case try reducing the dose next time.

Treatment options

Please see pages 96, 136 and 159 for herbal precautions.

- Take valerian tincture. **Adults:** 5ml diluted with some water, two to three times a day for two days only, tincture strength 1:2.
- Take crampbark tincture, by itself or in combination with valerian. **Adults:** 2ml diluted with some water, three to four times a day for two days only, tincture strength 1:2.
- Drink strong chamomile tea. **Adults:** 2–3 cups a day.
- Take the mix for reducing period pain (see box opposite).

Teenagers (11–16 years): 11–13 years, take half the adult dose; 14–16 years, take three-quarters of the adult dose.

Mix for reducing period pain

Please see pages 96, 136, 159 and 161 for herbal precautions.

INGREDIENTS

- 20ml valerian (tincture strength 1:2)
- 30ml chamomile (tincture strength 1:2)
- 20ml crampbark (tincture strength 1:2)
- 30ml yarrow (tincture strength 1:2)

METHOD

1. Mix the ingredients together.
2. Pour the mixture into a clean, dark glass bottle.
3. Label the bottle with the contents and the date.
4. Store at room temperature for up to 12 months.

ADULT DOSE: 5ml diluted with some water, two to three times a day for three to six months.

Premenstrual syndrome (PMS)

Practitioner treatment is recommended for this condition.

PMS is a combination of troublesome symptoms that some women experience before the onset of their period. These symptoms include nervous tension, irritability, anger, low mood, headache, sore breasts, bloated stomach, poor concentration, and cravings for sugar and chocolate. There are many herbs that can help, but they need to be matched carefully to your own particular symptoms. Evening primrose oil deserves special mention here. It is a great source of two essential fatty acids – linoleic acid and gamma-linolenic acid – which can correct any deficiency or imbalance of essential fatty acids, which can be a contributing factor in PMS.

Treatment options

Please see pages 96, 136 and 163 for herbal precautions.

- Take evening primrose oil as capsules. **Adults:** 3g daily from mid-cycle to the onset of your period.

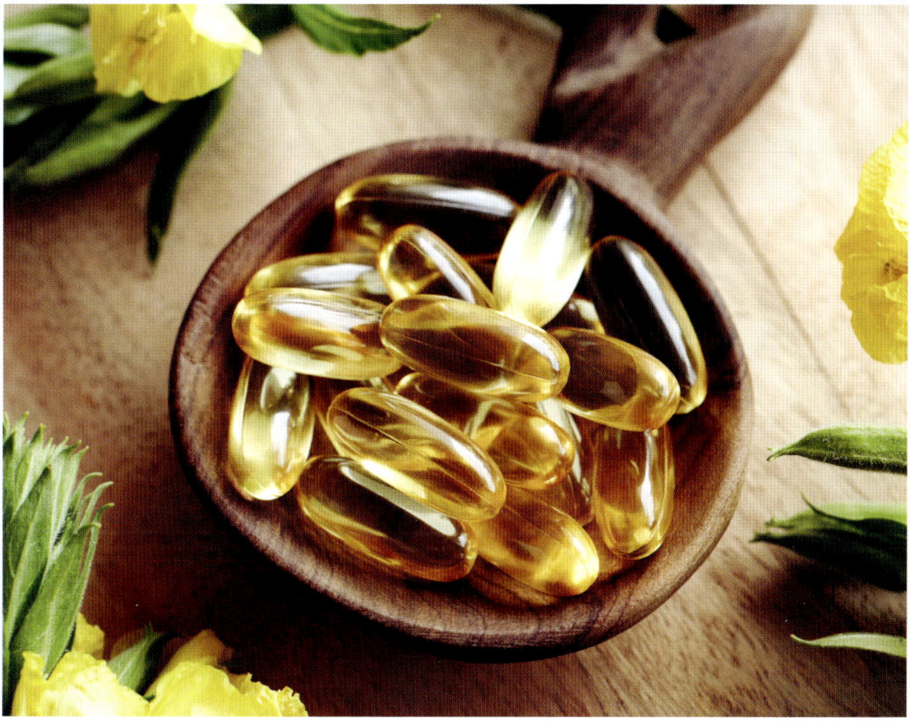

Above Evening primrose oil capsules.

- Take calming herbs such as valerian, chamomile or lemon balm, either singly or in combination (for dosages, see Chapter 10). Take the herbs from mid-cycle to the onset of your period, and throughout the period itself.
- If you suffer from symptoms of water retention (e.g. sore breasts, bloating) take dandelion leaf tea daily, starting 10 days before your period and stopping at the onset of the period. **Adults**: 1–2 cups a day. You can also take dandelion leaf tincture. **Adults:** 2–4ml, one to three times a day, tincture strength 1:1.

Teenagers (14–16 years): take three-quarters of the adult dose. Alternatively, you can adjust the dose according to the body weight of the person being treated (see page 33).

Prolapse

Practitioner treatment is recommended for this condition.

Uterine prolapse that is in its early stages and of recent origin can be improved with a simple herbal measure. There should normally be a rapid improvement within days to a couple of weeks, but to maintain the level of improvement achieved you may have to continue the treatment for many months. Medical supervision of this condition is recommended.

Treatment option

Please see page 163 for herbal precautions.

- Drink shepherd's purse tea on a daily basis until the symptoms improve. **Adults only:** 1–3 cups a day.

Thrush

Practitioner treatment is recommended for recurrent episodes of thrush.

Many women self-medicate for thrush with medicines available over the counter. Herbs can be very helpful, but if the problem frequently recurs, consult a medical herbalist who can prescribe a more individual approach. One helpful measure is to stop washing the genital area altogether for a few days, or only to use warm water without any products – this allows the natural bacterial population to multiply and compete with the thrush yeast.

Treatment options

Please see pages 135, 160 and 194 for herbal precautions.

- Take thyme tincture. **Adults:** 0.7–1.5ml, diluted with some water, one to three times a day, tincture strength 1:2.
- Take fresh garlic. **Adults:** one clove crushed and mixed with honey, once or twice a day.
- Have a 'sitz bath' in a strong marigold infusion (the term 'sitz' is derived from the German verb 'sitzen', meaning 'to sit'). The idea is that you sit in a basin filled with the herbal infusion so that the relevant parts of the body come into contact with the herbs for several minutes. **Adult dose:** one to three times a day, for 5–10 minutes each time.
- Use the cream for thrush (see box below, left).
- Take the mix for persistent thrush if it continues for longer than a week (see box below, right).

Teenagers (11–16 years): 11–13 years, take half the adult dose; 14–16 years, take three-quarters of the adult dose. Alternatively, you can adjust the dose according to the body weight of the person being treated (see page 33).

Cream for thrush

Please see pages 135 and 139 for herbal precautions.

INGREDIENTS

- 20g marigold ointment
- 2 drops tea tree essential oil

METHOD

1. Mix the ingredients well.
2. Transfer the mixture to a clean, dark glass jar, making sure that all air pockets are removed.
3. Store for up to 12 months.

ADULT DOSE: apply to the genital area, both internally and externally, two to three times a day.

Mix for persistent thrush

Please see pages 139, 160 and 164 for herbal precautions.

INGREDIENTS

- 30ml thyme (tincture strength 1:2)
- 30ml marigold (tincture strength 1:2)
- 40ml white deadnettle (tincture strength 1:2)

METHOD

1. Mix the ingredients together.
2. Pour the mixture into a clean, dark glass bottle.
3. Label the bottle with the contents and the date.
4. Store at room temperature for up to 12 months.

ADULT DOSE: 5ml diluted with some water, two to three times a day.

Conditions for which home treatment is not recommended

- Endometriosis: mild cases of this condition respond well to specific anti-inflammatory herbs.
- Severe menopausal symptoms: a combination of hormone-regulating herbs tailored to the individual is required.
- Major problems with periods and/or severe PMS: many other factors can be involved as well as hormonal imbalance, so careful assessment is needed.
- Polycystic ovary syndrome (PCOS): the treatment varies according to which particular symptoms are present in women with this condition.
- Kidney stones: if you have been diagnosed with kidney stones but don't need urgent treatment, it is worth trying specific herbs that are known to help to dissolve small stones; herbs can also be used to treat the colic caused by kidney stones, but such botanicals are available only to qualified practitioners.
- Low sex drive: often different herbs are used in men and women to treat this condition.
- Infertility and/or low sperm count: herbs can improve the ability to conceive, but prescriptions need to be tailored to the individual and their specific symptoms.
- Recurrent cystitis, interstitial cystitis and irritable bladder: these conditions may mimic each other, and the treatment may need to be continued for many months, with multiple adjustments to the prescription.
- Pelvic inflammatory disease: strong antibacterial and anti-inflammatory herbs are required, so this condition is best treated under supervision.

When to seek medical attention

- If you experience severe pain in your lower abdomen that does not go away.
- If you have a high temperature, above 39°C (102°F), and a dragging or stabbing pain in your lower abdomen (in women this is a possible symptom of ectopic pregnancy).
- If you have pain in the loin area, especially if you also have cystitis, general malaise or are running a high temperature (this combination of symptoms indicates a possible kidney infection).
- If you experience colicky pain in the loins (this could be a symptom of kidney stones).
- For women:
  - if there is a major change to your normal menstrual pattern or you experience severe bleeding during your period
  - if you experience an unusual discharge or bleeding, especially after the menopause.
- For men:
  - if you experience an unusual discharge from the urethra
  - if you have any enlargement of the testicles, or a lump.

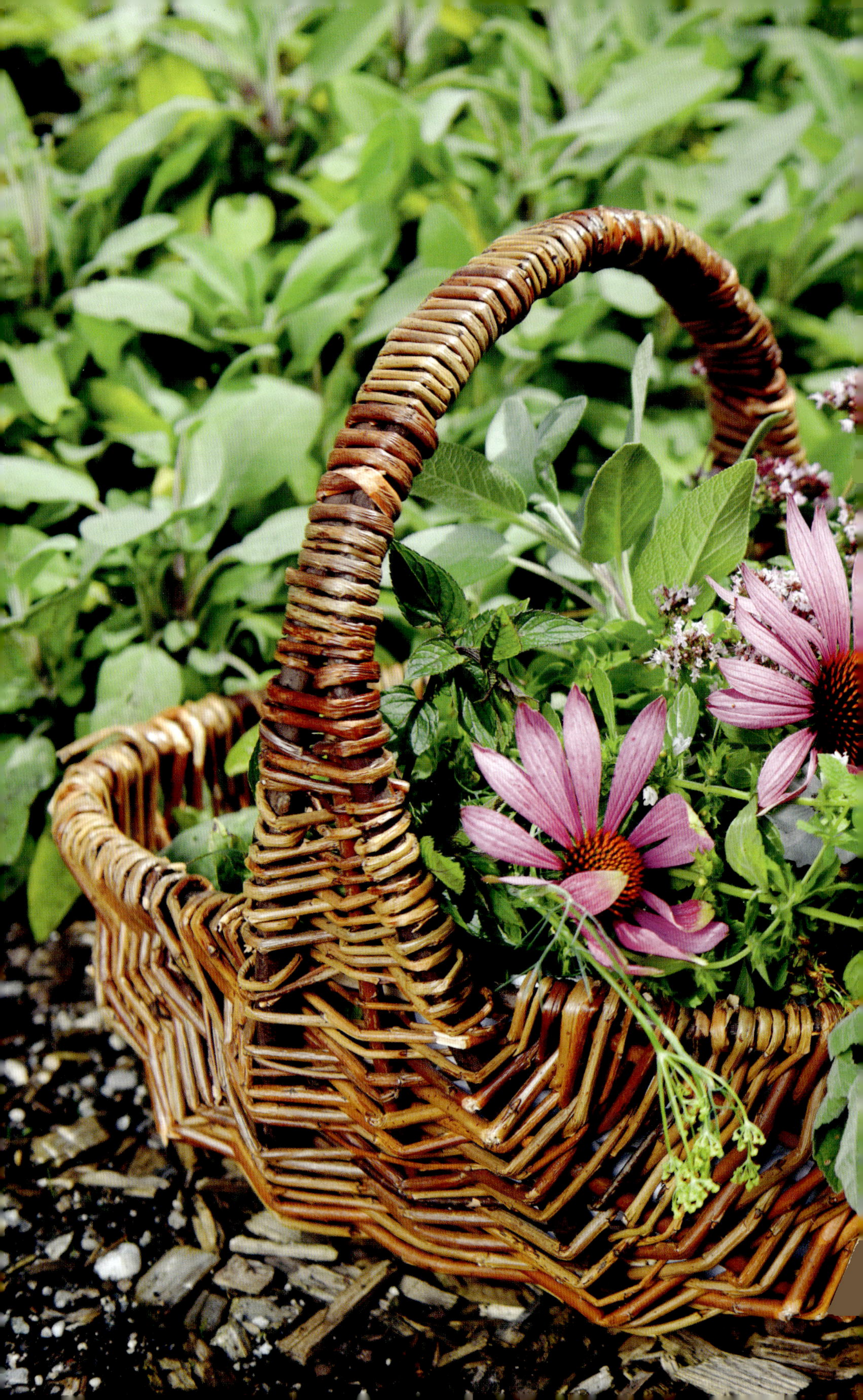

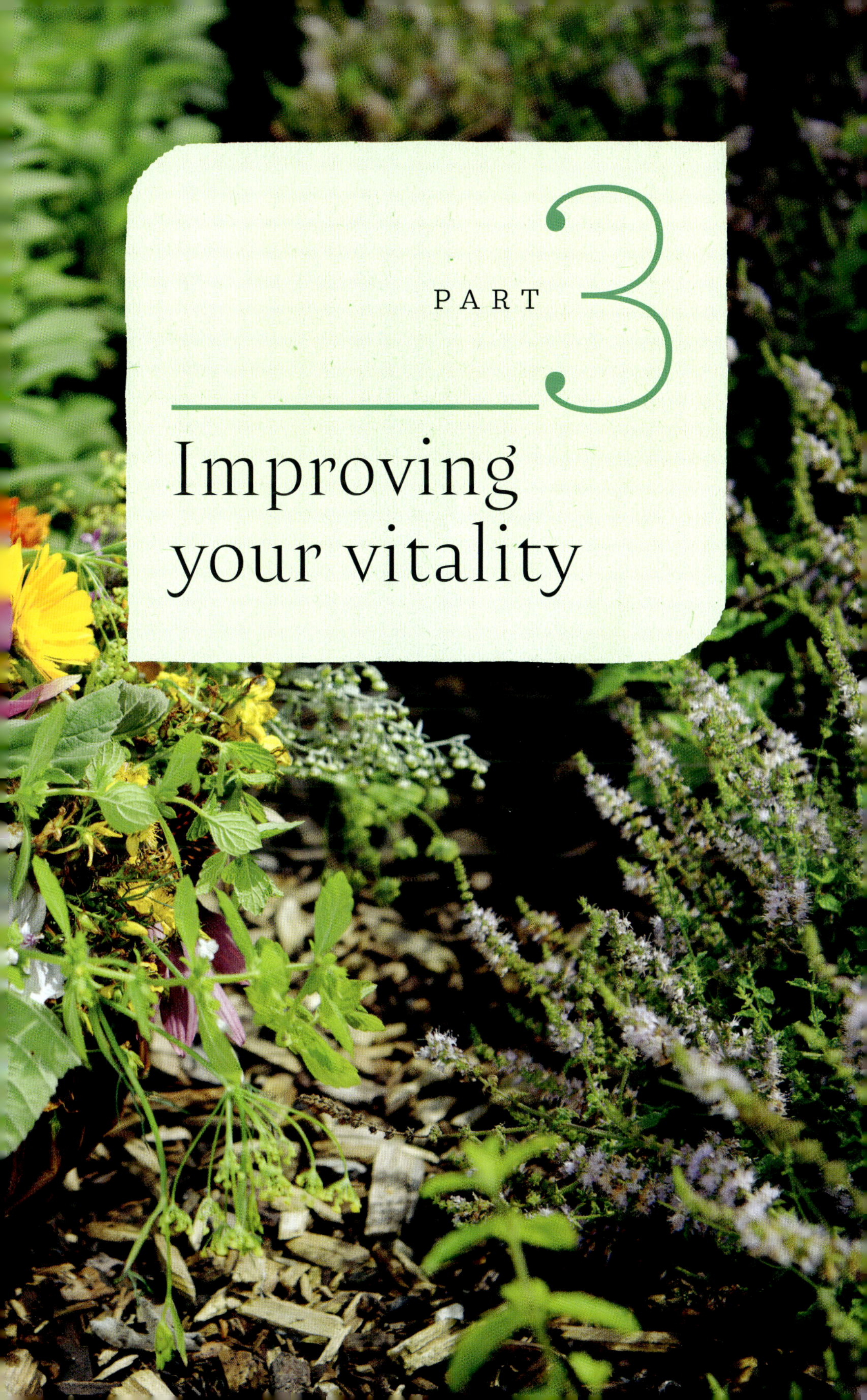

PART 3

Improving your vitality

CHAPTER 14

Maintain good energy levels

Changes in energy levels

Many people complain about lack of energy. Our capacity to maintain high energy levels decreases naturally with age, so it is unrealistic to expect a 60-year-old to have the same energy levels as a 20-year-old. You must make allowances for such a decrease, as well as for the fact that genetics partly explains why some people are more energetic than others. However, a drastic change in your normal energy levels does not occur without a reason.

Causes of low energy

- Overwork: this applies just as much to a mother looking after young children as it does to a busy company executive.
- Prolonged stress: stress that continues for a long time can exhaust the adrenal glands, which when healthy help our bodies to respond to stress.
- Lack of sleep: this should be rather obvious, but many people expect to function well despite having an inadequate amount of sleep. In fact, a good night's sleep is essential to allow the body and the brain to recuperate on a daily basis, and especially after a day that has been physically and mentally demanding.

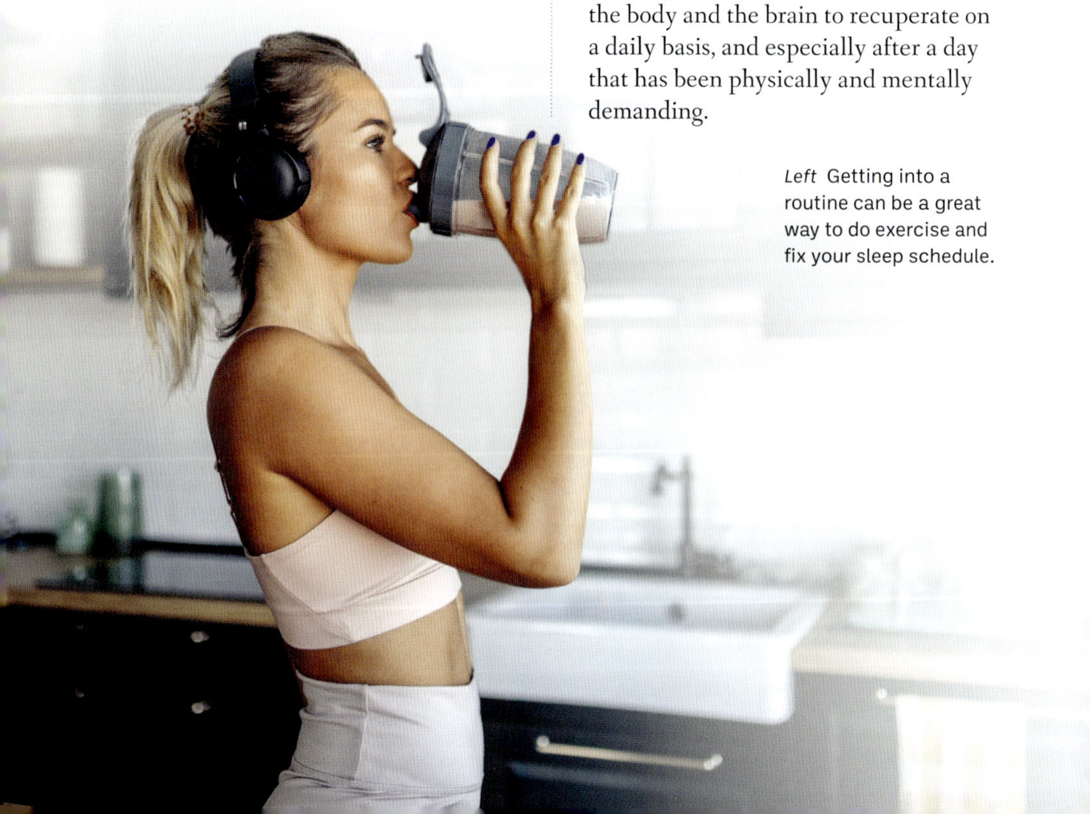

Left Getting into a routine can be a great way to do exercise and fix your sleep schedule.

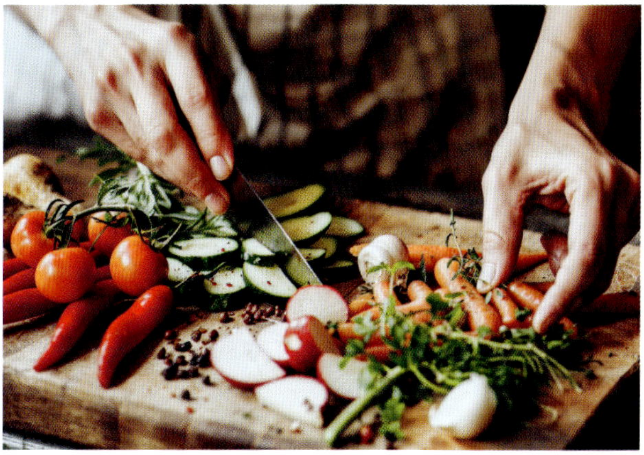

Right Fresh fruit and vegetables are important to stay healthy.

- Poor diet: food is literally the 'fuel' for the body – our energy comes mainly from oxidising (i.e. 'burning') glucose, which comes from the food we eat. However, to produce the molecules that are energy carriers, the cells of the body need many different vitamins and minerals. If some of these are lacking, which is often the case in a modern, highly processed diet, the body cannot maintain optimum energy levels.
- Depression: lack of energy, perhaps better described as lethargy, is one of the symptoms of depression.
- Disease: many diseases result in low energy levels – even a bad cold can leave you feeling exhausted for weeks. It is always worth having your thyroid hormone levels checked, as the thyroid plays an important part in determining your basal metabolic rate, which in turn affects your energy levels.
- Lack of exercise: exercise improves your circulation and hence the supply of oxygen and nutrients to your brain; it also makes your cardiovascular system work more efficiently. For these reasons, if you don't get enough exercise you will feel lethargic.

Identify the cause and treat it

The above list is not exhaustive – there can be many other reasons or combinations of reasons for low energy levels, and you need to identify precisely what the underlying problem is in your case. Some health conditions that cause low energy, such as depression, insomnia or post-viral fatigue, are discussed in other chapters, so please refer to these as necessary and treat the conditions with the suggested herbs. Attending to the possible causes should be your first line of approach, before you reach for energising herbs. For some ailments, such as impaired thyroid function, you will need to consult a health professional and take appropriate medication (herbal, conventional or both).

Herbs and lifestyle adjustments

The herbs discussed in the next section have energy-boosting effects and are suitable for people who need extra 'oomph' for a short period of time, from a few days to a few months.

However, there is no point in taking herbs to improve your energy levels if you do not make essential lifestyle adjustments. The herbs can prop you up for a while, but unless you deal with the root cause(s) of your tiredness the problem will come back.

Herbs are not a substitute for a healthy lifestyle, sensible working hours and a good diet. Energy-boosting herbs will work up to a point, but if you continually push your body to the verge of exhaustion and give it no chance to recover, even the best herbs will cease to be effective.

Choice of herbs

Siberian ginseng *Eleutherococcus senticosus*

Do not exceed the recommended dose of Siberian ginseng.

Uses

Siberian ginseng belongs to the group of herbs known as adaptogens. Such herbs help the body to adapt to stress, whether this is physical or mental. They do so by improving the functioning of all the body's systems, which makes both mind and body more resilient to stress. The result is an improvement in energy, functioning, concentration, memory, endurance and immune responses. This enhancement of physical and mental abilities leads to higher levels of efficiency in performing specific tasks, which should leave you with more time for proper rest. In fact, sleep becomes deeper and more refreshing as well. Overall, not only do you start to feel more energetic, but you can also achieve more in a shorter time.

Siberian ginseng is a true all-round tonic, suitable for adults and children, which can be taken for many months if necessary.

DOSAGE: **Adults:** 0.7–2.6ml diluted with some water, once or twice a day, tincture strength 1:2.

Ashwagandha *Withania somnifera*

Do not exceed the recommended dose.

Practitioner advice is recommended if you are taking thyroid medication.

Uses

Ashwagandha, an ayurvedic herb that can be cultivated in the UK, is also an adaptogen. It has a similar range of actions to Siberian ginseng, but it also has anti-inflammatory and mild sedative properties. This herb would be ideal in cases where low energy is a result of current or recent illness (e.g. depression, cancer, influenza, chronic fatigue syndrome, anaemia). It helps to rebuild muscle strength after a period of physical inactivity. You can use this herb on its own to improve your energy, or in a mix that will also address other aspects of your health. Ashwagandha can be taken for long periods of time.

COMBINATIONS: Siberian ginseng combines well with liquorice, with relaxing or antidepressant herbs (e.g. St John's wort, vervain, valerian, lemon balm) and with herbs that modulate the immune system (e.g. echinacea, astragalus). Refer to the appropriate chapters in this book for information on these herbs.

HOW TO TAKE IT: As a tincture or as tablets.

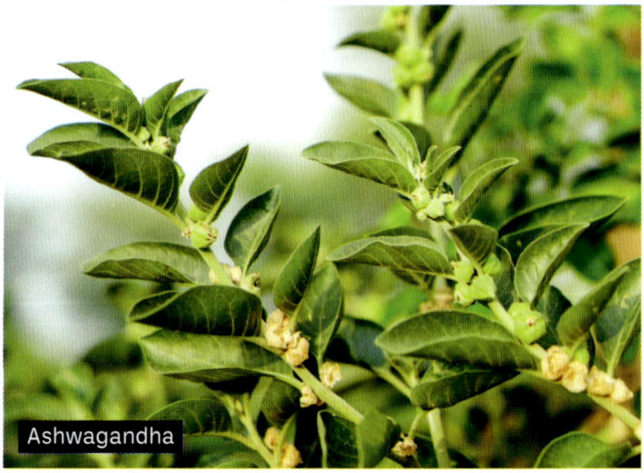

Ashwagandha

HOW TO TAKE IT: As a tincture or as tablets.
DOSAGE: Adults: 1.5–3.5ml diluted with some water, once or twice a day, tincture strength 1:2.

Korean ginseng *Panax ginseng*

Korean ginseng should not be used in people who are suffering from an acute disease, heavy periods, nose bleeds or high blood pressure.
This herb is not suitable for young people.

Korean ginseng is best avoided if you are taking warfarin, antidepressants, or coffee or other stimulants.

Uses

This tonic herb of Chinese origin should be used judiciously, as it can over-stimulate the body. Traditionally it was mainly given to men over 40 years of age in order to boost their energy and vitality. In my experience, Korean ginseng is more suitable for people over 40 years old rather than for individuals in their twenties or thirties, and it should only be taken for short periods of time, from a few days to a month. It is suitable for both men and women.

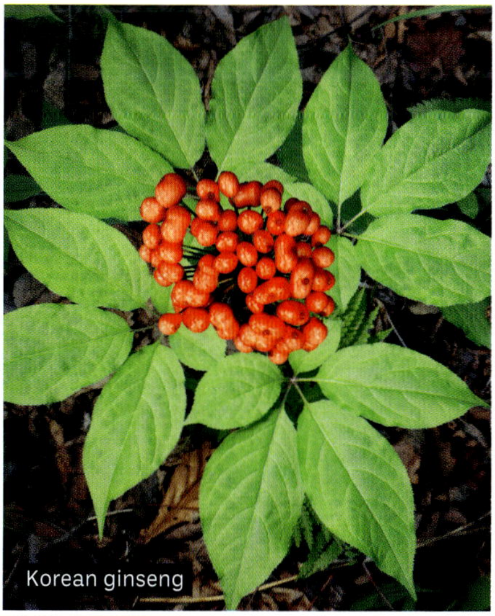
Korean ginseng

I recommend it for loss of energy related to ageing, but you can also use it as a stronger-acting substitute for Siberian ginseng or ashwagandha for short periods of time.

If you feel lightheaded or hyperactive and develop a fast heart rate while using this herb you must reduce the dose.

HOW TO TAKE IT: As tablets or as a tincture.
DOSAGE: Adults: 300–500mg a day in tablet form, or 0.5–2ml diluted with some water, twice a day, tincture strength 1:2.

Liquorice *Glycyrrhiza glabra*

Liquorice should not be taken during pregnancy, or by the elderly.
Do not take liquorice for a prolonged period if you have high blood pressure, low potassium levels, problems with your heart, kidneys or liver, or water retention.

Uses

Liquorice is an adrenal tonic, and is therefore a good choice for treating adrenal exhaustion due to continuous stress. It provides supportive treatment when lack of energy results from unrelenting stress, and is extremely useful if the stress has had a negative effect on the digestive system. I recommend it for people who work particularly long hours and are under constant pressure. It is also suitable for people with low energy levels as a result of disease (e.g. chronic fatigue syndrome).

COMBINATIONS: I recommend combining liquorice with a relaxing herb of your choice, such as lemon balm or passionflower. It also mixes well with Siberian ginseng or ashwagandha.
HOW TO TAKE IT: As a tincture.
DOSAGE: Adults: 0.5–2ml diluted with some water, one to three times a day, tincture strength 1:1.

Strategy for improving energy levels

- Treat the underlying health problem that is causing low energy (get adequate sleep, switch to a healthy balanced diet and take an enjoyable form of exercise).
- Add a herb or herbs that improve energy levels.
- Use restorative herbs that gradually restore health to a malfunctioning system or organ – for instance, green oats for the nervous system, or echinacea for the immune system.

The example mix in the box is one of the possible combinations for improving energy levels. Remember that this formula may not necessarily suit your own personal situation.

Example mix for improving energy levels

Please see pages 99–101 and 180 for herbal precautions.

INGREDIENTS

- 20ml St John's wort (tincture strength 1:2)
- 20ml Siberian ginseng (tincture strength 1:2)
- 20ml ashwagandha (tincture strength 1:2)
- 20ml green oats (tincture strength 1:2)
- 20ml vervain (tincture strength 1:2)

METHOD

1. Mix the ingredients together.
2. Pour the mixture into a clean, dark glass bottle.
3. Label the bottle with the contents and the date.
4. Store at room temperature for up to 12 months.

ADULT DOSE: 5ml, diluted with some water, two to three times a day.

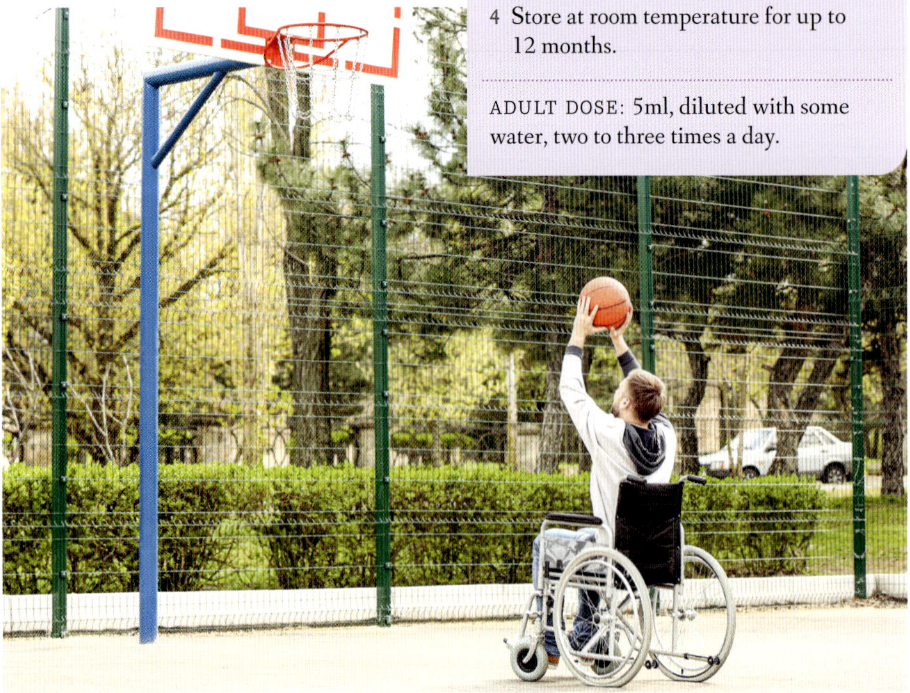

Below Remember exercise can take many forms – find one that you enjoy!

CHAPTER 15

Increase your mental and physical stamina

There is an overlap between the use of herbs to improve general energy levels and their use to improve levels of stamina and endurance, so Chapter 14 may also offer herbal strategies applicable to your circumstances.

When to use herbs

In this chapter I focus on a particular aspect of human functioning – that of mental and physical stamina. There are plenty of situations in modern life that require extra high levels of performance – for example, when we have exams, deadlines at work, sick children who won't sleep or an upcoming sports event. They all tap into our natural reserves of energy, but these reserves can be gently enhanced with the help of specific herbs. As a result, you will be able to study more intensively and for a longer period of time, concentrate on your task better or perform better in your chosen sport.

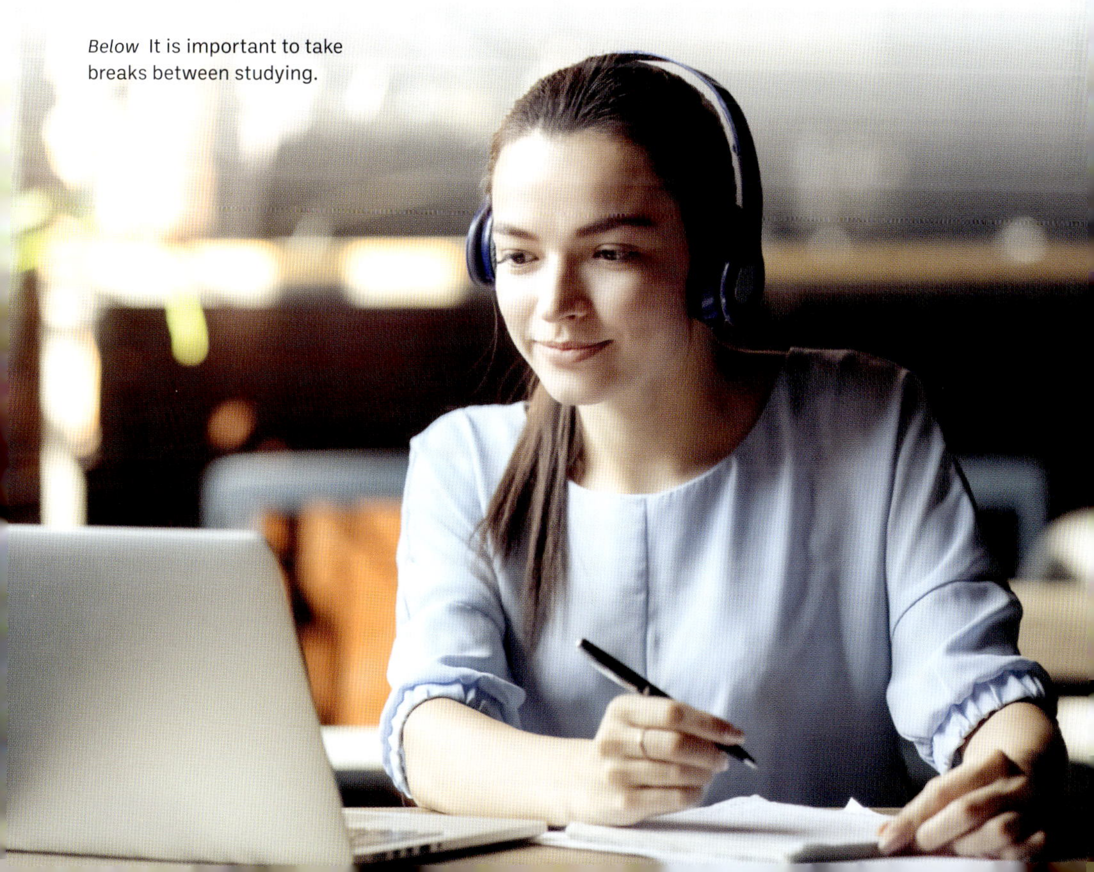

Below It is important to take breaks between studying.

Matching herbs to your situation

The underlying principle of using herbs for these purposes is to improve the general functioning of the body with the help of tonic herbs, and to improve the functioning of specific body systems involved in a particular activity that requires extra effort. For instance, if you have a very difficult exam coming up and you need to study exceptionally hard, you will want to combine energy boosters with herbs that improve circulation to the brain and improve the quality of sleep. To take another example, if you are going to trek for many days at high altitude, you will want a general tonic, warming herbs that improve the general circulation and herbs that aid the recovery of joints and muscles overnight.

Short-term versus long-term use

It is important to understand the difference between use of herbs to provide a short, intense boost and the prolonged, sustained use of herbs. Siberian ginseng and ashwagandha can be used long term for many months, whereas Korean ginseng should be a short-term treatment, taken for between a few days and a month. For short-term treatments use the maximum doses of these herbs, and for long-term treatments opt for the medium to low end of the recommended dose range. An intense boost should only be used in exceptional circumstances.

Choice of herbs

- Siberian ginseng, ashwagandha and Korean ginseng (see pages 180–181): these improve mental and physical performance and stamina.
- Liquorice (see page 181): this is suitable if you have been under a lot of stress for some time.
- Ginkgo and hawthorn (see pages 44 and 43): these improve the circulation.
- Arnica, comfrey and rosemary (see pages 81–83): these aid recovery from physical strain.

Example of a mix for improving physical stamina

INGREDIENTS

- 30ml Korean ginseng (tincture strength 1:2) (for precautions see page 181)
- 10ml ginger (tincture strength 1:2) (for precautions see page 45)
- 40ml ashwaganda (tincture strength 1:2) (for precautions see page 180)
- 20ml ginkgo (tincture strength 2:1) (for precautions see page 44)

METHOD

1. Mix the ingredients together.
2. Pour the mixture into a clean, dark glass bottle.
3. Label the bottle with the contents and the date.
4. Store at room temperature for up to 12 months.

ADULTS ONLY: 5ml diluted with some water, twice a day.

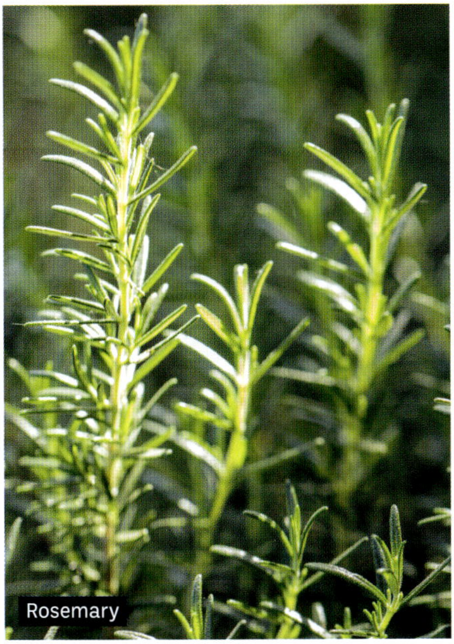

Rosemary

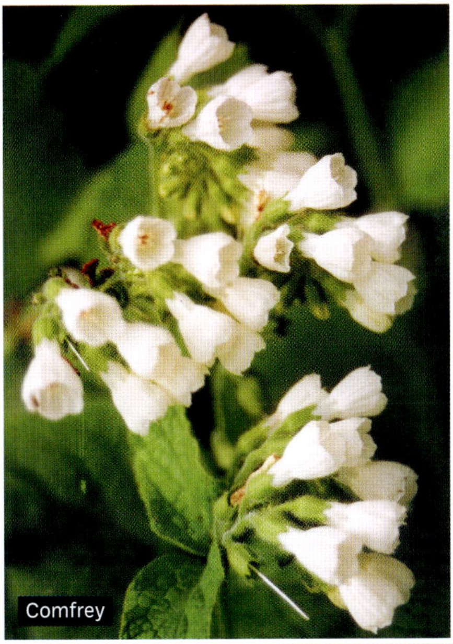

Comfrey

Example of a mix for improving mental performance

Please see pages 180–181 and 193 for herbal precautions.

INGREDIENTS

- 20ml ginkgo (tincture strength 2:1)
- 30ml Siberian ginseng (tincture strength 1:2)
- 30ml ashwagandha (tincture strength 1:2)
- 20ml liquorice (tincture strength 1:1)

METHOD

1. Mix the ingredients together.
2. Pour the mixture into a clean, dark glass bottle.
3. Label the bottle with the contents and the date.
4. Store at room temperature for up to 12 months.

ADULTS ONLY: 5ml diluted with some water, two to three times a day.

Example of a cream to aid muscle and joint recovery after strenuous exercise

Please see pages 81, 83, 87, 97, 136 and 137 for herbal precautions.

INGREDIENTS

- 20g comfrey cream
- 10g arnica cream
- 10ml willow bark tincture
- 10 drops rosemary essential oil
- 10 drops wintergreen essential oil
- 5 drops lavender essential oil

METHOD

1. Mix the ingredients well.
2. Transfer the mixture to a clean, dark glass jar, making sure that all air pockets are removed.
3. Store for up to 12 months.

ADULTS AND CHILDREN OVER FIVE YEARS OLD: apply to the aching muscles or joints once or twice a day or straight after exercise.

CHAPTER 16

Revive your libido

Causes of low libido

Low sex drive can result from many factors – for example, age, tiredness, illness or relationship problems. It is important to look at the possible reasons and address these before deciding to use aphrodisiac herbs. It is natural to lose some sex drive as we age, and as long as both partners are content with this decline it is not usually a problem.

Many illnesses and associated conventional treatments can reduce the libido, so make sure you are well informed about your symptoms and the side effects of your medication. Herbs are unlikely to override the effects of such medication, so you may want to ask your doctor about alternatives (or consider herbal treatment for your original ailment). The condition that most commonly has a negative effect on sex drive is depression. The second most common causes are overwork and lack of sleep!

What herbs can do

Herbs can help by putting you in a generally much more positive frame of mind, giving you more energy, relaxing you, improving the blood supply to your vital organs and gently stimulating your interest in sex.

Length of treatment

The treatment should be relatively short term – just a month or two. If you don't see any difference in your libido after that time, consider consulting a medical herbalist who may be able to identify the underlying causes, especially if these are related to hormonal imbalances.

Below Adequate sleep is linked to higher libido.

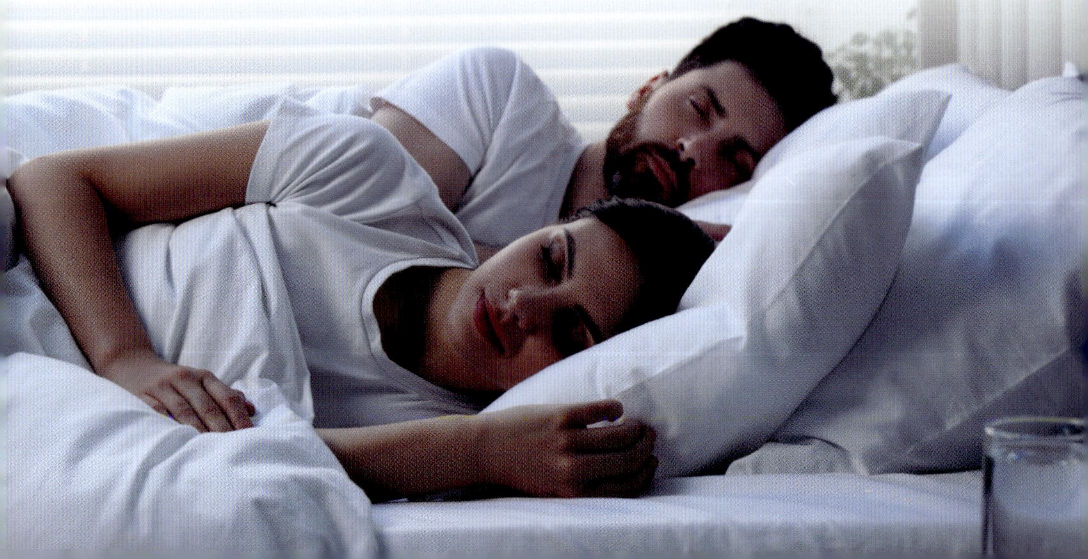

Choice of herbs

- Siberian ginseng and ashwagandha (see page 180): these are general energy improvers.
- Korean ginseng (see page 181): this improves libido in older people.
- Damiana (see page 162): this gently improves mood and libido in younger people.
- Vervain and St John's wort (see pages 101 and 100): these are antidepressants and mood improvers.
- Hawthorn, ginkgo and ginger (see pages 43, 44 and 45): these improve the circulation.
- Valerian, lemon balm and passionflower (see pages 47, 63 and 100): these are sleep-improving herbs.
- Essential oils with stimulating properties include nutmeg, labdanum, sandalwood, rose (page 100), cinnamon leaf, myrrh and cedar (for precautions see page 29).

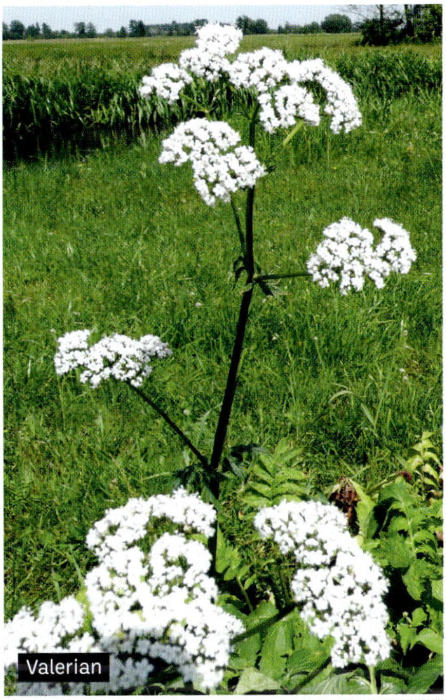

Valerian

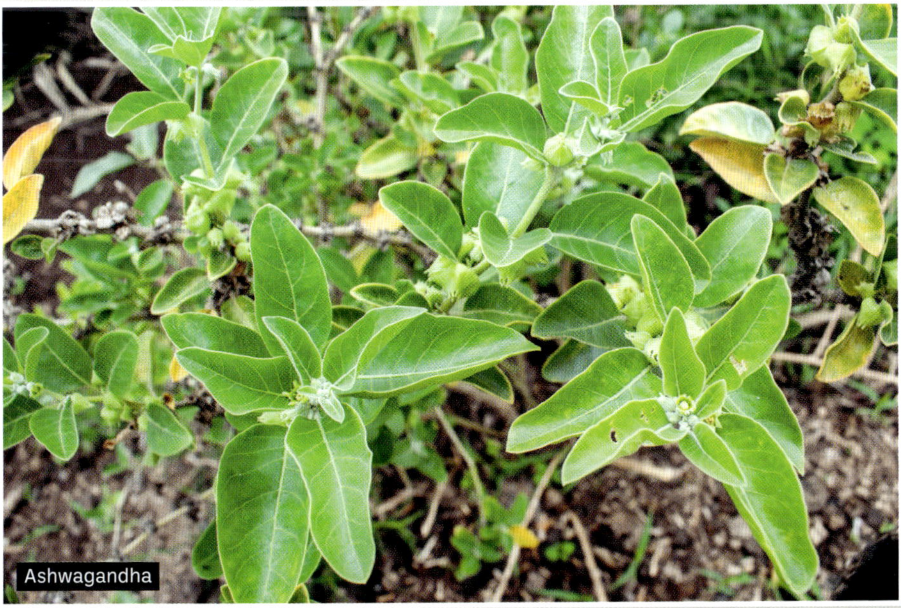

Ashwagandha

Herbal strategy to improve libido

- Combine one of the energy improvers with one of the libido improvers as a basic treatment.
- Add a relaxant or a mood improver if anxiety or low mood is a problem.
- Add a circulation-improving herb if you don't get much exercise or have problems with your blood circulation.
- Improve your sleep with a dedicated sleep mix.
- Invest in one or two good-quality essential oils that can put you and your partner in the right mood – use them in a relaxing bath or add them to a massage oil.

The mix in the box below is an example of one of the possible combinations.

Below Sandalwood essential oil.

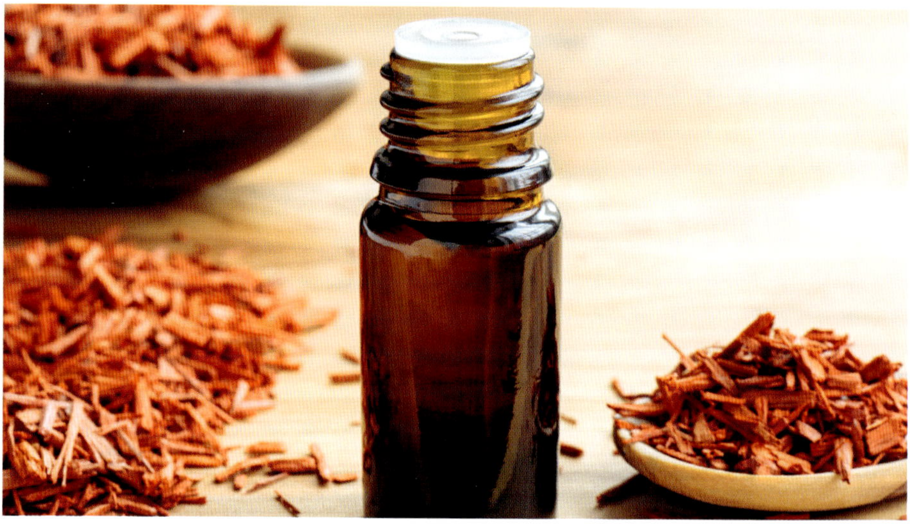

Example of a mix for improving libido

INGREDIENTS
- 20ml damiana (tincture strength 1:2) (for precautions see page 162)
- 20ml Korean ginseng (tincture strength 1:2) (for precautions see page 181)
- 20ml ashwaganda (tincture strength 1:2) (for precautions see page 180)
- 20ml hawthorn (tincture strength 1:2) (for precautions see page 43)
- 20ml lemon balm (tincture strength 1:2)

METHOD
1 Mix the ingredients together.
2 Pour the mixture into a clean, dark glass bottle.
3 Label the bottle with the contents and the date.
4 Store at room temperature for up to 12 months.

ADULTS ONLY: 5ml diluted with some water, two to three times a day.

CHAPTER 17

Feel motivated and happy

Causes of unhappiness

You don't need to be depressed in order to take steps to improve your mood and motivation – many herbs are gentle mood enhancers suitable for people whose enthusiasm for life is somewhat less than it used to be. I firmly believe that the natural state of mind is contentment. Of course there are objective reasons why we become unhappy, such as illness, job-related stress, relationship problems or financial worries, but there are also many other reasons, which are often not identified by the unhappy individual, such as lack of exercise, unhealthy diet or lifestyle, lack of contact with nature, lack of hobbies or interests, and fixed attitudes about what constitutes happiness.

Sometimes, however, we become dissatisfied with life for no apparent reason. Our zest for life diminishes and we don't feel like doing anything. If you feel that you are depressed and/or anxious, refer to Chapter 10 for specific advice on these conditions (see pages 103 and 102, respectively).

Long-term versus short-term treatment

If you are looking for long-term strategies write down the problems that you're facing or talk to a friend about them and, where possible, brainstorm ways to improve your situation. In addition, you could make small changes to your daily routine to improve your lifestyle, such as taking a 10-minute walk every day or learning how to cook. You can also take the herbs described overleaf while trying to sort things out. You may need to use these herbs for a longer period of time, from two to six months.

If you only require short-term treatment, from a few days to a couple of weeks, some of the herbs described below should restore your former enthusiasm for life. The herbs should put you in a positive frame of mind, and when that has been achieved it should be a self-perpetuating state. As a result, once you feel happier you will no longer need the herbs.

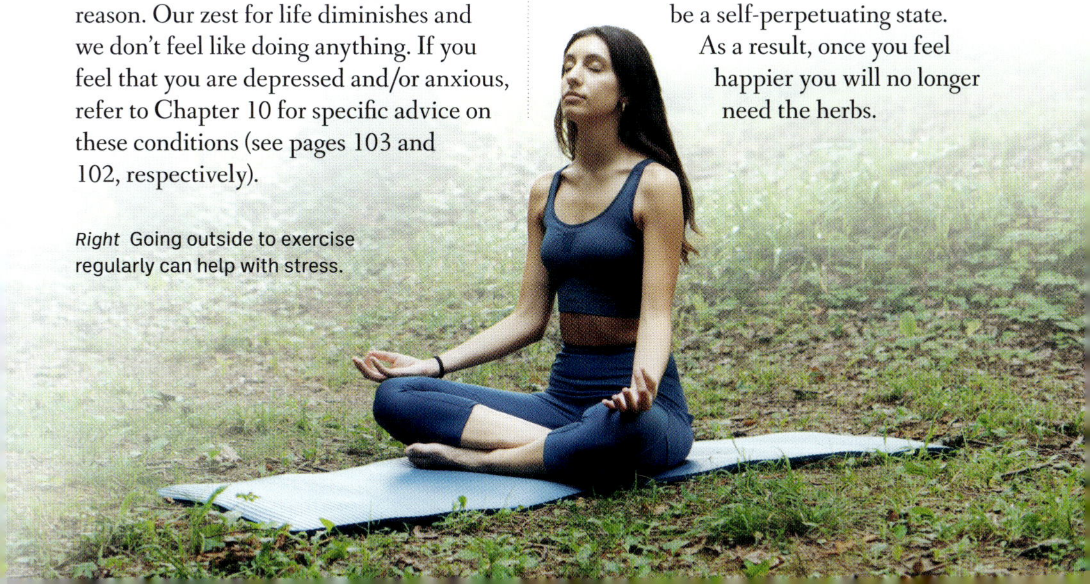

Right Going outside to exercise regularly can help with stress.

Choice of herbs

- Ashwagandha (see page 180): this herb puts you in a positive frame of mind and improves motivation.
- Rose, damiana and vervain (see pages 100, 162 and 101): these are gentle mood improvers.
- Green oats (see page 99): this is a restorative herb for the nervous system – it has energising effects and produces an improved sense of well-being.
- Ginkgo, ginger and hawthorn (see pages 44, 45 and 43): these improve the circulation.

The mix in the box shows an example of the possible combinations.

Example mix for improving the sense of well-being

INGREDIENTS

- 20ml rosemary (tincture strength 1:2) (for precautions see page 97)
- 20ml ashwaganda (tincture strength 1:2)
- 20ml green oats (tincture strength 1:2)
- 20ml vervain (tincture strength 1:2)
- 20ml damiana (tincture strength 1:2) (for precautions see page 162)

METHOD

1 Mix the ingredients together.
2 Pour the mixture into a clean, dark glass bottle.
3 Label the bottle with the contents and the date.
4 Store at room temperature for up to 12 months.

ADULTS ONLY: 5ml diluted with some water, two to three times a day.
Note: this mix is suitable for both short- and long-term use.

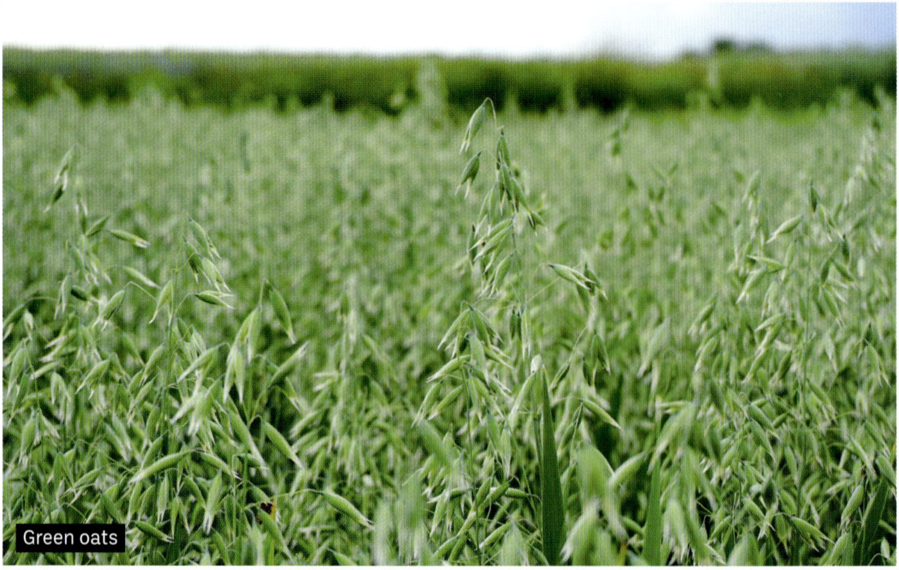

Green oats

CHAPTER 18

Healthy ageing

Ageing is a natural part of life and cannot be prevented. However, we all want to enjoy quality of life, including good health, for as long as possible. Herbs can significantly improve the chances of slowing down or preventing many of the degenerative conditions that are so common in older people, such as heart disease, stroke, cancer, dementia, and respiratory or arthritic inflammatory diseases.

Of course, taking care of your body and mind by having a healthy diet, taking regular exercise, keeping your weight down, avoiding stress and staying mentally active is vital. However, adding a few super-botanicals (including superfoods) to your health routine will substantially reduce the chances of developing a serious disease.

The choice of herbs offered here is for you to select from and introduce on a daily basis if possible. Each of these herbs has its own particular merits, and some of them may be more desirable than others for your particular situation – for instance, if there is a history of heart disease in your family you may consider taking garlic daily from the age of 30 onwards. Garlic supplements should be taken in an 'on-and-off' manner, with a month of supplementation being followed by a month off. Of course, garlic that has been cooked in your food can be eaten all the time.

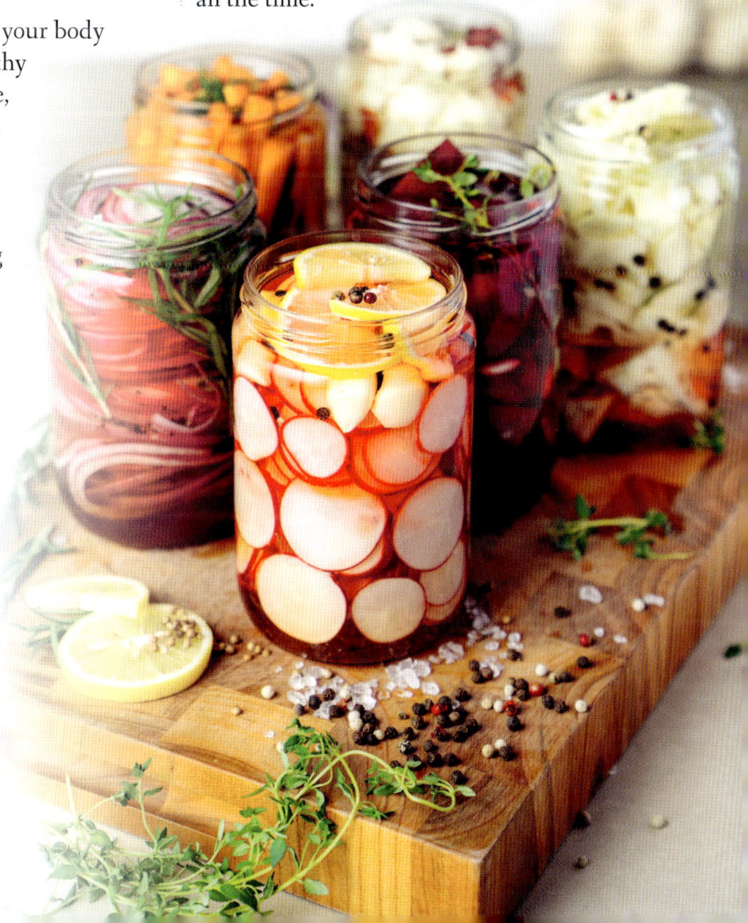

Right Fermented foods are great for healthy ageing.

Other foods and plants

Other foods that can help to slow down the ageing process include red grape juice, red wine, grape seed extract, turmeric, olive oil, hemp seed oil, nuts and seeds, dark-skinned berries, fermented foods, dark chocolate and coffee. The benefits of consuming these foods are linked to specific phytochemicals that are present in these plants. Foods that have dark pigments contain polyphenols – a diverse group of plant compounds that are known for their anti-oxidant action in the body. This category includes red wine (no more than one small glass a day), various berries, dark chocolate and coffee (1 cup a day, preferably in the morning). Foods that are rich in beneficial fats help to maintain a good balance of essential fatty acids in your body and hence have an anti-inflammatory effect. This category includes olive oil, hemp seed oil, and nuts and seeds. The next category, of which turmeric is a good example, is known specifically for its anti-inflammatory effects, and research has shown that chronic, low-grade inflammation is a major contributing factor in the development of a whole range of conditions, from osteoarthritis to Alzheimer's disease. Finally, fermented foods are beneficial for your microbiome, and the healthier your microbiome, the more effective your immune system will be, and hence your general health.[16]

Below Dark chocolate and coffee both have anti-ageing properties.

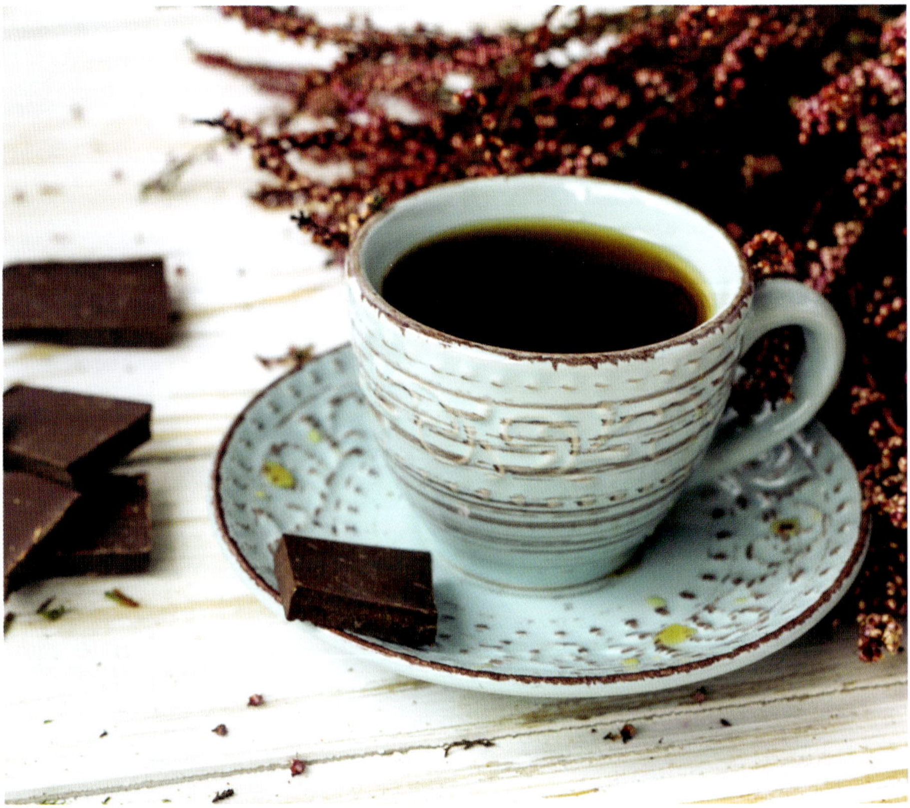

Choice of herbs and foods

Blueberries *Vaccinium corymbosum* or bilberries *Vaccinium myrtillus*

Benefits for healthy ageing

Due to their antioxidants, blueberries and bilberries help to prevent degenerative changes in the brain and circulatory system. Regular consumption of blueberries or bilberries can bring about an improvement in both night and day vision and possibly avert the degeneration of the retina. The constituents of blueberries/bilberries improve the microcirculation (the circulation in the smallest blood vessels), which in turn improves nourishment and repair of your brain and other vital organs, joints, bones and skin.

HOW TO TAKE THEM: As food in the form of either fresh or defrosted berries, or as a dried powder. You can also take a blueberry supplement in the form of tablets or capsules.

DOSAGE: **Adults**: 50–100g of berries a day, or the equivalent amount of dried powder. The supplement should be taken according to the manufacturer's instructions.

Ginkgo *Ginkgo biloba*

Caution is needed in people who are taking anticoagulant or antiplatelet medication, including aspirin. Discontinue ginkgo a week before surgery.

Benefits for healthy ageing

Ginkgo protects the nerve cells from oxidative damage, improves the supply of oxygen to the brain, has anti-inflammatory and anti-allergic properties, enhances concentration and memory in healthy older people, and may play a role in preventing the onset of dementia.

HOW TO TAKE IT: As a tincture.
DOSAGE: **Adults**: 1–2ml diluted with some water, one to three times a day, tincture strength 2:1.

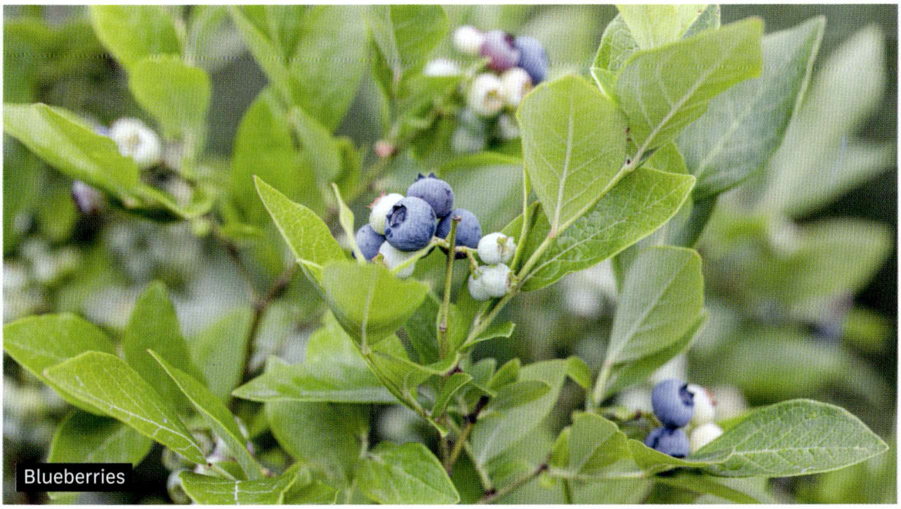

Blueberries

Korean ginseng *Panax ginseng*

Korean ginseng should not be used in people who are suffering from an acute disease, heavy periods, nose bleeds or high blood pressure.

This herb is not suitable for young people.

Korean ginseng is best avoided if you are taking warfarin, antidepressants, or coffee or other stimulants.

Benefits for healthy ageing

Korean ginseng has a protective effect against cancer and it improves survival rates once cancer is in remission. It also increases general vitality levels in older people.

HOW TO TAKE IT: As a tincture or as tablets.

DOSAGE: **Adults:** 300–500mg a day in tablet form, or 0.5–2.5ml diluted with some water, once or twice a day, tincture strength 1:2. I suggest taking it for a month on/month off basis.

Garlic *Allium sativum*

Do not take large doses for prolonged periods of time, or when pregnant or breastfeeding. Discontinue garlic 10 days before undergoing surgery. Medicinal use of garlic is not recommended for children under six years of age.

Caution is needed in people who are taking anticoagulant or antiplatelet medication.

Benefits for healthy ageing

Garlic reduces the risk of cardiovascular disease as it has a positive effect on many relevant factors – for example, it reduces the formation of fatty plaques in the arteries, preserves arterial wall elasticity, lowers blood pressure and cholesterol levels, and reduces the tendency for blood clot formation. It also decreases the frequency of viral infections.

HOW TO TAKE IT: As a food ingredient – fresh crushed garlic can be eaten in salads, or mixed with houmous or green smoothies. Alternatively, it can be taken as garlic juice (see page 114) or as a tablet.

DOSAGE: **Adults:** about 5g of fresh garlic a day, or one enteric-coated tablet containing 5.7mg of alliin a day.

Echinacea (purple coneflower) *Echinacea purpurea* and *Echinacea angustifolia*

Caution is needed in people who are allergic to plants belonging to the daisy family (the Asteraceae, formerly known as the Compositae). Not suitable for transplant patients and children under 12.

Benefits for healthy ageing

Echinacea reduces the number of viral and bacterial infections, which play a role in many degenerative illnesses.

HOW TO TAKE IT: As a tincture.

DOSAGE: **Adults:** 1.2–3ml diluted with some water, two to three times a day, tincture strength 1:2.

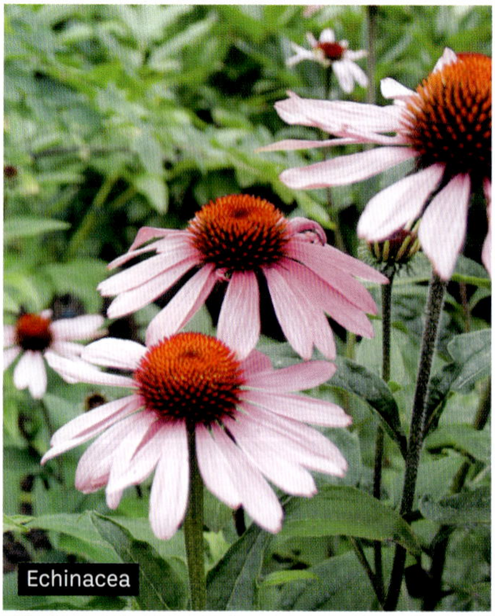

Echinacea

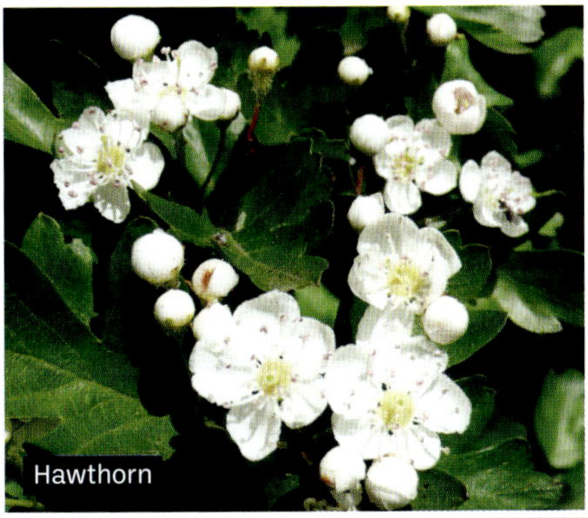

Hawthorn

Hawthorn *Crataegus monogyna* (common hawthorn) or *Crataegus laevigata* (Midland hawthorn)

Hawthorn is not recommended for people with low blood pressure. It is not always compatible with heart medication.

Benefits for healthy ageing

Hawthorn improves the functioning of the circulatory system, especially the circulation to the heart and brain, and it lowers blood pressure.

HOW TO TAKE IT: As a tincture.
DOSAGE: **Adults**: 1–2ml diluted with some water, one to three times a day, tincture strength 1:2.

Green tea *Camellia sinensis*

Tannins in green tea can interfere with the absorption of some medication.

Benefits for healthy ageing

Regular consumption of green tea is associated with a lower incidence of various cancers, the enhanced survival of cancer patients, a decreased risk of cardiovascular disease and prevention of memory decline in elderly people. If you are taking any prescribed medication it is best to either make a weak brew of tea or drink it 1–2 hours before or after your medication.

HOW TO TAKE IT: As a tea or as capsules.
DOSAGE: **Adults**: 3–5 cups a day – do not add milk, but a slice of lemon is fine. Alternatively, take it as capsules of green tea extract according to the manufacturer's instructions.

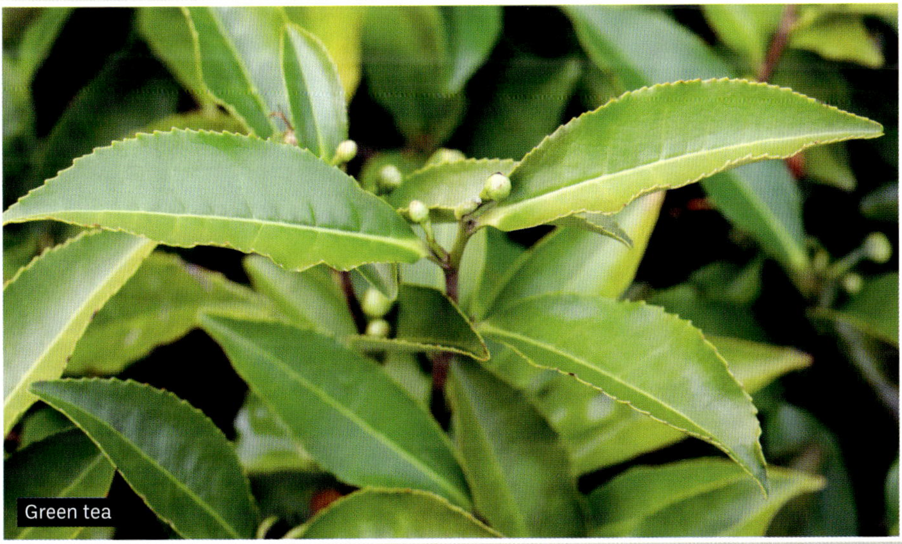

Green tea

CHAPTER 19

Improve the function of your immune system

A strong immune system is the basis of good health. When it is working well your immune system prevents you from getting minor infections and helps you to recover from illnesses quickly and completely. A well-functioning immune system surveys your body for potentially cancerous cells and destroys them before they have a chance to develop into a tumour. It controls the healing and repair of any damage to the huge variety of different tissues in your body. The immune system is immensely complicated and consists of highly specialised cells within your blood, digestive system and other tissues. It relies on a whole array of locally secreted hormones to coordinate its functions, and as a result it can be affected by your hormonal system, your brain and your emotions. Although it is an amazing defence mechanism, it can become impaired for a number of reasons – for example, it may be overwhelmed by an unknown pathogen, or it can start attacking specific tissues in your own body (as happens in autoimmune diseases) or it can get stuck in a constant inflammatory

Below Wild swimming is a great way to connect with nature.

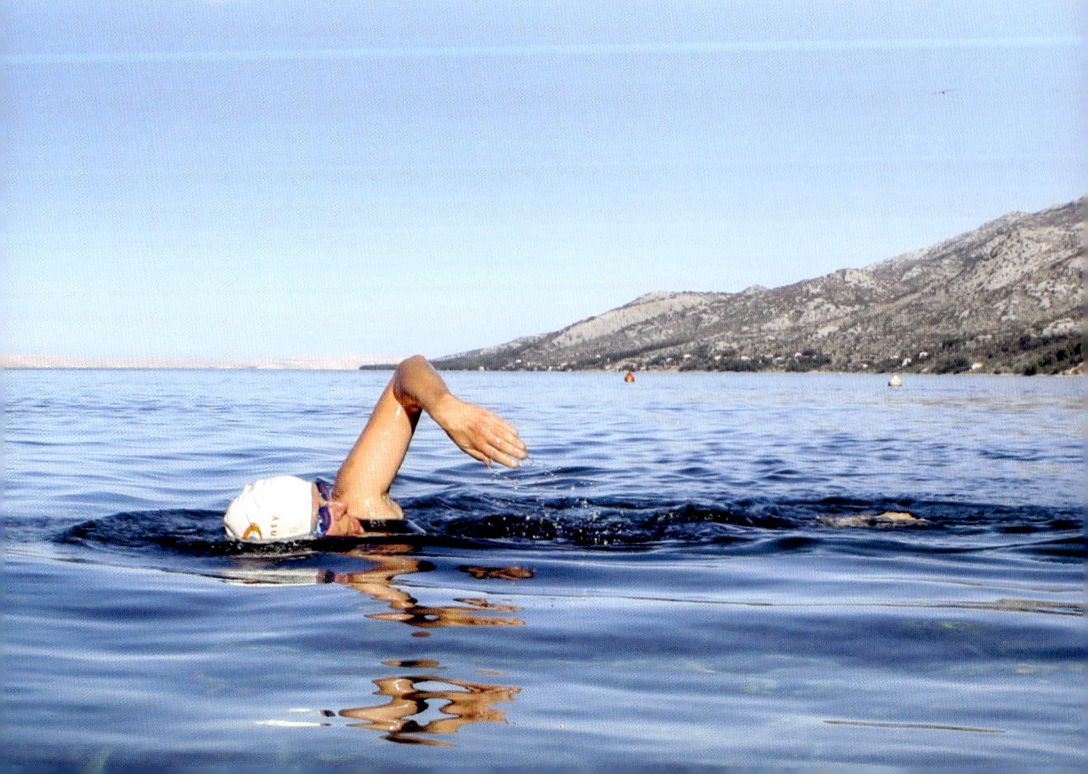

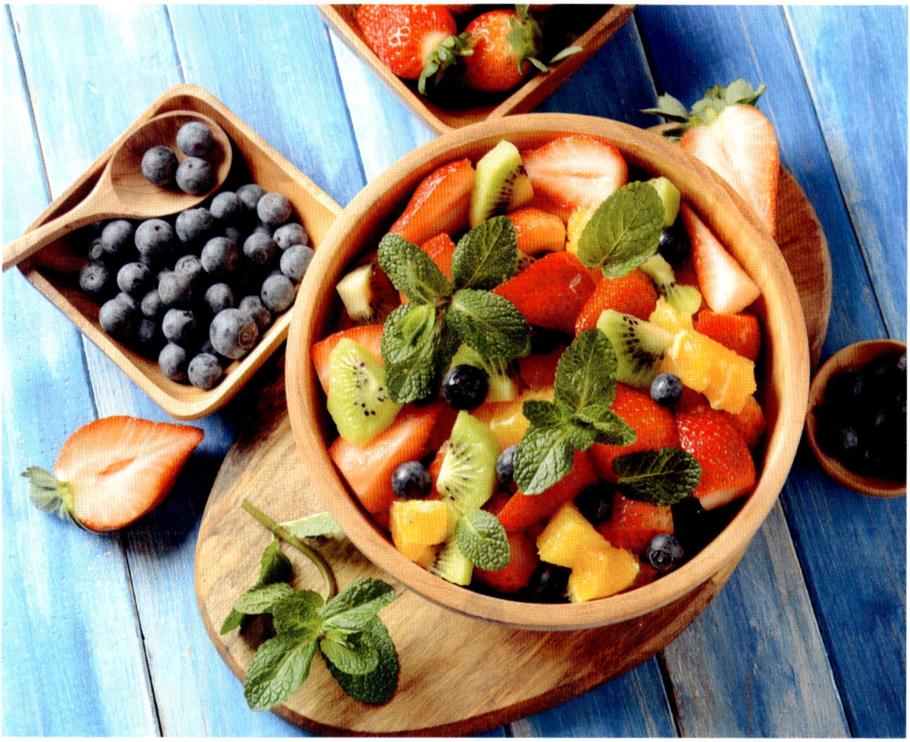

Above Try to eat a range of different fruits, vegetables and herbs to support your body.

state (as happens in chronic fatigue syndrome and post-viral fatigue).

There are a number of ways in which you can optimise the functioning of your immune system.

- Pay attention to your diet. Good nutrition is vital for the immune system to function properly. Make sure that you are getting enough vitamin D, vitamin C and zinc, eat a wide variety of fruit and vegetables, and make sure that you include good sources of healthy fats and protein. If possible, eat organically produced food, as your body (and immune system) won't then have to detoxify any pesticide residues, and you will be getting more nutrients in a natural way.
- Ensure that you get plenty of good-quality, restful sleep, as an inadequate amount of sleep weakens the immune system.
- Exercise regularly, preferably outdoors in a natural environment in fresh, unpolluted air, as nature boosts our immune system. Choose an exercise that you will enjoy, whether it is walking, running, cycling or even wild swimming. Note that excessive amounts of prolonged strenuous exercise can temporarily weaken some functions of the immune system.
- You can use botanicals to support, enhance and modify the immune system. There are many plants that can affect specific cells or communication pathways of the immune system, and in this book I recommend those that I use most often and have found to be most effective.

Choice of herbs

Echinacea (purple coneflower) *Echinacea purpurea* and *Echinacea angustifolia*

Caution is needed in people who are allergic to plants belonging to the daisy family (the Asteraceae, formerly known as the Compositae). Not suitable for transplant patients and children under 12.

Echinacea is not suitable for people who are taking immunosuppressive medication, such as transplant patients.

Currently, in the UK, the use of echinacea is not recommended for children under 12 years of age, due to the risk of an allergic reaction.

Uses

Echinacea is commonly known by its scientific name, and two distinct species are used medicinally – *Echinacea purpurea* (purple coneflower) and *Echinacea angustifolia* (narrow-leaved purple coneflower). The roots and aerial parts work best, based on current scientific research and a long history of traditional use of these preparations by Native Americans. Echinacea improves the functioning of the immune system and acts mainly on innate immunity, which is the first line of defence that your immune system mobilises against infections. This herb is used both to prevent and to treat a range of viral and bacterial infections, and to help to improve weakening or imbalance of the immune system. It is useful for many chronic conditions that involve inflammation and/or infections, such as wounds that don't heal, acne, abscesses and various allergies. Echinacea is also one of the most useful botanicals for treating post-viral syndrome and chronic fatigue syndrome.

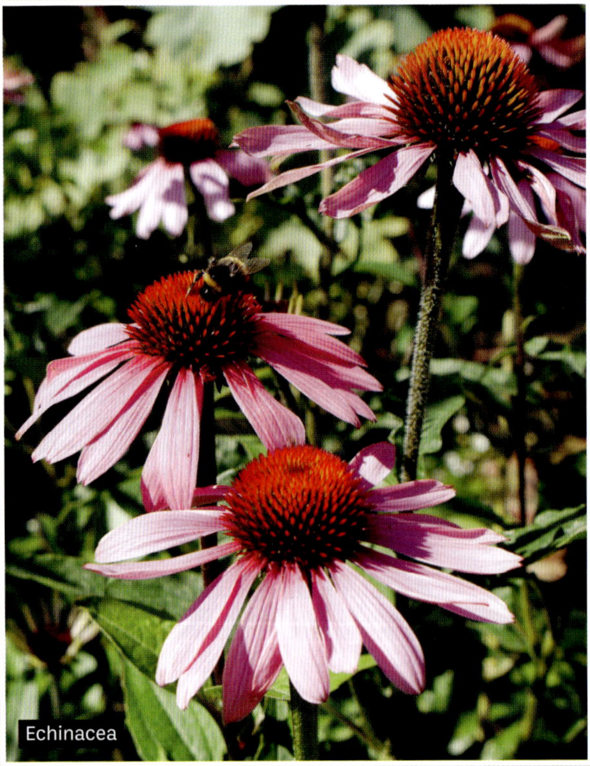

Echinacea

This herb is effective against a wide range of infections of the respiratory, digestive and urinary systems as well as the skin. Its most popular use is as a prophylactic measure to prevent the common cold, flu-like viruses and upper respiratory tract infections. There is no evidence that long-term use of echinacea is detrimental to the immune system, despite many claims to that effect on the internet and in some of the literature.

HOW TO TAKE IT: I would recommend that you source the tincture or tablets from accredited herbalists to ensure good quality. There is also a simple test to assess the quality of echinacea tincture. If you put one or two drops of the neat tincture on your tongue you should feel a strong tingling sensation that is caused by alkylamides, the most relevant active constituents of the plant. If you feel no tingling sensation, the tincture is unlikely to have medicinal properties.
COMBINATIONS: Herbal clinicians often combine echinacea with specific herbs that have additional supportive actions, such as antiviral or skin-regenerating properties.
DOSAGES:

Adults:

- For preventative and long-term use: 1.2–3ml, two to three times a day, tincture strength 1:2.
- As a first line of defence when the symptoms of a cold start to develop: 15ml/per day divided into three doses per day, tincture strength 1:2, for one or two days.

In my experience, taking echinacea in a large dose at the start of a cold will often prevent it from developing. However, if you do develop symptoms I would not recommend continuing with a large dose, especially if you are running a high temperature, though a small dose (3ml/day) is beneficial and will shorten the duration of the cold.

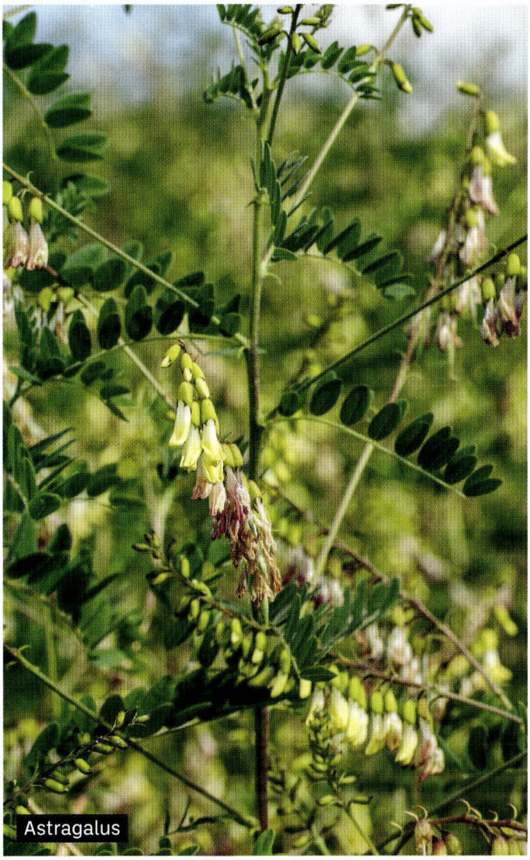

Astragalus

Astragalus *Astragalus mongholicus* (syn. *Astragalus membranaceus*)

Uses

This herb is commonly known as milk vetch. Its root has long been used in traditional Chinese medicine. Like echinacea, it can be cultivated in the UK or North America. It is a valuable enhancer and regulator of the immune system, with adaptogenic and tonic qualities. Astragalus can be used to treat a weakened or unbalanced immune system. It is also used for a range of viral infections, such as the common cold, flu-like viruses and recurrent cold sores.

I find this herb very useful for treating reduced vitality, general fatigue and post-viral or post-bacterial infections, or after a prolonged illness. It can be used both as a preventative botanical to reduce the likelihood of catching a cold, and as a treatment for colds. However, it is contraindicated during an acute phase of any infection if severe symptoms and a high temperature are present.

Additional benefits of astragalus include a positive effect on palpitations associated with viral infections, and a slight lowering of blood pressure.

I recommend its use as a prophylactic measure and a recovery aid, rather than as a treatment to be used during the infection.

Astragalus root can be used long term if necessary.

HOW TO TAKE IT: As a tincture.
DOSAGE: **Adult dose:** 4–8ml per day, tincture strength 1:2.

Example of a mix for supporting your immune system, to prevent an infection

INGREDIENTS

- 30ml echinacea root (tincture strength 1:2)
- 40ml elderflower or elderberry (tincture strength 1:2)
- 20ml astragalus (tincture strength 1:2)
- 10ml ginger (tincture strength 1:2)

METHOD

1. Mix the ingredients together.
2. Pour the mixture into a clean, dark glass bottle.
3. Label the bottle with the contents and the date.
4. Store at room temperature for up to 12 months.

ADULTS ONLY: 5ml diluted with some water, once or twice a day. Increase the dose to three to four times a day if you have been in close contact with anyone who has a cold or flu-like illness.

Example of a mix for supporting your immune system, to aid recovery after an infection

INGREDIENTS

- 20ml echinacea root (tincture strength 1:2)
- 20ml elderflower or elderberry (tincture strength 1:2)
- 20ml astragalus root (tincture strength 1:2)
- 20ml vervain (tincture strength 1:2)
- 20ml Siberian ginseng (tincture strength 1:2)

METHOD

1. Mix the ingredients together.
2. Pour the mixture into a clean, dark glass bottle.
3. Label the bottle with the contents and the date.
4. Store at room temperature for up to 12 months.

ADULTS ONLY: 5ml diluted with some water, two to three times a day.

CHAPTER 20

Make a full recovery from a serious illness

A serious illness can take a significant toll on the body, and it often takes weeks or months to achieve a full recovery. A suitable choice of herbs can greatly enhance the recovery process. You can speed up recovery by taking things easy, getting a lot of rest and eating nutritious food. Resist the temptation to start charging around as soon as you feel better after taking some herbs, and allow yourself plenty of rest for a few days or even weeks if your disease has been long-lasting.

The herbs listed below are those most commonly used for convalescence from a variety of conditions. You may look up other herbs that are recommended in relation to particular diseases and add these to your choice – for instance, after surgery you may want to use skin-healing herbs or arnica. Recovery from cancer is a special category and I recommend that you consult a medical herbalist about this. Always tell your doctor when you are taking herbal remedies to ensure that these do not interfere with any medication that you are taking already or are about to be prescribed.

Post-viral fatigue and chronic fatigue syndrome (often called myalgic encephalomyelitis, or ME) are both conditions characterised by symptoms of incomplete recovery from an illness. If your fatigue has been relatively short term (three to six months), follow the general strategy outlined below for two to three months. If you have been experiencing fatigue for more than six months I suggest that you consult a professional, as you will need a more complex, individualised treatment.

Below Sleep is vital for recovering from any illness.

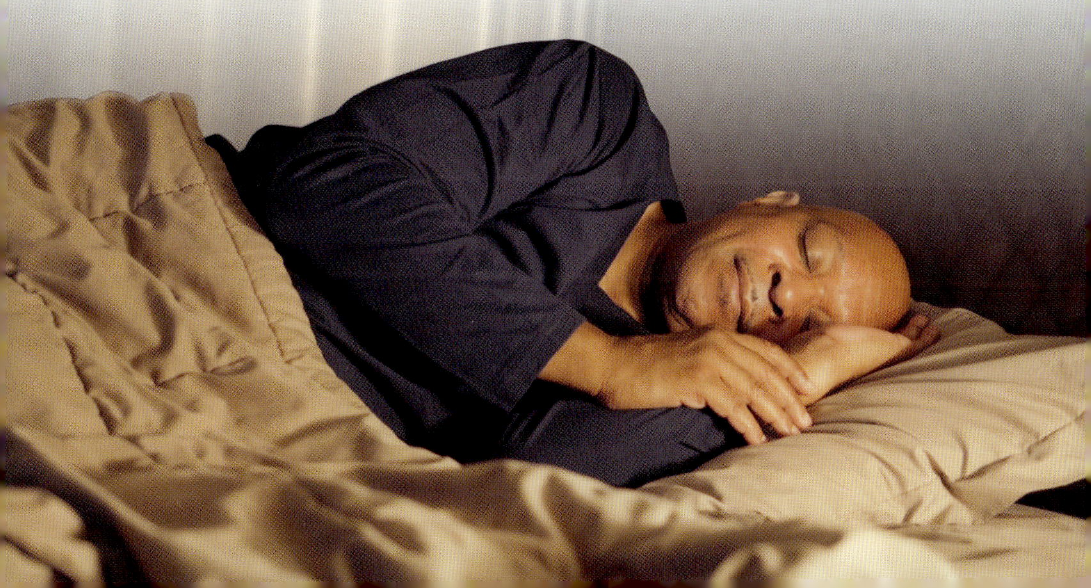

Choice of herbs

- Elderflower, marigold, andrographis, propolis and garlic (see pages 112, 135, 117, 116 and 194): these are antiviral herbs.
- Thyme, propolis, andrographis and garlic (see pages 121, 116, 117 and 194): these are antibacterial herbs.
- Echinacea and astragalus (see pages 198 and 199): these are immune modulators.
- Ashwagandha (see page 180): use this herb if you have experienced some weight loss or muscle wasting as a result of disease, and your general levels of vitality are low.
- Liquorice (see page 99): this is the herb to take for adrenal exhaustion.
- Vervain, St John's wort, rose and green oats (see pages 99–101): these are antidepressants and have a restorative effect on the nervous system.
- Siberian ginseng (see page 180): this herb improves vitality and energy.

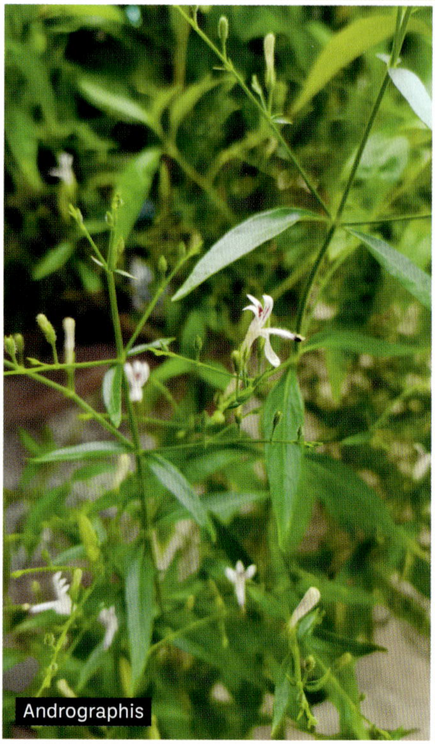

Andrographis

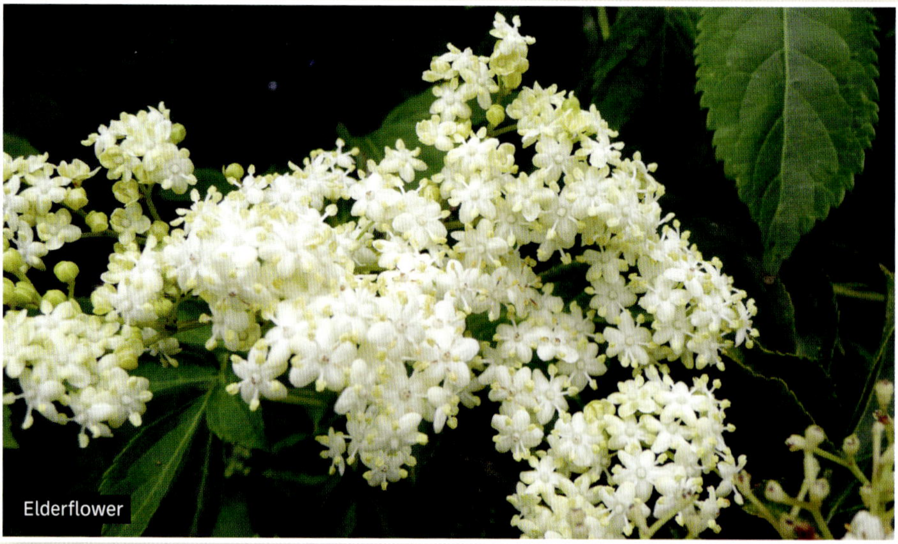

Elderflower

Herbal strategy to aid recovery from illness

- If you are suffering from an infectious illness, choose one or two antiviral or antibacterial herbs and start taking these at the maximum recommended dose for 7–10 days.
- If you have had an infectious illness it is still worth taking one or two antiviral or antibacterial herbs at the medium recommended dose for 7–10 days to eradicate the pathogen.
- Support your immune system with echinacea or astragalus if you are over the acute phase of your illness.
- Take ashwagandha if you have lost too much weight due to illness.
- Take ashwagandha and/or Siberian ginseng if your energy levels are low (but do not take these if you are still very ill).
- Take liquorice if your disease has been long-lasting and has left you mentally and physically exhausted.
- Take one or two herbs that improve mood if your illness has left you feeling low, lethargic or depressed.

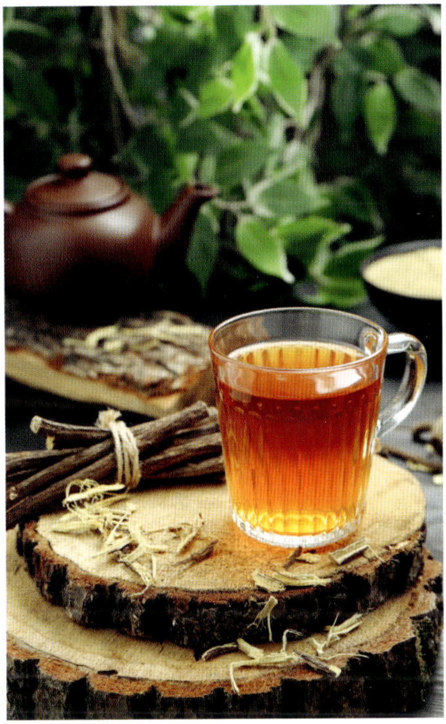

Above Liquorice tea.

Example of a mix for improving recovery from infectious illness

INGREDIENTS

- 20ml St John's wort (tincture strength 1:2) (for precautions see page 100)
- 20ml Siberian ginseng (tincture strength 1:2) (for precautions see page 180)
- 20ml ashwaganda (tincture strength 1:2) (for precautions see page 180)
- 20ml propolis (tincture strength 1:5) (for precautions see page 116)
- 20ml vervain (tincture strength 1:2) (for precautions see page 101)

METHOD

1 Mix the ingredients together.
2 Pour the mixture into a clean, dark glass bottle.
3 Label the bottle with the contents and the date.
4 Store at room temperature for up to 12 months.

ADULTS: 5ml diluted with some water, two to three times a day.

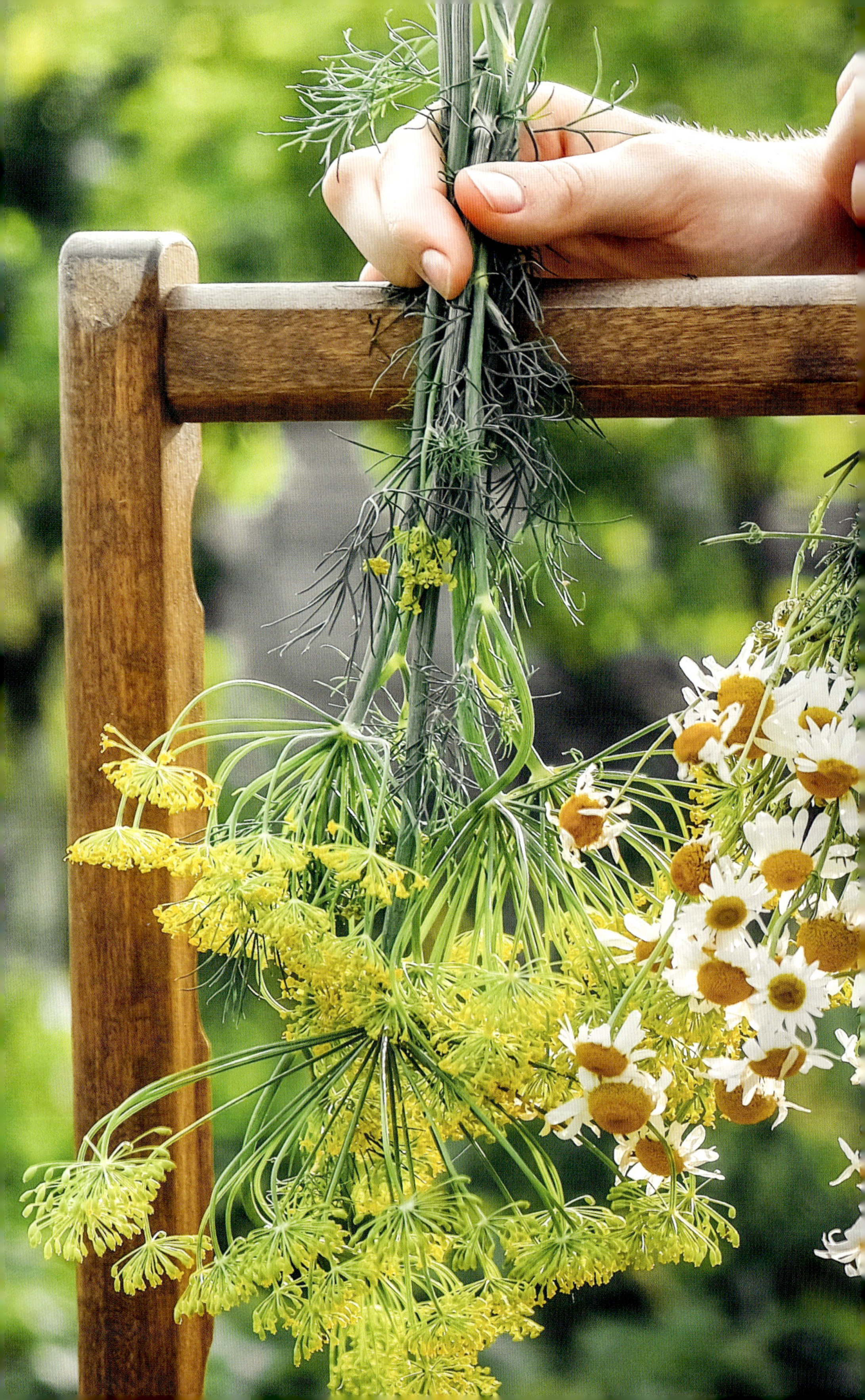

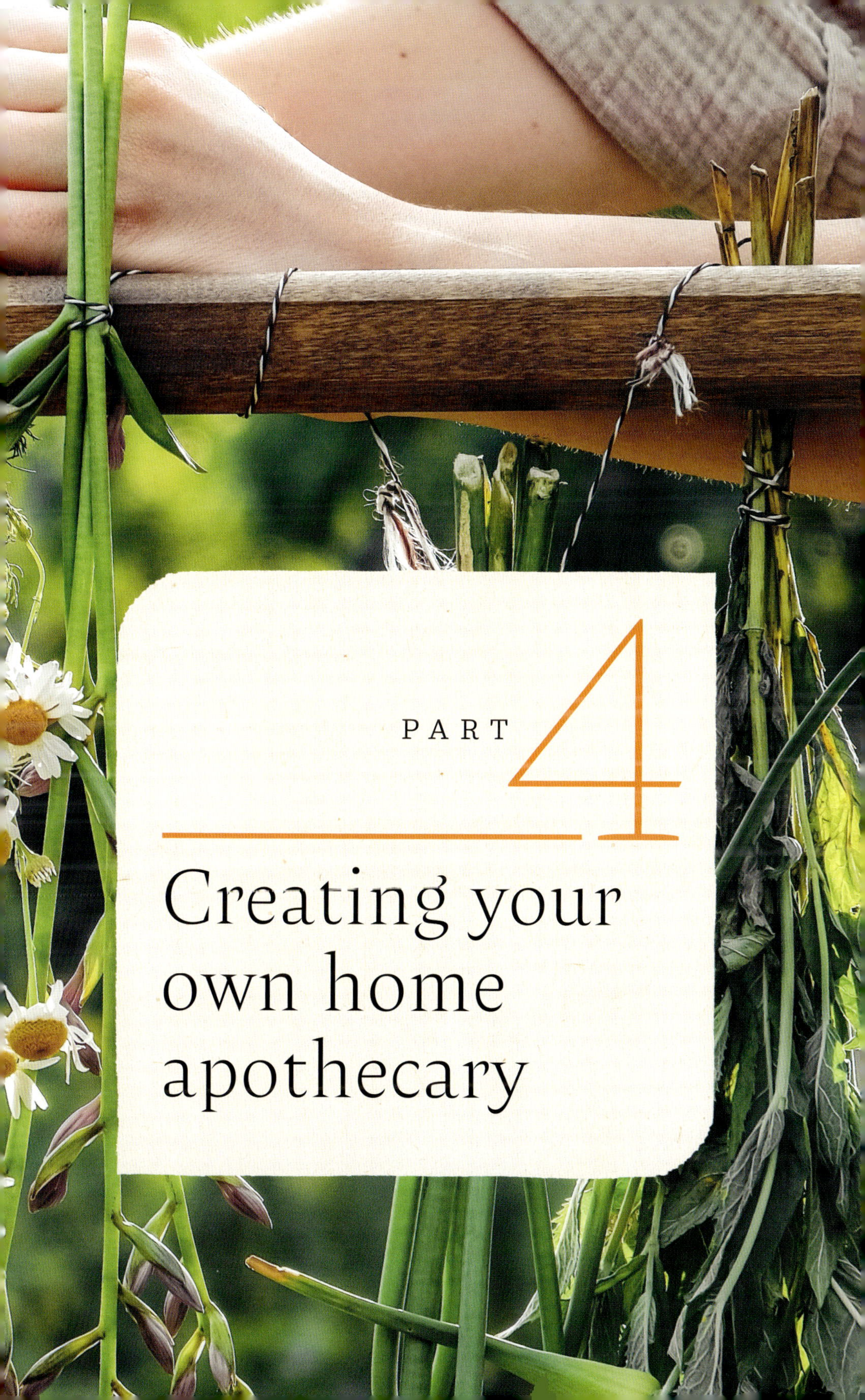

PART 4

Creating your own home apothecary

CHAPTER 21

Buying from reputable sources

Buying versus growing

If you want to stock herbs for regular use you have two options – you can either grow your own or buy from herbal suppliers.

I would encourage you to grow your own, but I recognise that most people are too busy to dry their own medicinal plants or to make their own tinctures. I think that for the majority of people a compromise solution will work best – you may want to grow a few herbs that are easy to cultivate and versatile in use, to perhaps make a herbal syrup or ointment, but otherwise you may prefer to buy ready-made herbal products.

Whichever option you choose, there are some important issues associated with both growing and buying. The pros and cons of buying will be discussed in this chapter, while the advantages of growing your own and suggestions on which herbs to grow are provided in Chapter 22.

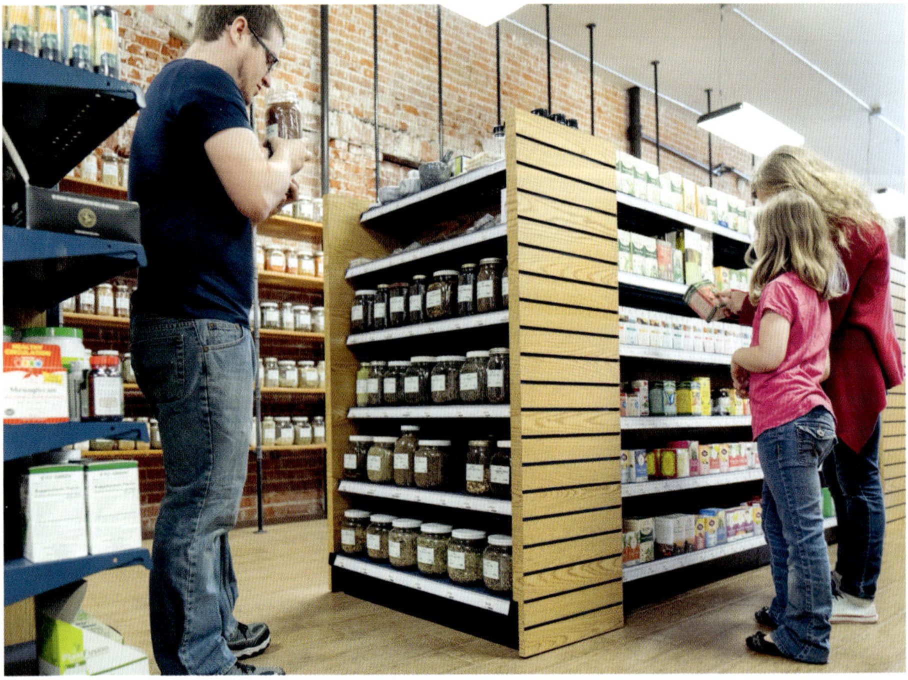

Buying ready-made products

The main advantages of buying from herbal suppliers are as follows:

- Ready-made tinctures are often superior in quality to home-made versions (some manufacturers will check the actual biochemical composition of each batch to ensure consistent quality).
- You can buy larger quantities if necessary.
- You can buy herbs in tablet form that cannot be made at home.
- You have access to a wide variety of herbs, some of which cannot be grown in the UK climate.

However, there are also some problems associated with ready-made herbal products:

- Unscrupulous traders will sell adulterated products, where one plant species has been substituted for another. Such adulteration can be seriously harmful if potentially toxic plants are used as substitutes.
- Some herbal preparations on the market are of poor quality and will have little therapeutic value.
- Others herbal preparations are artificially 'strengthened' with a particular constituent, and the safety of such products is not known.

If you decide to buy ready-processed herbs, consider the following points to ensure your safety and avoid wasting your money.

Buy from reputable suppliers only

This is of paramount importance. You should only buy from suppliers who can guarantee the quality of their products. Please refer to the Useful resources chapter for a list of recommended retailers and suppliers.

Unfortunately, not all health food shops can be relied upon to offer consistently high quality across the herbal product range. As a rule of thumb, obtain your herbs from well-known companies – the European and Australian companies that make herbal products have the best reputation. Look for symbols that denote good manufacturing quality on the labels of ready-made herbal products, or ask your local herbal practitioner about recommended suppliers.

Buy directly from herbal apothecaries

Many accredited herbal clinicians run their own apothecaries, and these are the best sources from which to buy your herbs, as the products will be guaranteed to be of good quality, and you will also receive advice on the appropriate dosage. To find such apothecaries, contact the organisations listed on page 247.

Buy either native herbs or non-native ones that are cultivated locally

Remember that the herbs that are most prone to adulteration are the imported, rare and exotic ones. At the time of writing there is hardly any quality control of Chinese and ayurvedic preparations, and there are frequent cases of herb adulteration in China and India. Buying native herbs or those that are non-native but cultivated in the UK reduces the risk of buying the wrong (and possibly harmful) species.

Price and quality

Price is often a reflection of quality, so beware of exceptionally cheap products. However, an exorbitant price is not a guarantee of extra quality, and is much more likely to mean that the herb you are buying is rare and endangered.

CHAPTER 22

Growing your own herbs

Before you start growing your own herbs, ask yourself which ones you will actually use and what quantities of them you will need. Do you want to have just a few fragrant leaves to pick for a summer tea, or do you want to make your own tinctures and creams?

How much and what to grow

In general, I recommend cultivating about 8–11 different herbs that are exceptionally versatile, are available fresh for most of the year or are easy to dry. These herbs are included in List 1 on page 212. For an average family you will not need many plants for each herb species – perhaps one lemon balm plant, one elderflower bush, four or five meadowsweet plants and a total of one square metre sown with chamomile or marigold. Many herbs, including lemon balm, peppermint and marigold, can be harvested throughout the season, and harvesting will encourage new growth.

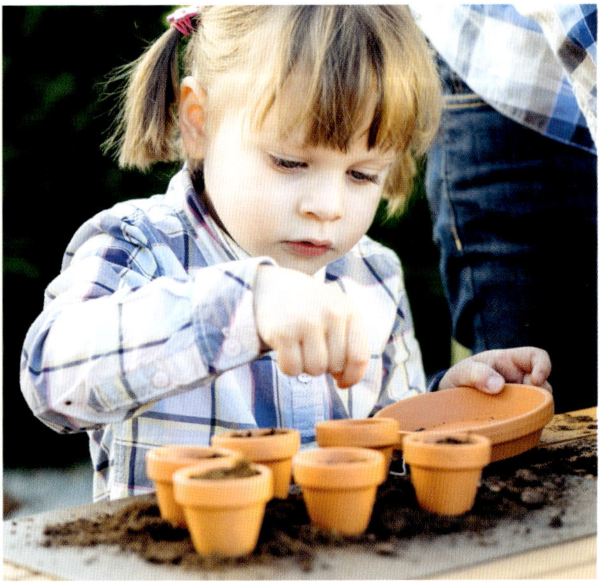

Right Growing from seed is good fun for children too.

It is difficult to recommend a specific quantity to grow, as needs will vary from household to household. As a general rule, plants that are evergreen and can be harvested all year round can be planted in small numbers, whereas plants that need to be dried or made into tinctures will be required in larger amounts.

Of course there is also an overlap between culinary and medicinal herbs. You may grow certain herbs primarily for cooking and only occasionally use them medicinally. Herbs in this category include garlic, dill, fennel, sage, thyme, peppermint, lavender and rosemary.

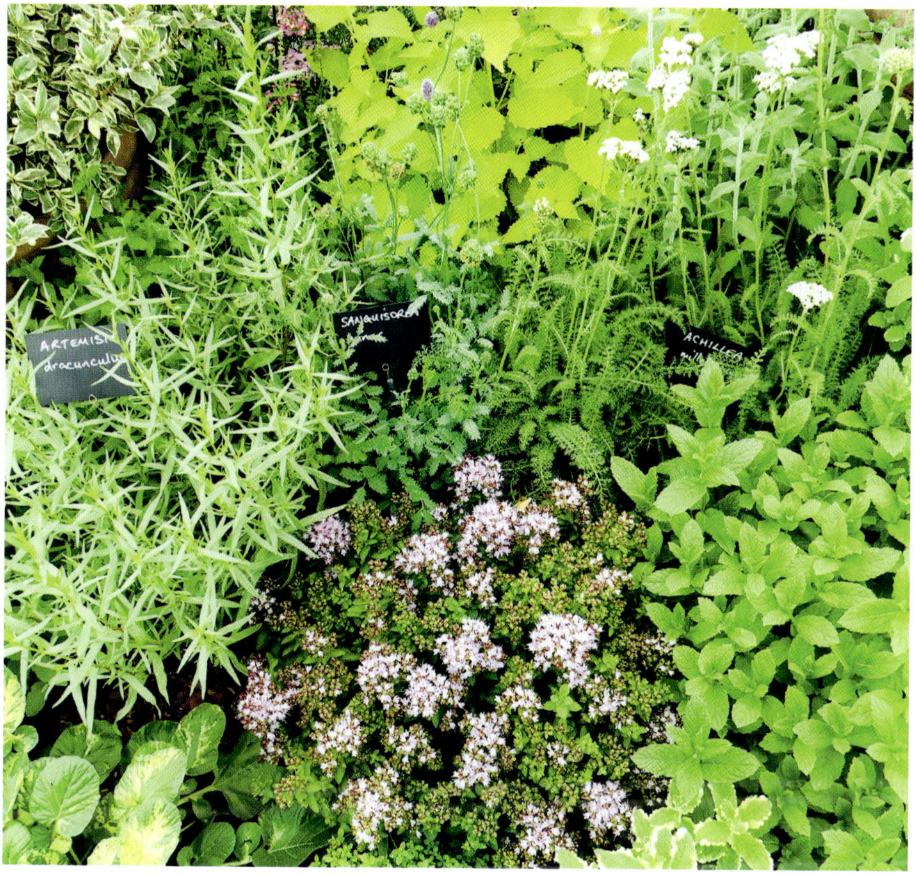

Above There are lots of delicious and helpful herbs to consider for your garden.

Easy to grow

Herbs are the easiest plants to grow. They are generally undemanding, thrive in a range of soil types, and are robust and resistant to pests. Most are perennials, one or two are biennials and there are a few reliably self-seeding annuals. It is a joy to have your own lemon balm or peppermint from which to harvest leaves to make a refreshing and relaxing summer tea, and it is a pleasure to see the cheerful flowers of marigold open and close daily. Hawthorn and elderflower make particularly graceful hedges that will be a magnet for wildlife.

Organic or biodynamic?

Herbs should be grown organically, which means that they are not sprayed with pesticides or treated with any other kind of chemical. The herbs listed in this chapter don't need any kind of fertiliser – in fact many favourites, including thyme and sage, prefer poor soil. Make sure that the soil has not been contaminated with any chemicals beforehand. If you intend to harvest the herbs from your garden for your own use it is worth reading up on biodynamic gardening and following the advice given, as medicinal plants that are grown and harvested using a biodynamic approach contain higher levels of active constituents.

Attracting wildlife

Flowering herbs provide a rich source of nectar for bees and butterflies, and some flower late in the season when food for insects is scarce. Bushes that are used medicinally have both attractive flowers and valuable berries for the birds. You will be growing plants that happen to have medicinal value, while at the same time creating a wildlife garden.

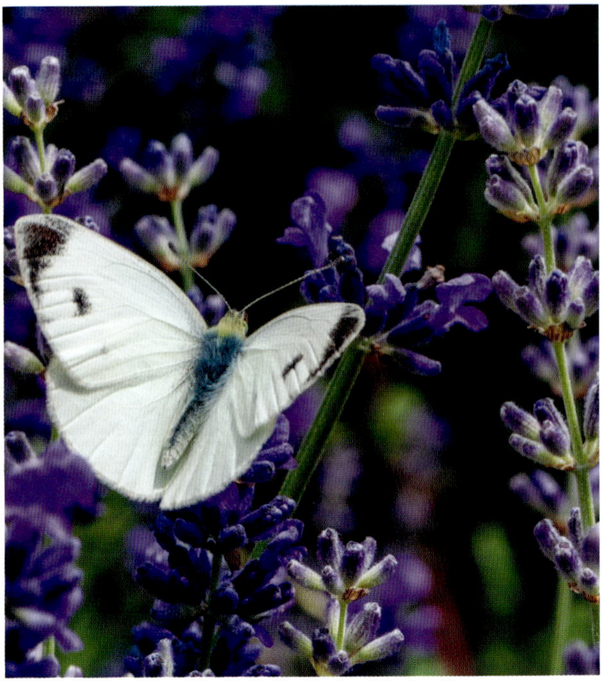

Ways to grow herbs

You can grow your herbs in an organised way in a flowerbed fashion, or in containers, or you can dot them around your garden or allotment between other flowering plants and vegetables. In fact they will be happiest when squeezed among other plants and made to struggle

Above Herbs such as lavender are fabulous food for pollinators.

Below For those without a garden, consider transforming a sunny windowsill into a herb garden.

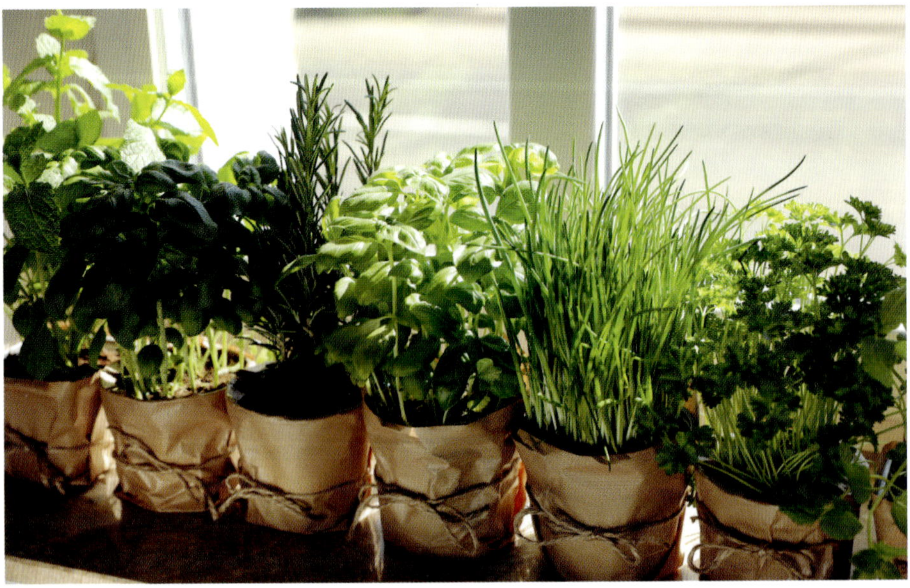

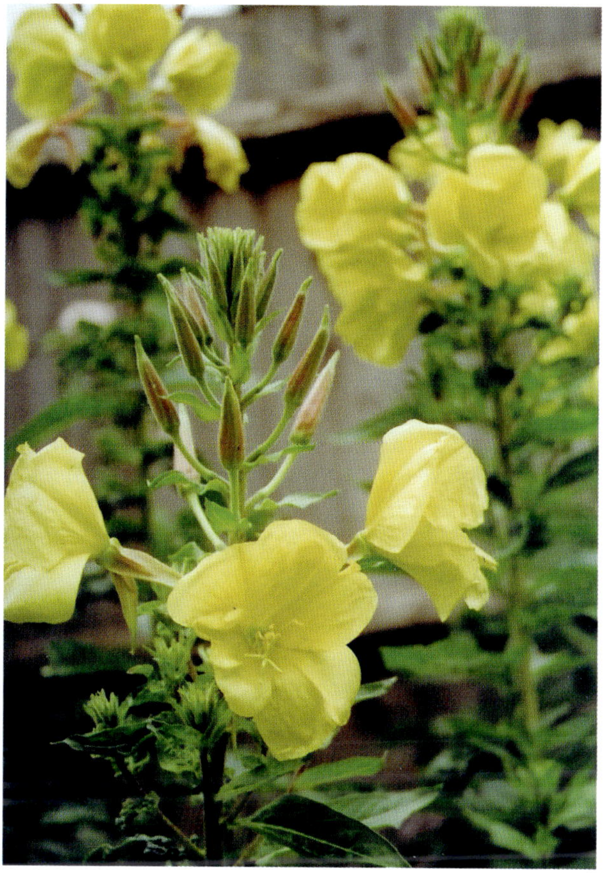

Right Evening primrose is a lovely plant to have in the garden.

a bit – this is how they have to survive in their native habitat. You can grow most of the herbs recommended in this book in the UK, apart from one or two which require a hot climate. And you do not need to grow them just to use them – many medicinal plants can be grown for their beauty or for their attractiveness to wildlife.

I prefer to grow herbs mixed with other plants, either in the borders or in the vegetable plot. I grow marigold and chamomile between rows of carrots and radishes, I let the peppermint grow through the flower bed (but thin the runners in early spring) and I plant black cohosh for its beautiful, scented flowers which brighten the beds in late autumn. I have never planted St John's wort, elderflower, evening primrose, hawthorn, dandelion, nettles or ribwort plantain in my garden – they all arrived of their own accord, with the help of wind and birds, and I let most of them be, occasionally shifting a particular plant to a different place.

Growing from seed and buying plants from nurseries

It is easy to grow herbs from seed, which you should source from specialist seed producers. You can also purchase mature plants from specialist nurseries (see the Useful resources chapter for a list of these nurseries). The herb varieties that are found in general garden centres are often modified garden cultivars, which are also often incorrectly labelled. Always check the scientific name on the seed packet or plant label. Once you start growing annual herbs, either collect the seeds or let the plants seed naturally. Some herbs (including lemon balm and peppermint) need to be divided or thinned out every few years, but most will live happily if left undisturbed in the same place, without any need for watering or fertiliser. However, herbs that are cultivated in containers will need watering and an occasional feed (comfrey liquid manure is particularly suitable for this).

Recommended selection of herbs

Below I recommend a number of different herbs to grow in your garden. The first list includes those that are easy to harvest fresh and to dry. The second list gives you a choice of pretty herbs with attractive flowers that can be incorporated into a perennial border or hedging – all of these have the added benefit of attracting pollinators. The third list consists of herbs that have to be dug out to harvest the roots, so they may need a dedicated place in your garden. The final list includes those herbs that will appear uninvited in your lawn or in a neglected corner of your garden, and which you should cherish and leave alone – once you know that these are valuable medicinal plants that you can use if needed, you will no longer perceive them as useless weeds!

For harvesting times, see the list of common and scientific names of herbs on pages 230–237.

List 1: Must-haves

These herbs are nice to have fresh, easy to harvest and dry, and versatile in use.

- Chamomile
- Elderflower
- Lavender
- Lemon balm
- Marigold
- Meadowsweet
- Peppermint
- Rose
- Rosemary
- Sage
- Thyme

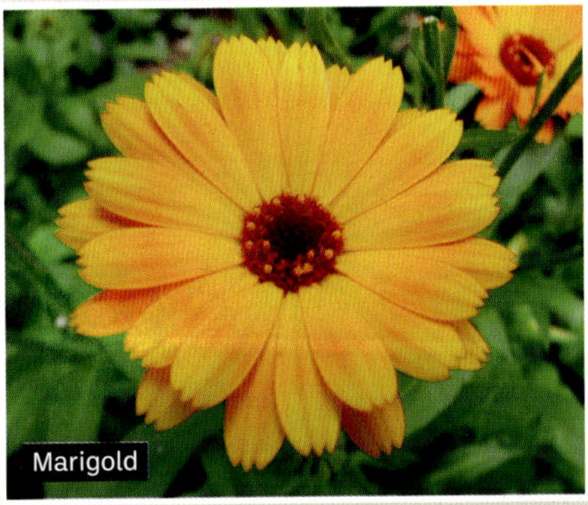

Marigold

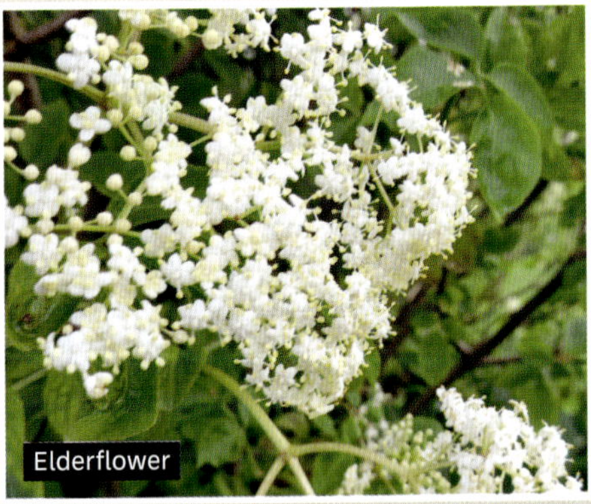

Elderflower

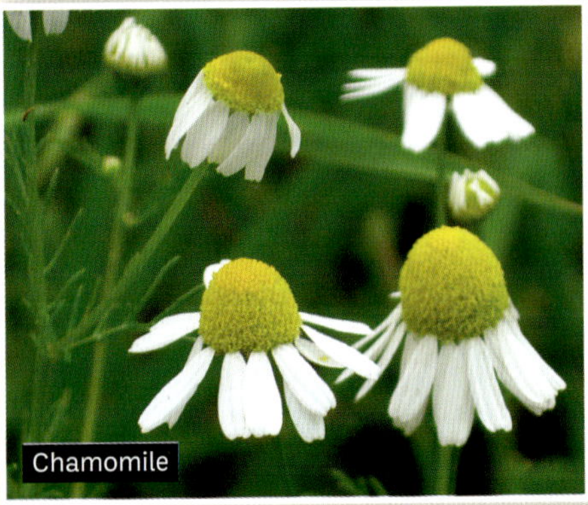

Chamomile

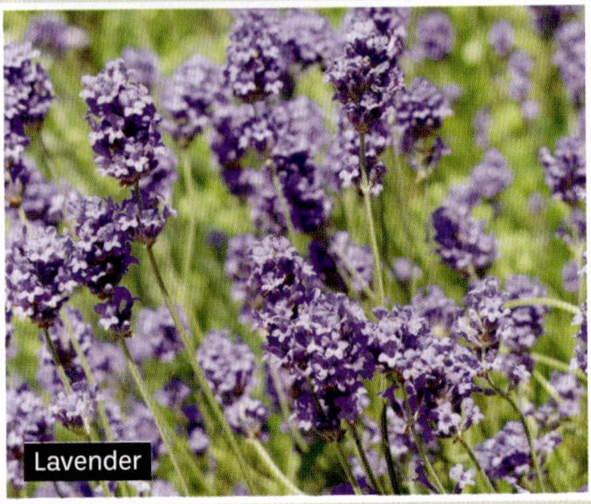

Lavender

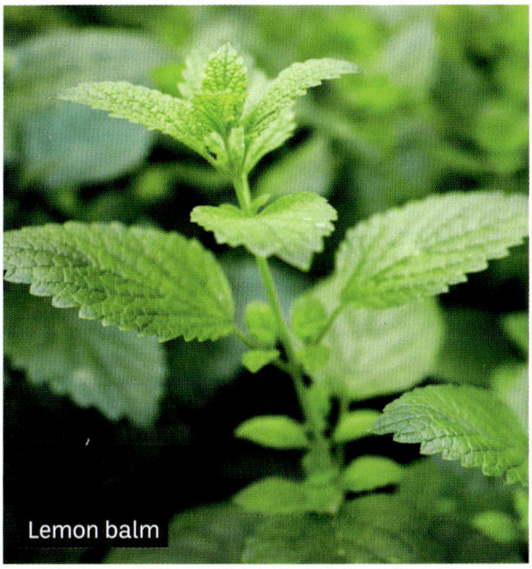
Lemon balm

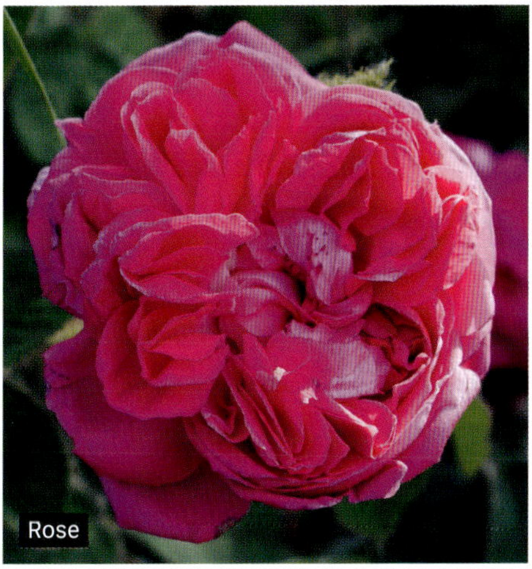
Rose

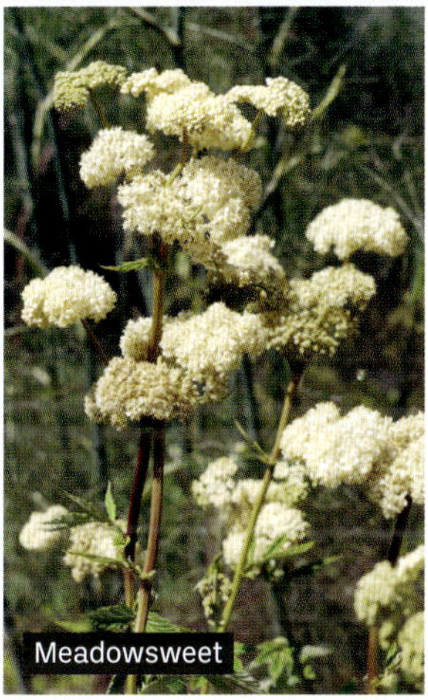
Meadowsweet

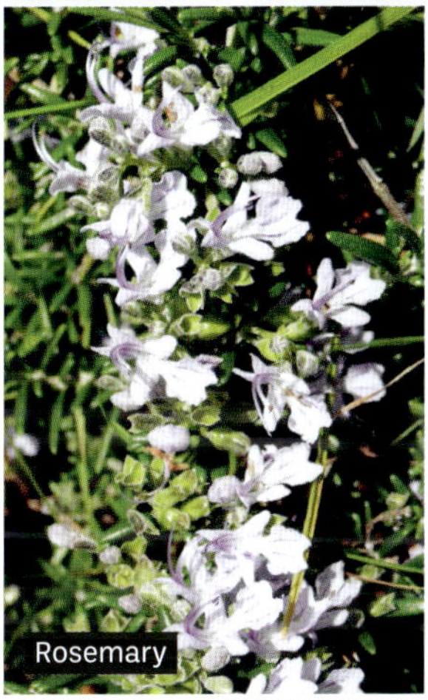
Rosemary

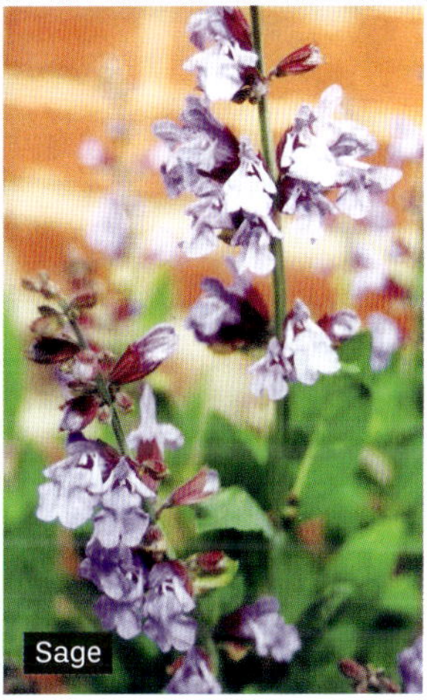
Sage

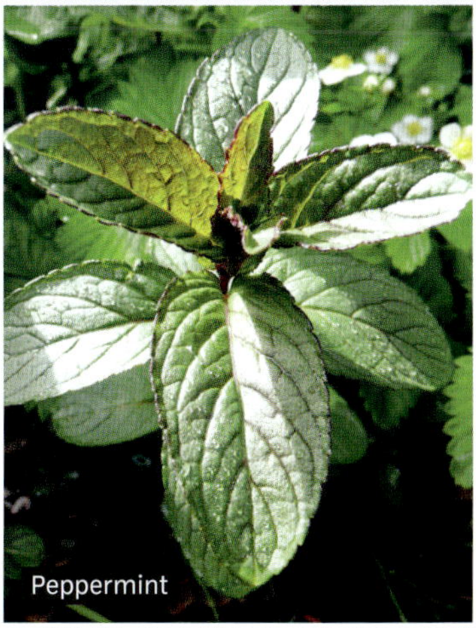
Peppermint

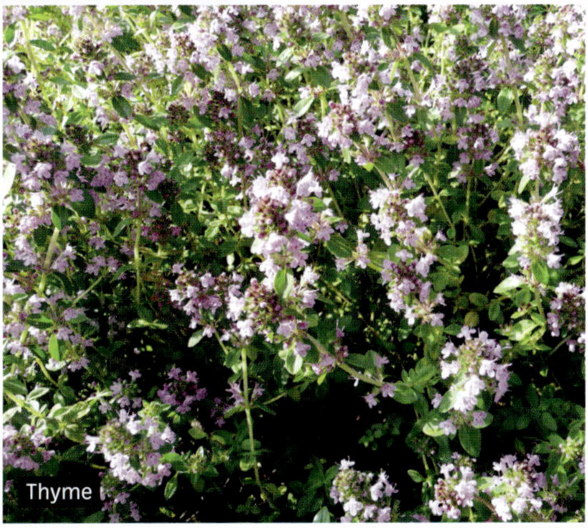
Thyme

List 2: Pretty plants with attractive flowers

The herbs in this list can be incorporated into a perennial border or hedging, and will attract wildlife.

- Barberry
- Comfrey
- Crampbark bush
- Echinacea
- Elecampane
- Evening primrose
- Eyebright
- Fennel
- Flax (linseed)
- Ginkgo
- Hawthorn
- Lime tree
- Marigold
- Marshmallow
- Milk thistle
- Sage
- St John's wort
- Valerian
- Wintergreen
- Witch hazel

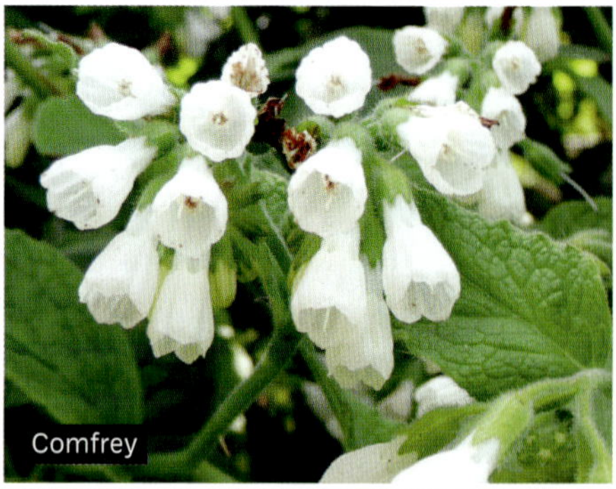

Comfrey

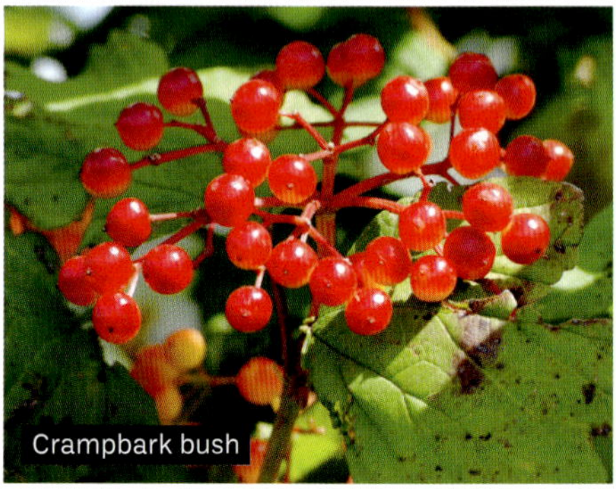

Crampbark bush

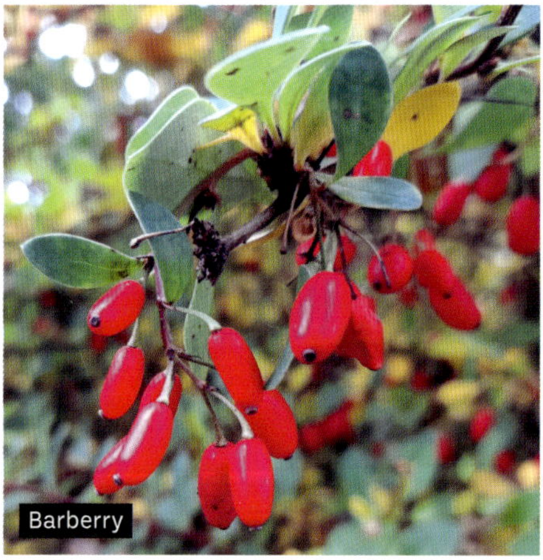

Barberry

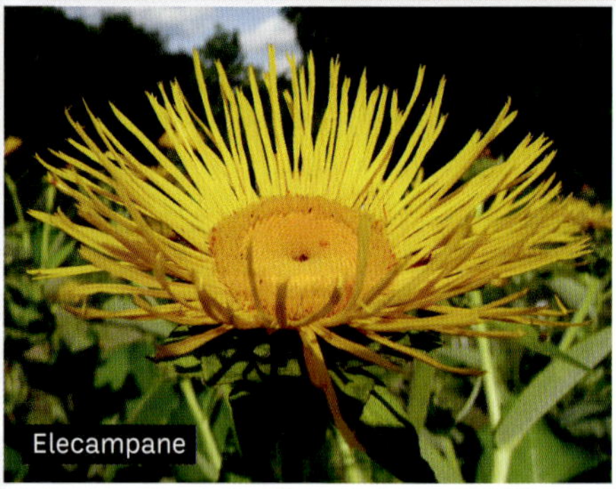

Elecampane

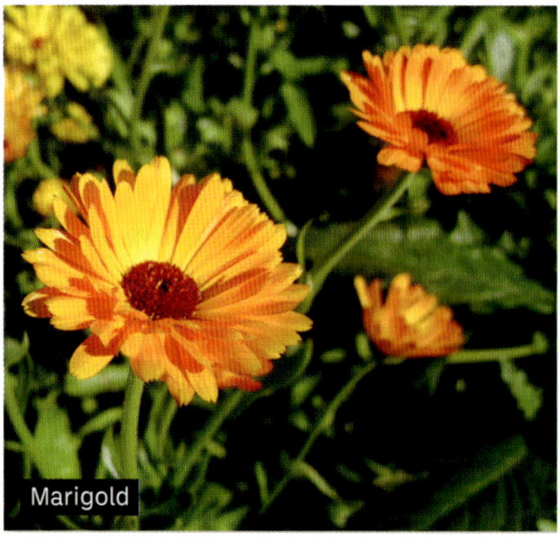

Marigold

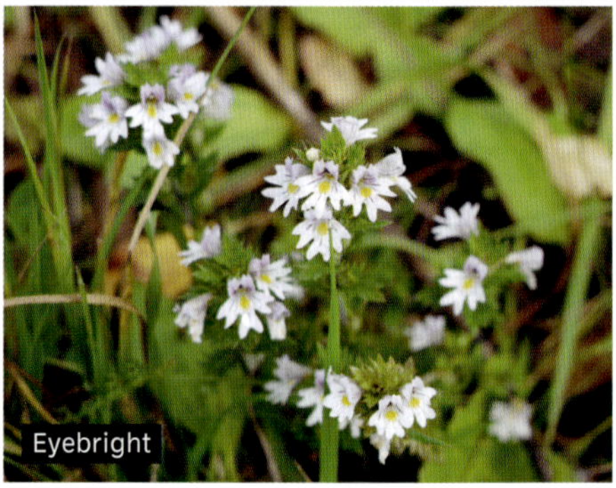

Eyebright

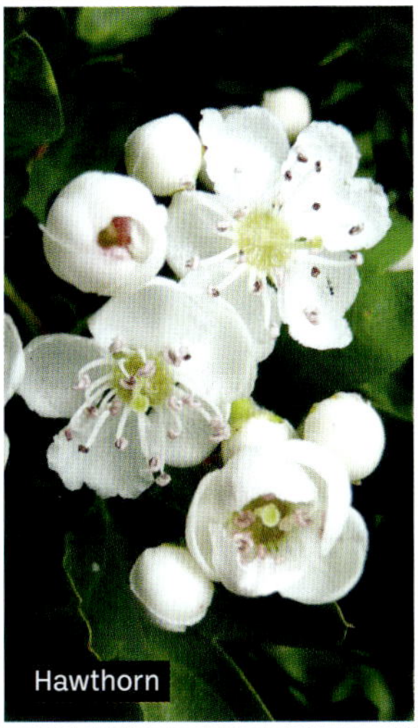
Hawthorn

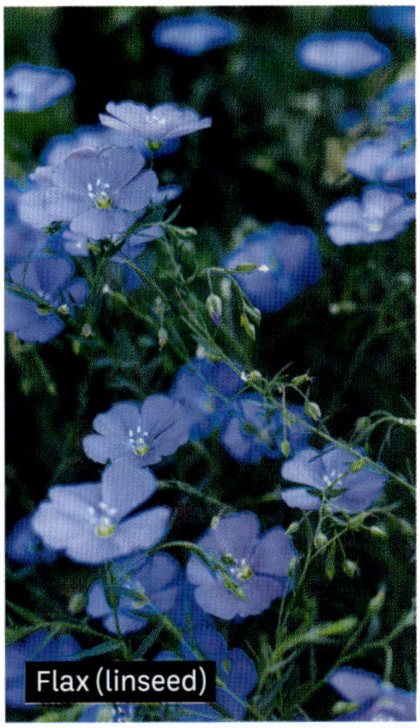
Flax (linseed)

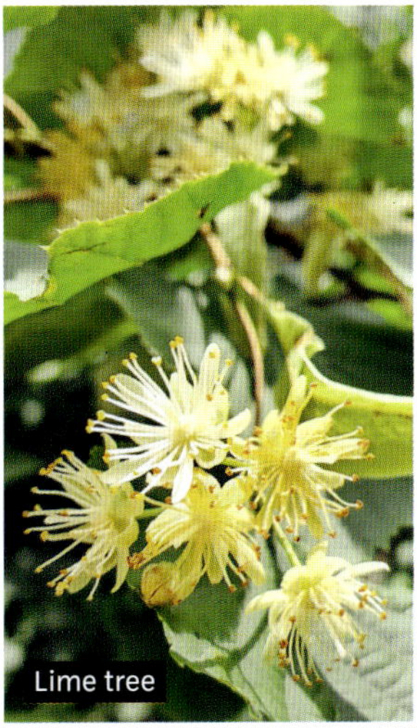
Lime tree

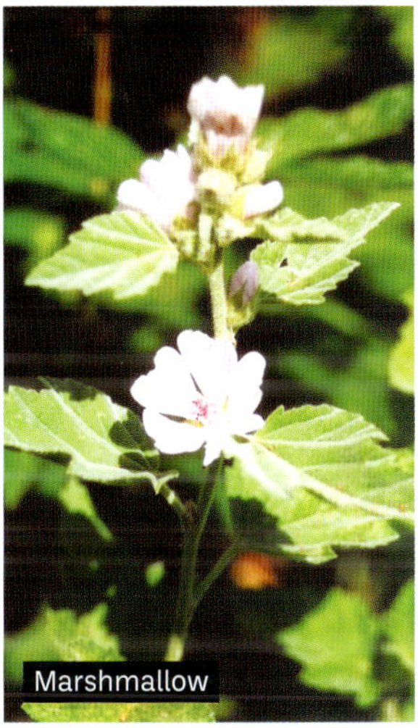
Marshmallow

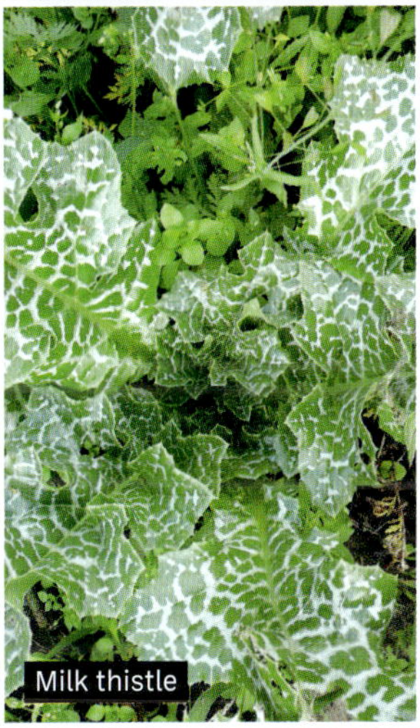
Milk thistle

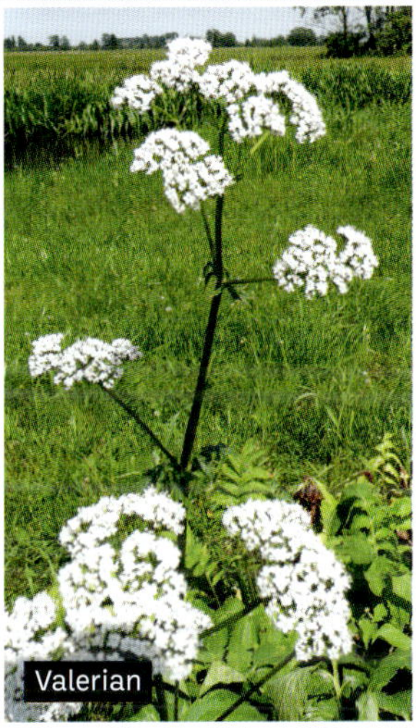
Valerian

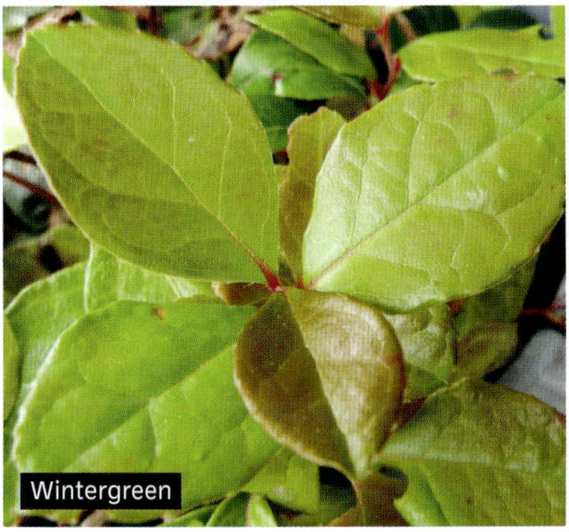
Wintergreen

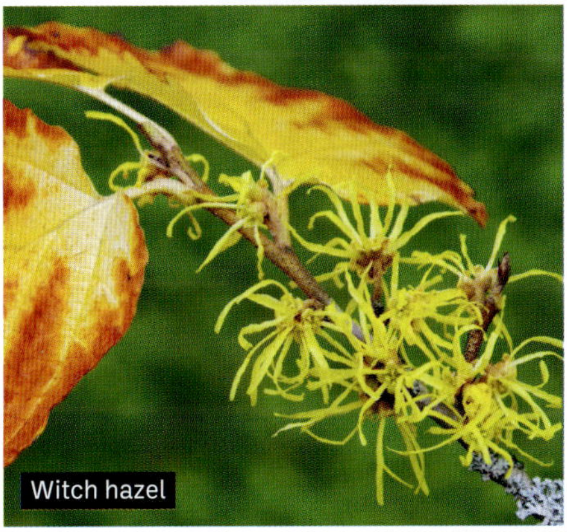
Witch hazel

List 3: Root herbs

These herbs may need a dedicated place in your garden, as you will be harvesting their roots.

- Dandelion
- Echinacea
- Elecampane
- Valerian
- Yellow dock

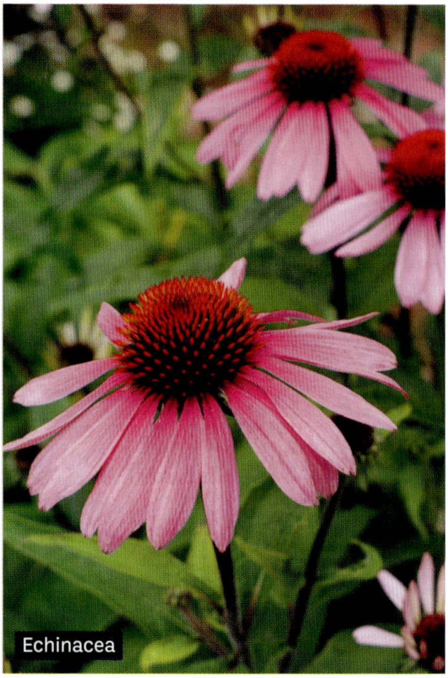

Echinacea

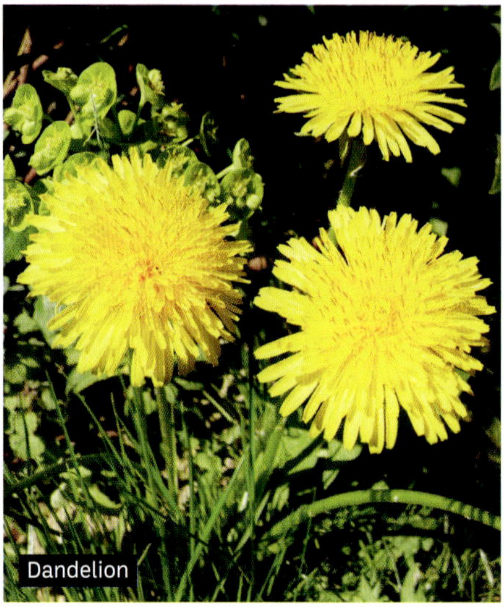

Dandelion

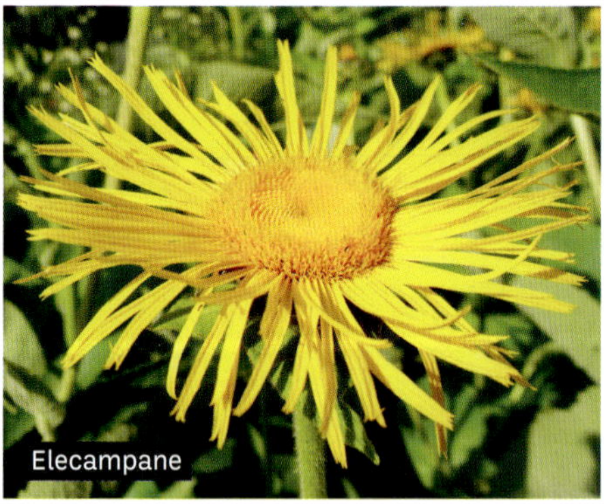

Elecampane

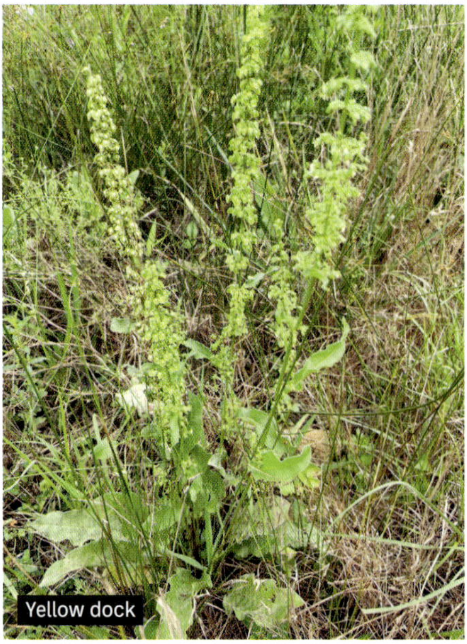

Yellow dock

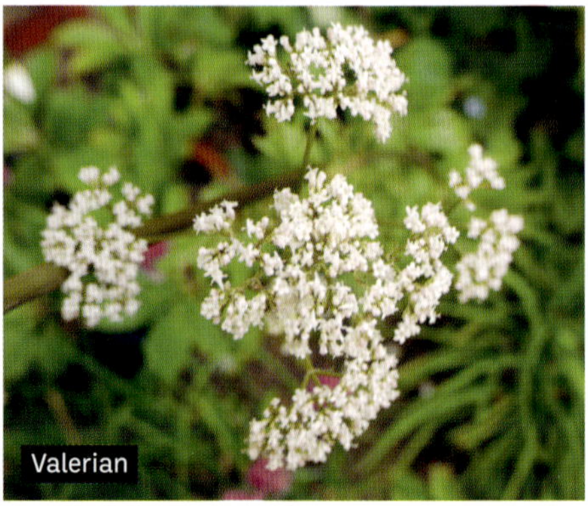

Valerian

List 4: Weeds that are also medicinal herbs

These common garden weeds that will appear uninvited in your garden are also valuable medicinal plants that you should cherish – perhaps by allowing them to grow in less conspicuous places with a view to occasional medicinal use.

- Dandelion
- Ground ivy
- Nettles
- Oats
- Red clover
- Ribwort plantain
- Shepherd's purse
- Vervain
- White deadnettle
- Yarrow

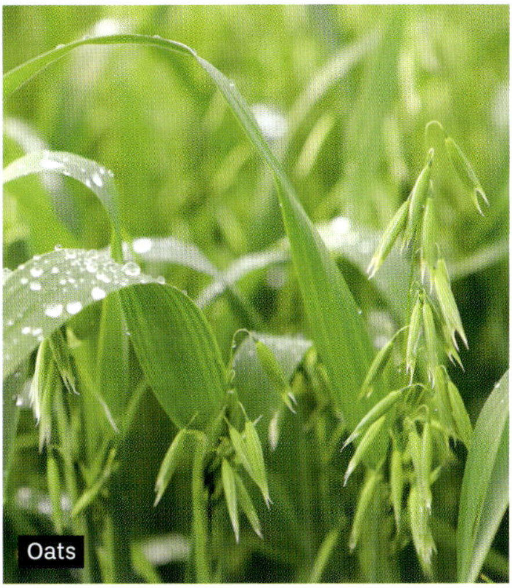
Oats

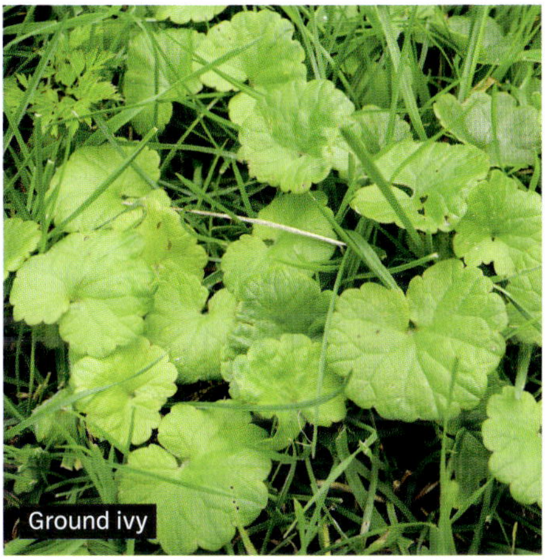
Ground ivy

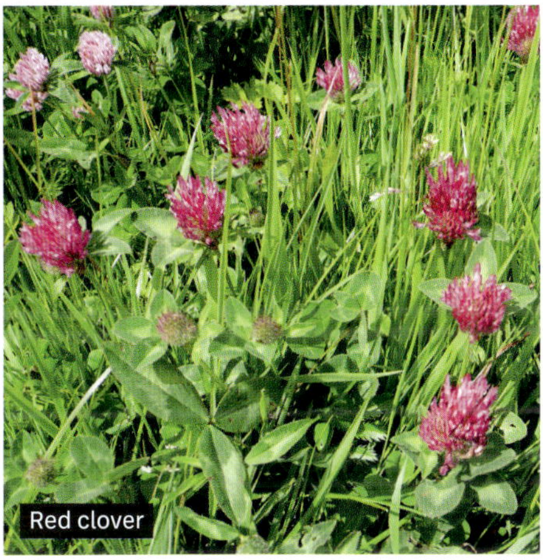
Red clover

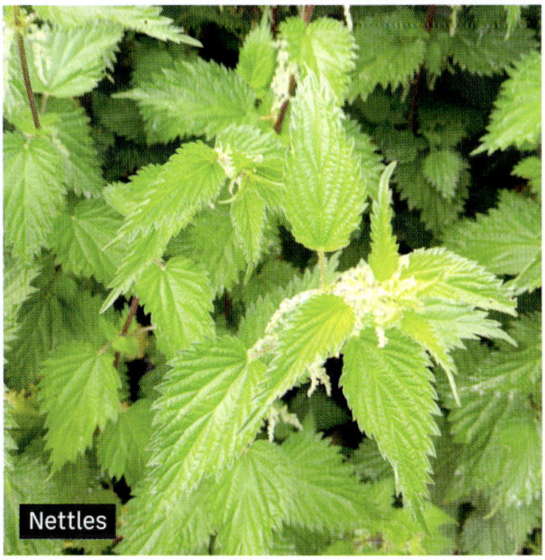
Nettles

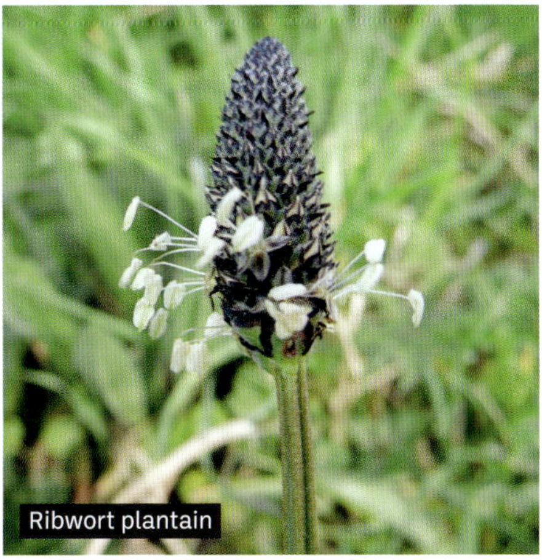
Ribwort plantain

Drying herbs

Make sure that you identify plants correctly before drying them, and then label them for storage with the plant name and the date. Always store them out of reach of children.

Drying herbs is the simplest way to preserve them. There are different ways to dry different parts of the plant, but the underlying process is the same – you expose cut herbs to heat so that their natural water content can evaporate. Because the UK climate is so humid, I recommend that you use only the oven method, otherwise you are likely to end up with a half-mouldy product. Herbs need to be dried quickly, at a reasonably high temperature and away from sunlight. Bunches of herbs hanging in the kitchen or attic look picturesque, but this is not an ideal way to dry them – not enough air can circulate around the herbs and

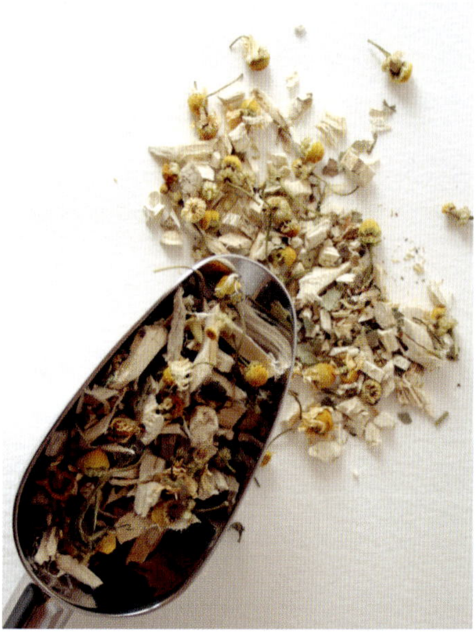

Above A scoop can be useful if you've got lots of dried herbs.

Below Dried herbs stored in paper bags.

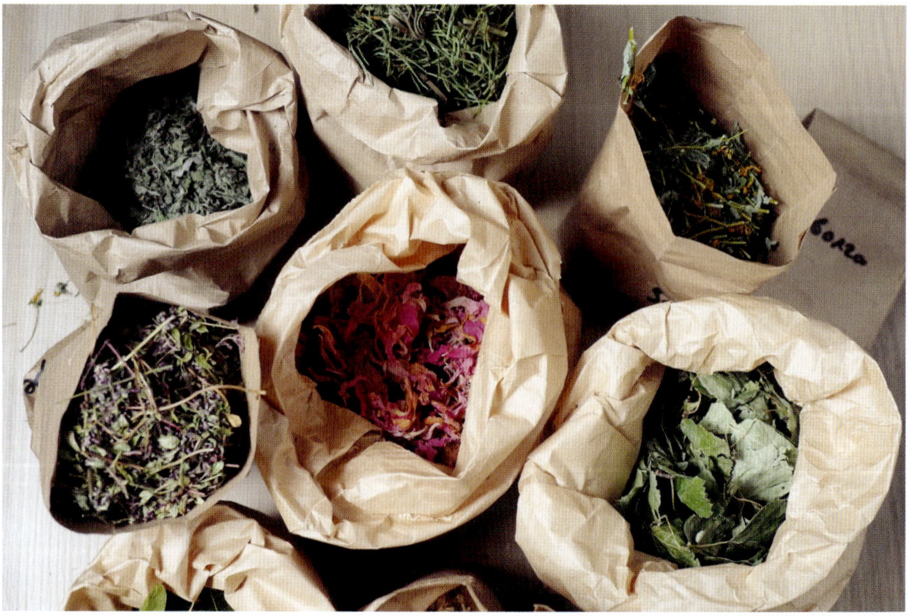

they will take too long to dry, providing an opportunity for fungal infections to develop on the leaves.

If you intend to dry herbs you must collect the aerial (above-ground) parts such as leaves and flowers on a dry, sunny day, ideally after several consecutive days without rain. However, it is not so important to collect the roots on a dry day, as you will still need to wash them. When gathering the aerial parts of herbs make sure that they look healthy, without any visible disease or insect damage, and that they are free from dirt so that you don't need to wash them.

Different herbs have different optimum times for harvesting, and following biodynamic principles of sowing and harvesting will yield better-quality herbs. See the list of common herbs on pages 230–237 for harvesting times.

Below Getting elderflower ready for drying.

Prepare the appropriate part

- Aerial parts of the plant should be left for a while after harvesting to give any small insects and other invertebrates a chance to crawl away. Then chop the leaves and stems roughly with a sharp knife or rocking herb knife.
- Single flowers should be cut off the stems. In the case of marigold and rose, strip the petals from the flowers. Flowers that produce large umbels, such as elderflower, should be dried while attached to the stems but then shaken off. Small flowers such as chamomile should be dried whole with a small amount of stem left attached.
- Berries must be detached from the plant, although sometimes it is easier to leave part of the stem attached. For example, hawthorn berries and elderberries disintegrate if you try to pull them off the stems.

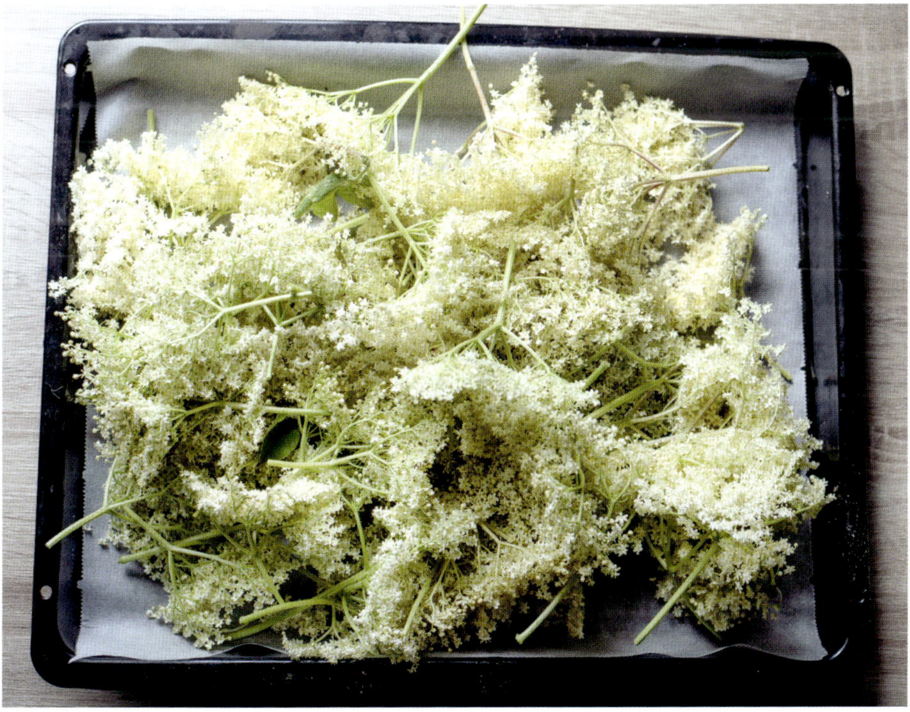

- Roots must be cleaned thoroughly under running water with a nail brush or a toothbrush, patted dry with a clean cloth and then chopped into small pieces (not more than 1cm in length).

Drying in the oven

Only electric ovens are suitable for this method of drying. If possible, avoid using a fan oven.

- Line a baking tray with greaseproof paper.
- Spread your herbs in a thin layer – the root pieces need to be in a single layer, with individual pieces just touching each other.
- Set the oven temperature to 40°C (104°F).
- The time needed for drying will depend on the herb – the more delicate the plant, the less time it will take to dry. As a rule of thumb, leafy plants such as lemon balm take about an hour, whereas roots and berries take two to three hours. Check the herbs periodically. If they look dry and are easily crushed in your fingers they are ready.

Storing dried herbs

There are a number of ways to store dried herbs so as to preserve their medicinal properties. The most important point is to keep them in dry, dark conditions.

- The simplest method is to put your herbs in two brown paper bags, one inside the other. The bags should be folded at the top to the level of the herbs and kept tightly closed with a large paper clip or clothes peg. Keep the bags in a dry cupboard or a drawer.
- An even better method is to put the dry herbs in a paper bag and then place this in another container that can be tightly closed, such as a tin or a glass jar. Storing herbs in this way gives them the chance to breathe and at the same time minimises the effect of seasonal changes in temperature and humidity. Keep the container in a dry cupboard or a drawer away from any sources of excessive heat.

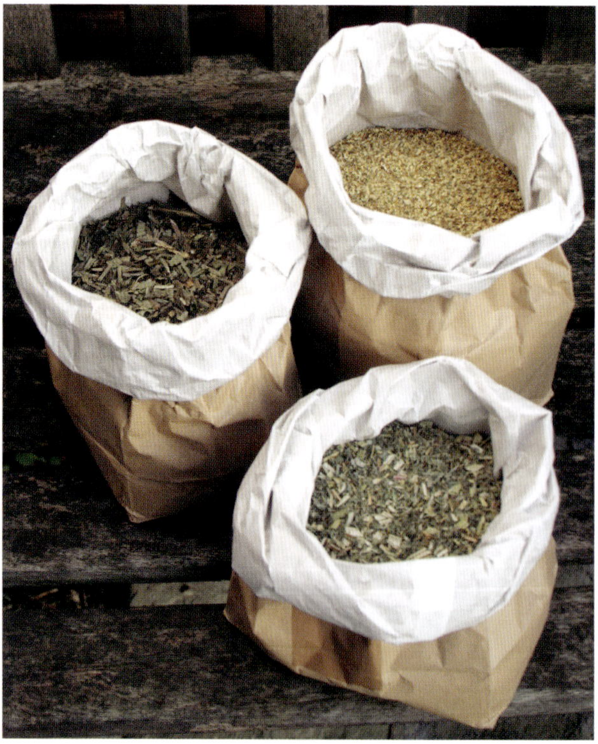

Left Paper bags are the best way to store dried herbs.

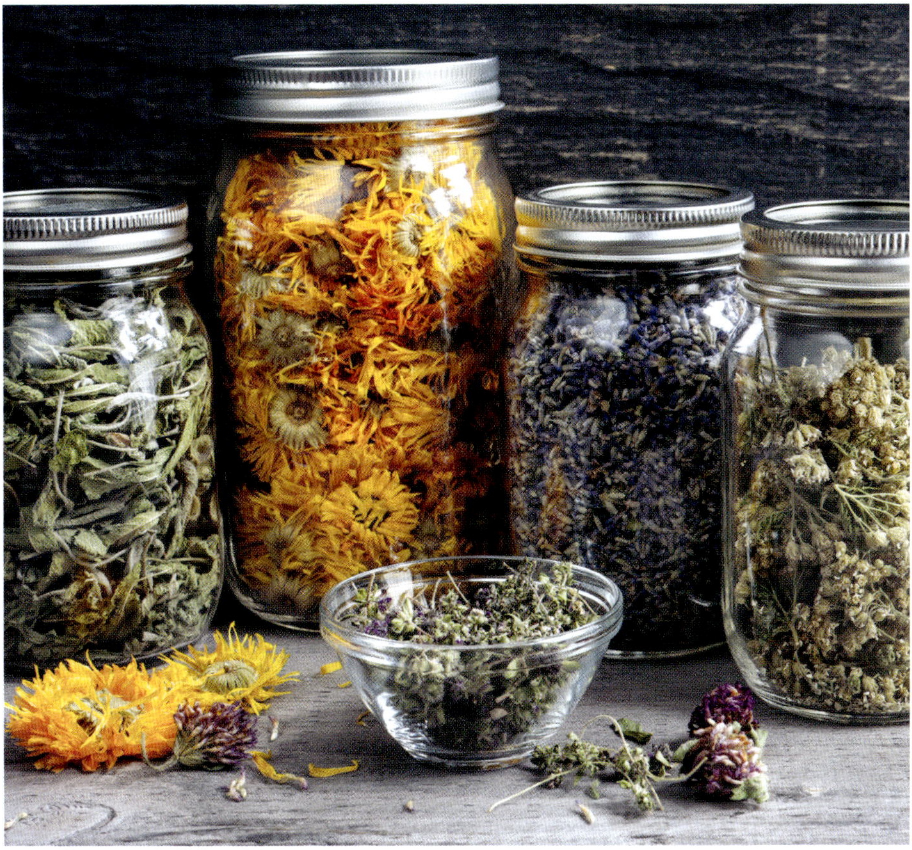

Above When storing dried herbs, try to fill as much of the container as possible.

- You can store your herbs in glass or ceramic jars. Match the size of the jar to the amount of herbs – try to fill the jar almost to the top, leaving a small gap of empty space. If there is a lot of empty space in your container the herbs will lose their fragrance to the air. Also, if the jar is transparent, keep it away from the light or the colour of your herbs will fade and they will lose their medicinal properties.
- I do not recommend storing dried herbs in a plastic bag unless this is for a short period of time – for instance, if you want to take dried herbs with you on holiday. If you do use a plastic bag it should be fully compostable.

Shelf life of dried herbs

- Leaves, flowers, and mixed leaves and stems will keep for up to two years, but from time to time check carefully that their colour and smell are not fading. It is also worth checking for any pests, as occasionally some eggs or larvae may survive the drying process.
- Roots, seeds and berries will keep for up to four years.
- Some authorities recommend much shorter periods of storage, but in my experience if herbs are stored well their medicinal properties will last well, too.

CHAPTER 23

Making your own tinctures, infused oils, syrups and ointments

Make sure that you identify plants correctly before processing them, and then label them for storage with the plant name and date. Always store them out of reach of children.

Extracting and preserving

Making your own medicine is great fun and quite easy. The basic principle is that you extract the active constituents from the plant material with a suitable medium, and then preserve the product in a suitable way. The medium for extraction is water, alcohol or oil. The preserving substances are alcohol, oil, sugar, honey or emulsifying ointment (available from chemists). Alcohol and oil act as both extraction media and preserving substances.

In this chapter I provide you with general instructions for making tinctures, infused oils, syrups and ointments. There are many books available that will give you more detailed instructions on making tinctures, especially in terms of alcohol strength and the required period of steeping. However, as we are talking here about small-scale domestic products, the basic instructions given in this chapter will be adequate. In general, fresh herbs make better products, but using dried herbs (see Chapter 22) is quite traditional and perfectly acceptable, too.

Making tinctures

All of the herbs recommended in this book can be made into tinctures using 40% clear vodka. You can use either fresh or dried herbs. If you opt for fresh ones, your final product will contain a lower percentage of alcohol, as the water content of the fresh

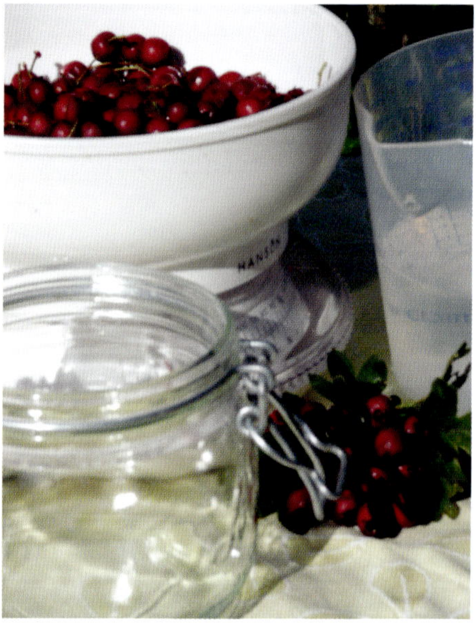

Above Making hawthorn tincture.

plant will dilute the alcohol. Each tincture should be made from a single herb. These can then be used to make specific tincture combinations.

Storage

Tinctures should be stored in dark glass bottles with screw-on caps, and kept away from light and heat. Sterilise the bottles before use.

Shelf life

The shelf life of tinctures is, on average, three to five years.

The herb-to-alcohol ratio

I follow a traditional method of making tinctures, whereas some modern manufacturers have developed specialised methods for making more concentrated ones.

The crucial point about making a tincture is to preserve the right proportion of herbs to alcohol. The herb-to-alcohol ratio, known as the tincture strength, is expressed in numbers (e.g. 1:2, 1:5, 1:10, etc.), where the first number refers to the amount (number of parts) of herbs and the second number refers to the amount (number of parts) of alcohol used to make the tincture (e.g. 1 part herbs to 2, 5 or 10 parts alcohol). Most of the tinctures referred to in this book have a strength of 1:2, which means that you take one part of herbs (in weight) and mix it with two parts of alcohol (in weight or volume). For instance, if you have 100g of herbs you will need 200ml (or 200g) of alcohol (for the sake of simplicity you can assume that 1ml is equivalent to 1g of alcohol). Please refer to the individual herb descriptions to check the correct tincture strength. Tinctures made from fresh herbs often require more alcohol than those made from dried herbs, because you need to submerge a larger bulk of herbs in the alcohol. Therefore fresh herb tinctures have lower strengths, and the dosage may need to be adjusted upwards. On the other hand, I have found that tinctures made from fresh herbs are more effective, perhaps because they preserve more of a fresh plant's 'bouquet' of volatile constituents.

For homemade tinctures you can use any vodka that is made from grain. The strength of alcohol is about 40%, which is adequate for most herbs.

How to make a tincture

1. Weigh the herbs if you are using dried ones.
2. If you are using fresh herbs, prepare them by chopping them into small pieces, and then weigh them.
3. Put the herbs in a large, sterilised glass jar with a screw-on lid – jars that are normally used for storing preserves are fine for this.
4. Measure out the correct amount of vodka in a measuring jug.
5. Pour the alcohol over the herbs, making sure that all of them are covered with it – if necessary, press down on the herbs with a clean spoon.
6. Screw the lid on and give the jar a good shake.
7. Leave the mixture to macerate for two weeks in a dark place. Shake the jar vigorously every day if possible to disperse the extract evenly throughout the jar.
8. Strain the herbs through a jelly bag or cheesecloth and squeeze them manually to extract all of the liquid. You can use a wine press for straining if you have one. The used herbs can be composted.
9. Pour the tincture into dark glass bottles and label them with the name of the herb, the tincture strength, the dosage and the date.

Making infused oils

Infused oils can be used on their own for external applications or they can be added to various creams or ointments. You can use any good-quality organic oil – sunflower oil and olive oil are the ones most often used. You can use fresh or dried herbs. The herbs most often used for infused oils are marigold (petals), comfrey (leaf) and St John's wort (flowers). If you are using fresh plant parts you can crush them slightly beforehand with a rolling pin to aid the extraction process.

I recommend making small amounts of infused oils, as generally these are used in small quantities and have a short shelf life. The ratio of plant material to oil is not as crucial as in the case of tinctures, as infused oils are intended only for external use.

It is difficult to give the exact proportions of plant material to oil, as the volumes of herbs will differ depending on which part of the plant you are using (petals, leaves or flowerheads). You should aim to cover the tightly packed herbs with the oil, and you can repeatedly strain the oil and add more fresh herbs to produce a more concentrated infused oil. Look for a change in colour of the original oil – for instance, St John's wort infused oil should be red, and marigold infused oil should be orange. *Bartram's Encyclopaedia of Herbal Medicine* suggests that 250g of dried herbs (or 750g of fresh herbs) should be used per 500ml of oil, but I recommend that you aim to make about 100ml of any infused oil, as it is unlikely that you will need more than this.

Storage

Infused oils should be stored in dark glass bottles with screw-on lids, away from light and heat. Sterilise the bottles before use.

Shelf life

Infused oils can be stored for up to two years.

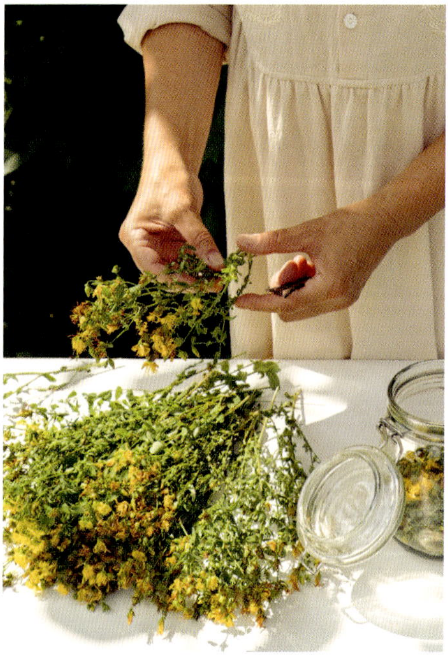

Above Preparing St John's wort flowers.

How to make an infused oil

1. Prepare fresh herbs by stripping the petals from marigold, chopping the leaves of comfrey or cutting off the flowers of St John's wort.
2. Fill a sterilised glass jar with the herbs, packing them as tightly as possible.
3. Pour the oil in slowly until all of the herbs are covered and no air pockets are left. Screw the lid on.
4. Put the jar on a sunny windowsill to infuse for two to four weeks. Shake the jar regularly (daily if possible). You are looking for a definite change of colour in the oil.
5. Strain the oil through a jelly bag into a jug.
6. Pour the infused oil into a sterilised dark glass bottle, and label it with the name of the herb and the date.

Making ointments

Ointments can be made in a variety of ways, but I have found the following recipe the easiest to use. Fresh or dried herbs are suitable, and emulsifying ointment and glycerol can be obtained from a chemist. You can use a variety of herbs in ointments, the most common ones being marigold and comfrey leaf.

Shelf life

Ointment can be stored in dark glass jars for up to two years.

How to make an ointment

1. Prepare the herbs. Weigh the dried herbs, or chop the fresh ones and then weigh them (if you are using marigold, strip the petals off the flowers and weigh them).
2. Melt 600g of emulsifying ointment (a ready-made ointment base) in a glass dish that has been placed in a saucepan half-filled with water on a low heat.
3. Add 270ml glycerol.
4. Add 330ml water.
5. Add 120g herbs.
6. Simmer for three hours while stirring occasionally, topping up the saucepan with water if necessary.
7. Strain the mixture through a jelly bag into a glass bowl while it is still hot (be very careful!).
8. Stir continually until it is cold.
9. Transfer the ointment into sterilised dark glass jars using a palette knife, making sure that all air pockets are removed.
10. Label the jars with the name of the herb and the date.

Below Comfrey ointment.

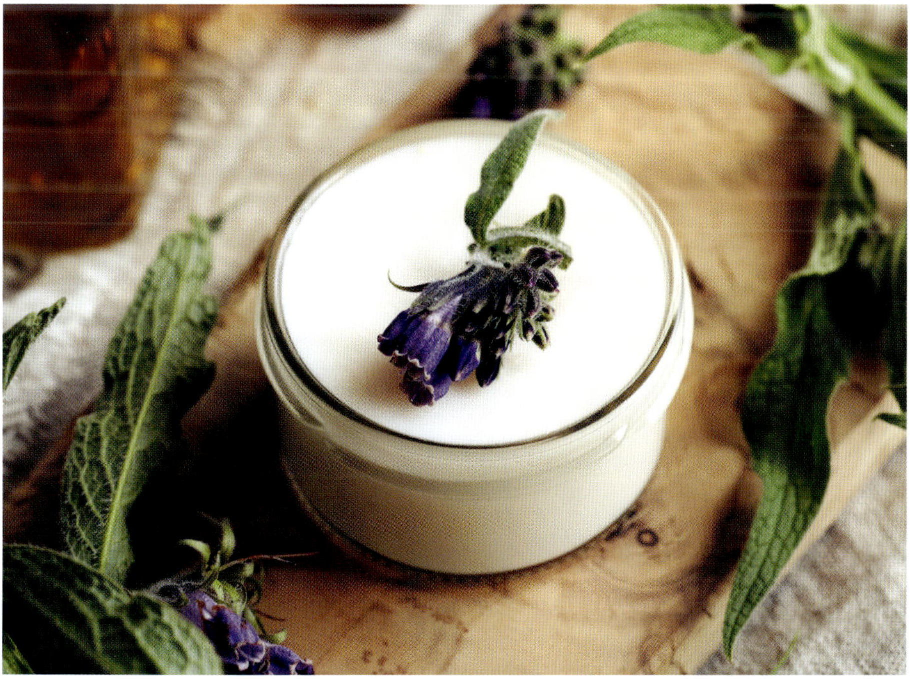

Making syrups

Syrups are the best way to administer cough medicine. Typical herbs used for making syrups are liquorice, thyme, marshmallow root, rose, mullein, hyssop, and the young shoots of fir tree or spruce. You can use either dried or fresh herbs, or a mixture of the two. I recommend using a single herb per syrup, except for thyme and liquorice, which can be mixed in equal proportions.

Young shoots of fir tree are processed differently (see the instructions in box opposite). It is crucial that you are able to identify the right species, as some conifers are unsuitable (e.g. yew, cedar). You are essentially looking for a 'Christmas tree' type of fir growing wild in a forest and belonging to one of two species – Norway spruce (*Picea abies*) or silver fir (*Abies alba*). You can also use new growth of Scots pine (*Pinus sylvestris*). You are looking for the young, soft, bright green new shoots that appears at the tips of the branches in the spring. Ideally you should collect them when they are about 2–3cm long.

Storage

Syrups should be stored in dark glass bottles, away from light and heat. Syrups made with honey may occasionally ferment, so keep the bottle sealed with a cork to prevent an explosion!

Shelf life

Most syrups can be stored for two to three years. For fir tree and pine tree syrups the recommended shelf life is 12 months. Watch out for any signs of mould, and discard any syrup that looks suspect.

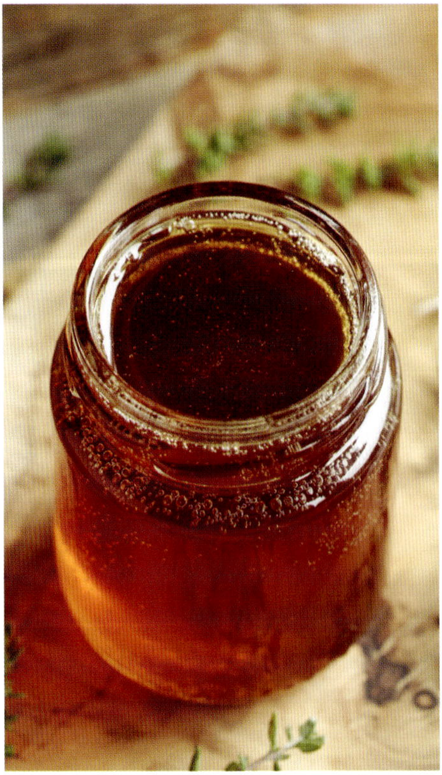

Left Thyme syrup is good for a cough.

How to make a herbal syrup

1. Prepare 500ml of a suitable infusion or decoction using 25g of dried herbs or 75g of fresh herbs per 500ml of water.
2. Strain the herbs through a cheesecloth into a saucepan and add 500g of honey or unrefined sugar. Mix well until the honey or sugar has dissolved.
3. Simmer on a low heat, stirring all the time until the syrup thickens.
4. Leave the syrup to cool down, and then pour it into sterilised glass bottles, being careful not to overfill them, and use corks to seal the bottles.
5. Label the bottles with the plant name, dosage and date.

How to make a syrup from fir tree young shoots

1. First, identify a suitable species (*Picea abies, Abies alba or Pinus sylvestris*), being careful not to confuse these with yew or other conifers.
2. Collect the very soft, bright green new shoots from the tips of fir tree branches when they are about 2–3cm long (see the photograph for reference) (the time of year for collection varies from one year to the next, but new growth usually appears sometime between March and early May). You will need enough shoots to fill a jam jar. Pine tree shoots should be cut into small pieces.
3. Place a layer of plant material 1cm deep at the bottom of the jar.
4. Place a 1cm layer of white or brown sugar on top of this.
5. Repeat the process with alternating layers until you have filled the jar, finishing with a layer of sugar at the top.
6. Screw on the lid and leave the jar on a sunny windowsill for two to three weeks. Shake the jar daily, and add more sugar if the top layer becomes exposed to the air.
7. Strain the syrup through a fine cloth.
8. Transfer it to a new jar and sterilise it in an oven in the same way as you would jams or any other preserves.
9. You can add some vodka (about a third of the volume) to the syrup as an additional preservative after sterilising and cooling.
10. Label the jar with the plant name, dosage and date.

Below Norway spruce (*Picea abies*) with new growth.

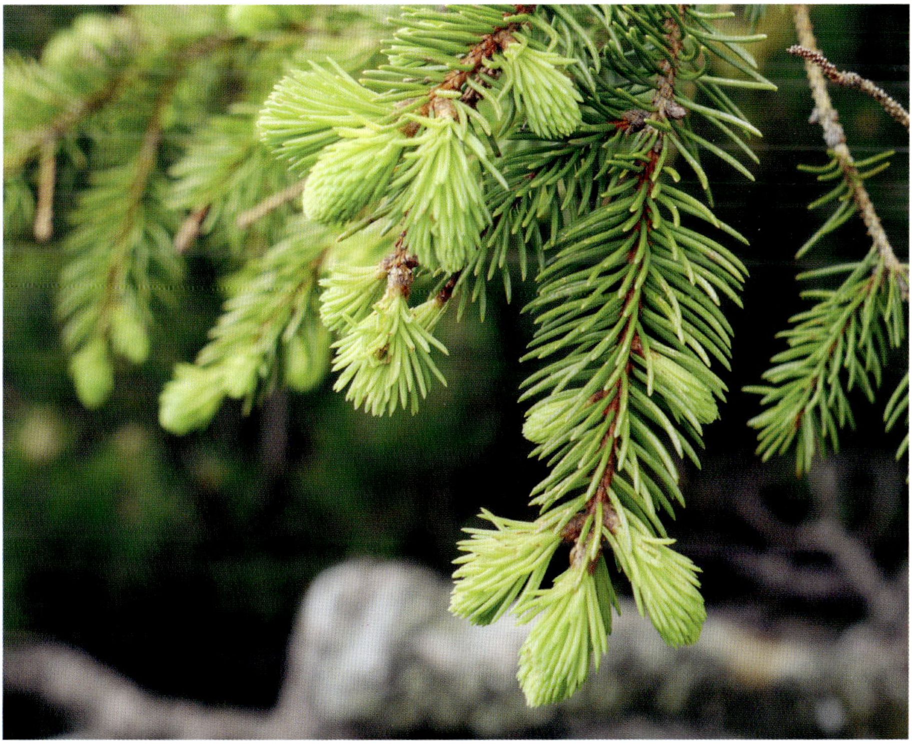

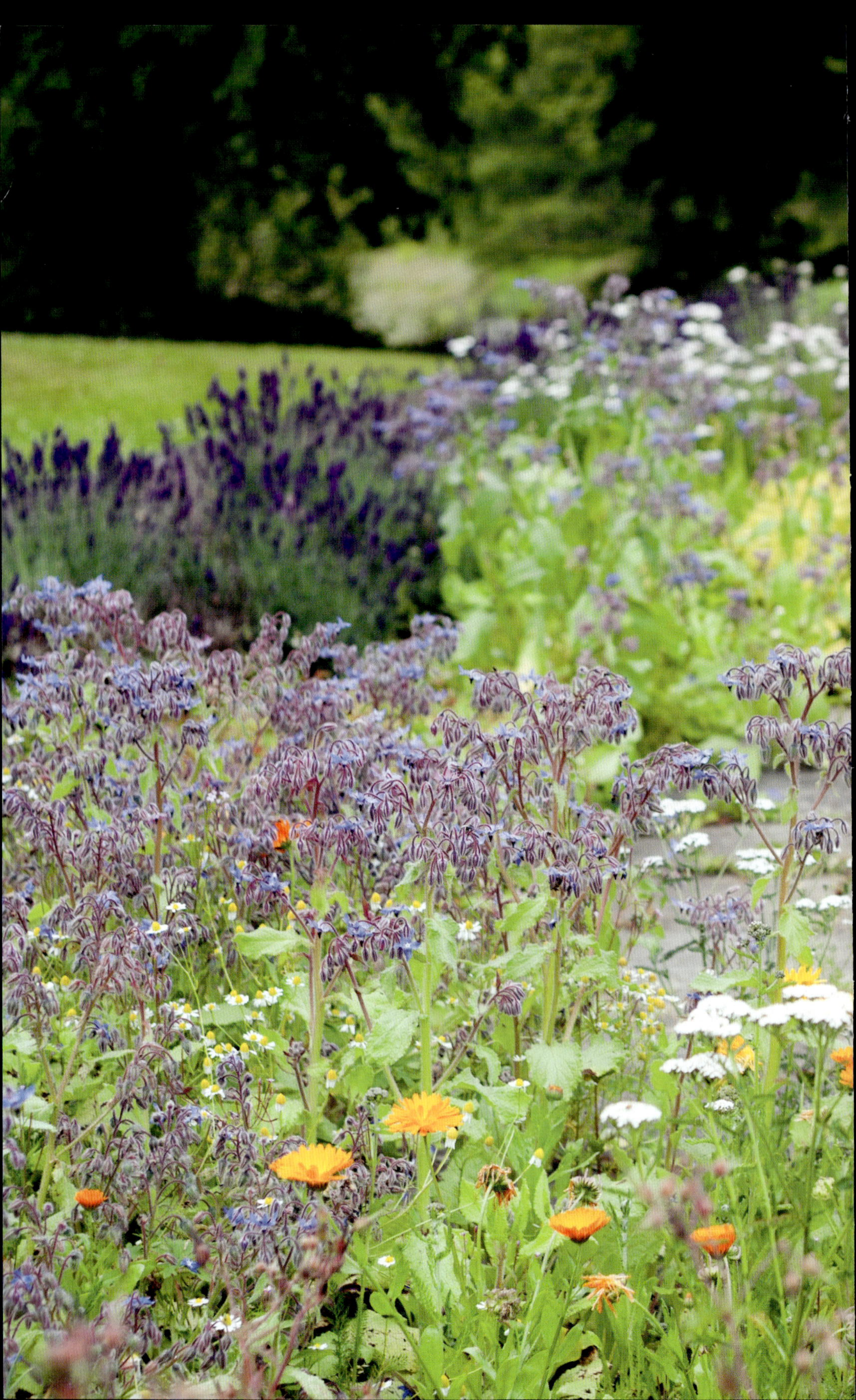

Appendices

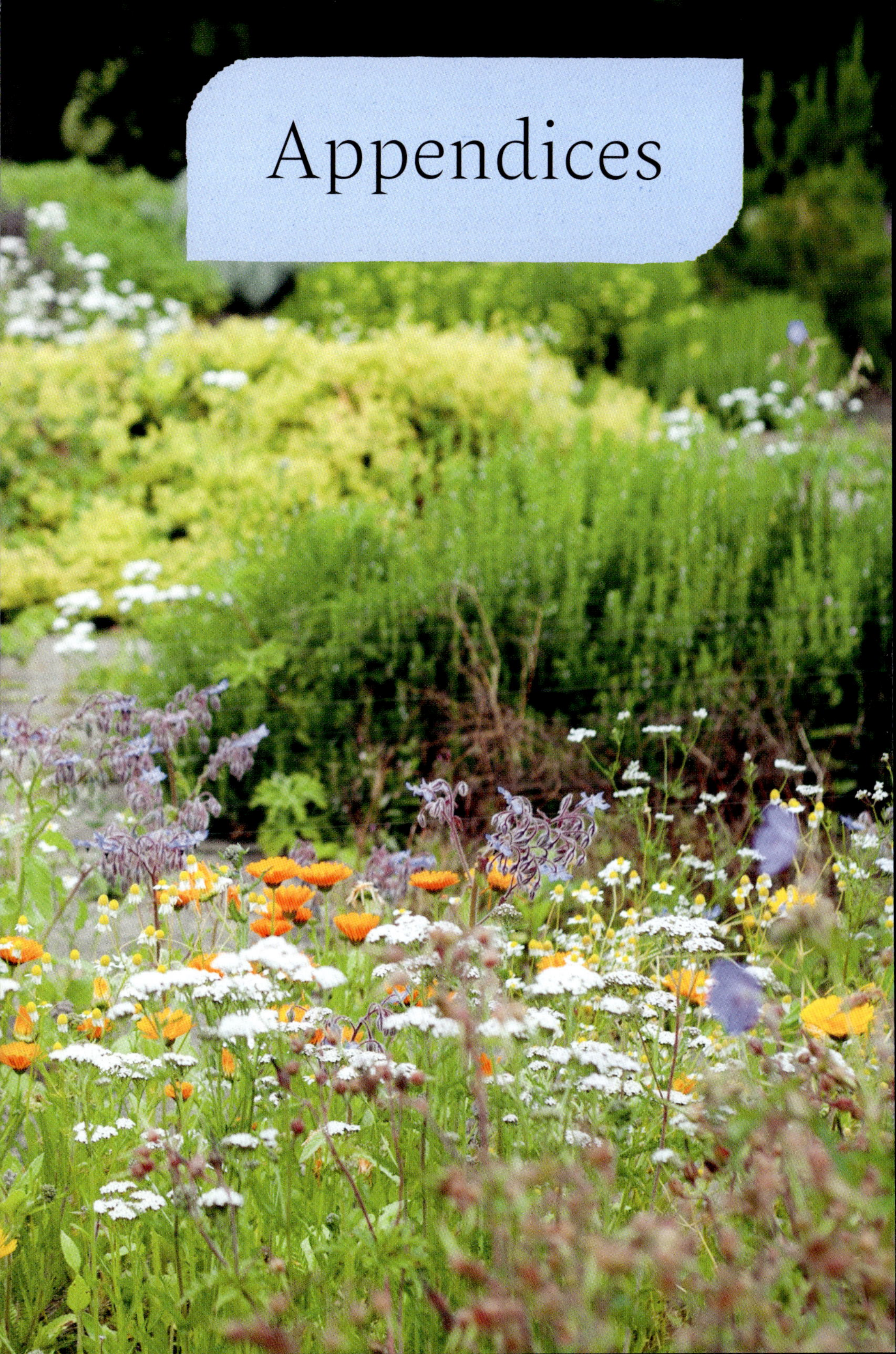

List of common and scientific names of herbs

Most of these common herbs can be grown in the UK. Unless otherwise stated, the harvest times given are for the UK.

Herb	Part used	Harvest	Uses	Page
Andrographis *Andrographis paniculata*	Leaf	When the plant is in bloom	Prevention of colds, treatment of colds, viral or bacterial infections, cold sore, tonsillitis, cystitis and urethritis, aid to recovery from illness	117
Aniseed *Pimpinella anisum*	Seed	When seeds are ripe	Digestive problems, gas, bloating	60–61
Arnica *Arnica montana*	Flower	When flowers are fully open	Bruises, sprains, broken bones, other injuries (if skin is intact), back pain, recovery from strenuous exercise	81
Ashwagandha *Withania somnifera*	Root	Late summer	Adaptogenic herb for improving energy levels, increasing physical stamina, improving mental performance, treating low libido and low mood, aid to recovery from illness and loss of muscle due to illness	180
Astragalus *Astragalus mongholicus* (syn. *Astragalus membranaceus*)	Root	Late summer or autumn	Modulator of immune function, prophylactic for infections (especially viral ones), aid to recovery from illness, treatment of palpitations (after viral infections)	199
Barberry *Berberis vulgaris*	Root and/ or stem bark	Autumn	Modulating the microbiome, treatment of food poisoning, gastritis, diarrhoea, lack of appetite, food intolerances and weak stomach acid	61, 214
Bilberries *Vaccinium myrtillus* **Blueberries** *Vaccinium corymbosum*	Fruit	Summer, when fruits are ripe	Improving microcirculation and eye health, treatment of bruising, nose bleed and erectile dysfunction, aid to healthy ageing	45, 193

Herb	Part used	Harvest	Uses	Page
Birch *Betula pendula* (syn. *Betula alba*)	Leaves, buds	May to July	Arthritis, gout, urinary tract infections (as a diuretic) including cystitis and urethritis	86
Calendula *Calendula officinalis*	See Marigold	See Marigold	See Marigold	135, 212, 214
Celery seed *Apium graveolens*	Fruit	When ripe	Osteoarthritis, rheumatoid arthritis, muscular and rheumatic pains, gout prevention, detoxification, urinary tract infections	84, 162
Chamomile (German) *Matricaria recutita* (syn. *Chamomilla recutita*)	Flower	June to August	Indigestion (especially related to anxiety), stomach ache (especially in children), infant colic, IBS, bloating, nausea, morning sickness, mild diarrhoea, food poisoning, vomiting, lack of appetite, regulating stomach acidity, problems with sleeping, mild anxiety, mouth ulcers, eczema and acne, insect bites, period pain and PMS, tired and/or puffy eyes	57–58, 97, 136, 212
Chilli (cayenne pepper) *Capsicum annuum*	Fruit	When fully ripe	Poor circulation, chilblains, low blood pressure, rheumatic pains	84
Comfrey *Symphytum officinale*	Leaves and flowering stems (avoid first leaves and those produced after early October)	Spring to summer	Injuries, cuts, skin healing, painful and/or swollen joints, sprains, bone fractures, muscular pain (*external treatment only*)	82, 136, 214
Couch grass *Elymus repens* (syn. *Agropyron repens*)	Rhizome	March to May, or September to October	Infections of the urinary tract (cystitis and urethritis)	160
Crampbark (also called guelder rose) *Viburnum opulus*	Bark	No critical time	Muscle relaxant, treatment for high blood pressure, period cramps, muscle spasm and tension, bed wetting	82, 159, 214
Damiana *Turnera diffusa* (syn. *Turnera aphrodisiaca*)	Leaf	When flowering	Mood improver, improves low libido, tonic for male and female reproductive systems	162

Herb	Part used	Harvest	Uses	Page
Dandelion *Taraxacum officinale*	Leaf	April to May	Whenever diuretic action is required (e.g. to treat water retention in PMS)	163, 216, 217
Dandelion *Taraxacum officinale*	Root	Autumn	Improves liver function, stimulates release of bile, digestive aid, treatment for lack of appetite, constipation, low stomach acidity	61, 216, 217
Echinacea (purple coneflower) *Echinacea purpurea* and *Echinacea angustifolia*	Root and aerial parts	Autumn, when in flower	Immune modulator, prevention of colds, treatment of colds, viral and bacterial infections, wound healing, shingles, ear infection, skin problems, recurring episodes of cystitis or thrush, recovery from illness, aid to healthy ageing	115, 137, 160, 194, 198, 214, 216
Elderflower *Sambucus nigra*	Flowers	May to June	Prevention of colds, treatment of colds, flu, viral infections, runny nose, reduction of fever, productive cold, ear infection, hay fever, cold sore and sore throat	112, 212
Elecampane *Inula helenium*	Root	Spring and autumn	Chest infections, cough	118, 214, 216
Evening primrose *Oenothera biennis*	Pressed oil from the seed	When ripe, usually in September or October	PMS	172, 214
Eyebright *Euphrasia* species	Aerial parts when in flower	July to September	Eye irritation or mild infection, stye, conjunctivitis	137, 214
Fennel *Foeniculum vulgare*	Leaves, fruit	Leaves in summer, fruit in autumn	Indigestion, bloating, excess gas, infant colic	62, 215
Garlic *Allium sativum*	Bulb (cloves)	August	Improving circulation, prevention of colds, treatment of colds, viral and bacterial infections, raised blood pressure, high cholesterol levels, food poisoning, diarrhoea, intestinal parasites, sinusitis, runny nose, sore throat, warts, verrucas and thrush, aid to recovery from illness, aid to healthy ageing	43–44, 62–63, 113–114, 194

Herb	Part used	Harvest	Uses	Page
Ginger *Zingiber officinale*	Rhizome	When plants are 10 months old (grown in tropical regions)	Improving circulation, digestive stimulant, treatment of chilblains, low blood pressure, morning sickness, nausea, lack of appetite, muscular pain, common cold	45, 63
Ginkgo *Ginkgo biloba*	Leaf	Early summer	Improving peripheral circulation (including blood supply to the brain), treatment of chilblains, low blood pressure, muscular pain, aid to healthy ageing	44, 193, 214
Green tea *Camellia sinensis*	Leaf	When leaves are young (grown mainly in Asia)	Antioxidant action, aid to healthy ageing	195
Ground ivy *Glechoma hederacea*	Leaves and flowering tops	May	Infections of the respiratory tract, cough	118, 217
Hawthorn *Crataegus monogyna* (common hawthorn) or *Crataegus laevigata* (Midland hawthorn)	Leaves with flowers or berries	May to June, or September to October	Improving functioning of the heart, treatment of poor circulation, high blood pressure, muscular pain, erectile dysfunction, hot flushes, aid to healthy ageing	43, 195, 215
Horse chestnut *Aesculus hippocastanum*	Seed	September	Varicose veins and related leg swelling, haemorrhoids	46
Lavender *Lavandula angustifolia* (syn. *Lavandula officinalis*)	Flower	June to August	Gentle relaxant, treatment of insomnia, non-specific rheumatic and muscular pain, tension headache, back pain, eczema, muscular tension	85, 96–97, 137–138, 212
Lemon balm *Melissa officinalis*	Aerial parts	May to October (before flowering)	Relaxant, digestive aid, treatment of anxiety, panic attacks, insomnia, exam nerves, tension headache, heartburn (stress related), cold sore (external treatment)	63, 98, 213
Lime tree flowers *Tilia cordata*, *Tilia platyphyllos* and *Tilia × europaea*	Flower	Early in flowering period	Relaxant, digestive aid, mood improver, treatment for high blood pressure, high cholesterol levels, stress-induced indigestion, tension headache, fever reduction	46, 98–99, 119, 215

Herb	Part used	Harvest	Uses	Page
Linseed *Linum usitatissimum*	Seed	September	Digestive aid, a source of phytoestrogens, treatment for constipation, diarrhoea, diverticular disease, IBS, gastritis, peptic ulcers, irritation of the digestive tract after gall-bladder removal	64, 215
Liquorice (licorice) *Glycyrrhiza glabra*	Root	Late autumn, when plants are three to four years old (grown in southern Europe)	Treatment for adrenal exhaustion, prolonged stress, emotional fragility, mild depression, nervous exhaustion, digestive problems, diarrhoea, heartburn, stomach ache, cough, chest infection, general anti-inflammatory, aids recovery from illness	65, 99, 119, 181
Korean ginseng *Panax ginseng*	Root	Cultivated in China, Korea and Japan and harvested when plants are 5–6 years old	General tonic, improves libido/ vitality/energy, improves physical performance and stamina, protective against cancer	181, 194
Marigold (calendula, common marigold or pot marigold) *Calendula officinalis*	Flower petals	In full flower, in the middle of the day, from June to September	Skin problems, cuts, grazes, sunburn, heat burns, insect stings, dry lips, various skin rashes, eczema, chilblains, haemorrhoids, mouth ulcers, nappy rash, shingles, acne, fungal infections (including thrush), dandruff, itchy skin and scalp, puffy eyes, stye	135, 212, 214
Marshmallow *Althaea officinalis*	Leaf	June to July	Soothing diuretic, treatment of infections and irritation of the urinary tract, cystitis, urethritis, benign prostatic enlargement, incontinence, bedwetting, heartburn, beneficial after gall-bladder removal	159, 215
Marshmallow *Althaea officinalis*	Root (from plants at least two years old)	Early autumn	Digestive problems, gastritis, heartburn, burning diarrhoea, diverticular disease, peptic ulcer, IBS, inflammatory bowel disease, drawing splinters out	59, 120, 159
Meadowsweet *Filipendula ulmaria*	Aerial parts	June to July (early in flowering period)	Indigestion, any inflammation in the digestive tract, reflux (heartburn), hiatus hernia, stomach over-acidity, recovering from a stomach ulcer, joint or muscle pain	57, 86, 213

Herb	Part used	Harvest	Uses	Page
Milk thistle (St Mary's thistle) *Silybum marianum* (syn. *Carduus marianus*)	Seed	When ripe, autumn	Improves liver function and protects liver from toxicity, improves bile flow (prophylactic against gallstone formation), aids recovery from liver disease	65, 215
Nettle *Urtica dioica*	Leaf	May to June	Allergies, hay fever, eczema, urticaria (hives), gout prevention, detoxifying action	138, 217
Oats (green oats) *Avena sativa*	Green aerial parts	Before seeds ripen	Low mood, mild depression, lack of energy, prolonged stress, nervous exhaustion, anxiety, insomnia	99, 217
Onion *Allium cepa*	Bulb	Autumn	Infections of the respiratory tract, cough, common cold	114
Passionflower *Passiflora incarnata*	Aerial parts	When flowering (grows in hot, sunny countries or in a heated greenhouse)	Relaxant effect on the nervous system, treatment of insomnia, anxiety, exam nerves, neuralgia	100
Peppermint *Mentha × piperita*	Leaf	May to September	Indigestion, bloating, excess wind, IBS, nausea, cooling effect (external application), runny nose (inhalation)	58–59, 86, 213
Raspberry *Rubus idaeus*	Leaf	August to September	Diarrhoea of various causes, stomach bug, IBS	66
Red clover *Trifolium pratense*	Flower	Summer (when flowering)	Detoxifying effect, skin disorders, eczema, acne, psoriasis, menopausal problems	138–139, 217
Ribwort plantain *Plantago lanceolata*	Leaf	May (when flowering)	Skin irritation and/or inflammation, eczema, aids skin healing	139, 217
Rose *Rosa × damascena*, *Rosa gallica* and *Rosa × centifolia*	Petals from newly open flowers	June to July	Mild depression, bereavement, menopausal mood swings	100, 213
Rosemary *Salvia rosmarinus* (syn. *Rosmarinus officinalis*)	Leaf, young twigs	March to October	Muscle relaxant, treatment of muscular pain and tension, poor concentration and memory, tension headache, mild depression, blocked nose, aids recovery from strenuous exercise	83, 97, 213

Herb	Part used	Harvest	Uses	Page
Sage *Salvia officinalis*	Leaf	Just before flowering	Hot flushes, sore throat	120, 163, 213
Saw palmetto *Serenoa repens* (syn. *Serenoa serrulata*)	Fruit	Autumn (grows in North America)	Benign prostatic hypertrophy (enlargement), male urethritis, orchitis	161
Shepherd's purse *Capsella bursa-pastoris*	Aerial parts	April to June	Heavy periods, weak uterine tone or prolapse, incontinence	163, 217
Siberian ginseng *Eleutherococcus senticosus*	Root	Autumn (grows in eastern Russia, China, Korea and Japan)	Adaptogen, all-round tonic, improves mental and physical performance and stamina, resilience to stress, energy levels, recovery from illness	180
St John's wort *Hypericum perforatum*	Aerial parts	During flowering	Mild to moderate depression, post-viral depression and fatigue, menopausal mood swings, injury to nervous tissue, neuralgia, common cold (treatment and recovery), ear infection (infused oil), psoriasis (infused oil), menopausal low mood, recovery from illness	100–101, 121, 214
Tea tree *Melaleuca alternifolia*	Leaf	All year round (grows in Australia)	Antiseptic for external use, fungal or bacterial skin infections, sinusitis, acne, drawing out splinters and boils	139–140
Thyme *Thymus vulgaris*	Leaf and flower	April to September	Chest infections, dry cough, blocked nose, fungal and bacterial skin infections, sunburn, a variety of itchy skin conditions, urinary tract infections, thrush	121, 136, 160–161, 213
Turmeric *Curcuma longa*	Rhizome	Winter (grown in South Asia)	General anti-inflammatory (especially for chronic, low-grade inflammation), reduces blood clotting, treatment of osteoarthritis, rheumatoid arthritis, back pain, muscle pain	87

Herb	Part used	Harvest	Uses	Page
Valerian *Valeriana officinalis*	Root	September to October	Relaxant effect on the nervous system, supports coping with stress, treatment of raised pulse rate, heart palpitations caused by stress, mildly raised blood pressure, anxiety, panic attacks, insomnia, exam nerves, nervous indigestion, irritability, PMS, tension headache, period pain, ear ache	47, 96, 215, 216
Vervain *Verbena officinalis*	Aerial parts	Early stages of flowering	Relaxant, antidepressant, treatment of stress, irritability, low energy, menopausal mood swings, aids recovery from illness	101, 217
White deadnettle *Lamium album*	Flowering tops	April to July	Vaginal discharge, thrush	164, 217
Wild yam *Dioscorea villosa*	Rhizome	Autumn (grown in sunny regions, both tropical and temperate)	Osteoarthritis, rheumatoid arthritis, joint pain associated with the menopause, other menopausal symptoms (e.g. hot flushes)	87, 164
Willow *Salix alba* (white willow) and *Salix purpurea* (purple willow)	Bark from two- to five-year-old trees	April to May	Any type of arthritis, inflammation of the joints, muscle ache (especially if secondary to joint ache), muscle tension, tension headache, backache	83
Wintergreen *Gaultheria procumbens*	Leaf	Leaves may be collected at any time (for essential oil only)	Joint ache, back pain (external treatment)	87, 215
Witch hazel *Hamamelis virginiana*	Leaf, bark	Autumn	Diarrhoea, haemorrhoids	66, 215
Yarrow *Achillea millefolium*	Aerial parts	Late summer, when in full flower	Poor circulation, chilblains, nosebleeds, bruising easily, varicose veins, bleeding haemorrhoids, heavy periods, bleeding cuts, elevated blood pressure, muscular pain, aid to digestion	47, 161, 217
Yellow dock (curled dock) *Rumex crispus*	Root	October	Detoxifier, treatment for constipation, eczema, acne, psoriasis	140, 216

Glossary

Adaptogen – helps the body to cope with physical or mental stress

Adrenal tonic – improves the function of the adrenal glands (which regulate the body's responses to stress and can become exhausted by prolonged stress)

Anaesthetic, local – brings about a reversible numbness in a part of the body or skin

Analgesic – relieves pain

Antacid – neutralises acidity in the stomach

Anti-allergic – reduces the intensity or frequency of allergic reactions

Anti-anxiety – reduces the symptoms of anxiety, and has a relaxant effect on the nervous system

Anti-arthritic – reduces joint inflammation

Antibacterial – destroys bacteria or inhibits their growth

Anti-catarrhal – reduces catarrh (the accumulation of mucus or phlegm in the airways)

Anticoagulant – prevents the formation of blood clots

Antidepressant – alleviates depression

Anti-diarrhoeal – stops diarrhoea

Antifungal – destroys fungi or inhibits their growth

Anti-inflammatory – reduces inflammation

Anti-irritant – reduces local surface inflammation (internal or external)

Antimicrobial – destroys micro-organisms or inhibits their growth (this term is usually used when referring to internal use; see also 'Antiseptic')

Antioxidant – capable of slowing down or preventing the damaging effects of oxidation and free radicals

Anti-platelet – reduces the clumping together of platelets (small blood cells that play a part in the formation of blood clots)

Anti-rheumatic – alleviates rheumatic complaints

Antiseptic – destroys microorganisms or inhibits their growth (this term is usually used when referring to external use; see also 'Antimicrobial')

Antiviral – inhibits virus replication or destroys viruses

Aphrodisiac – stimulates the libido or sex drive

Astringent – causes shrinkage of mucous membranes or exposed tissues, thus creating a surface barrier

Bitter (tonic) – stimulates the whole of the digestive system through its bitter taste in the mouth

Carminative – alleviates flatulence (excessive gas) and relieves bowel spasms

Circulatory stimulant – improves the circulation of the blood, either to specific parts of the body or to all tissues

Cooling – reduces the sensation of feeling hot, either of a particular body part or of the whole body

Demulcent – reduces irritation and has a soothing effect on the mucous membranes of the digestive, respiratory and urinary systems

Detoxifying – improves the elimination of metabolic waste from the body (the terms 'depurative', 'blood purifying' or 'alterative' have been used in the past)

Digestive – improves or stimulates the digestion

Disinfectant – capable of destroying microorganisms on contact; in connection with living tissue the term 'antiseptic' is normally used

Diuretic – increases the production of urine

Expectorant – improves the clearing of excess mucus from the airways

Healing – stimulates tissue repair

Immune modulator – balances the functioning of the immune system

Immune stimulant – stimulates the activity of a particular set of immune system cells

Laxative – induces a bowel movement or loosens the stool

Male tonic – improves the function of the male reproductive system

Mucous membrane restorative – facilitates the repair of damaged or inflamed mucous membrane

Relaxant, muscle – decreases the tone of muscles, especially if the muscles are in spasm

Relaxant, nerve – has a calming effect on the nervous system

Restorative – restores optimal function to a body organ or tissue

Sedative – reduces nervous tension, in order to relieve anxiety or induce sleep

Stimulant – increases the activity of a particular organ or system, or of the whole body

Tonic – improves the function and vigour of a particular organ or system, or of the whole body

Warming – increases the sensation of feeling warm, either of a particular body part or of the whole body

Endnotes

1 Zbiorowe, O. (2001). *Ziołolecznictwo Amazońskie i Andyjskie*. Edited by K. Zurowskiej. Tower Press.

Kujawska, M. and Albán-Castillo, J. (2025). Wild-grown medicinal plants used by the Asháninka people from the Tambo River, Peruvian Amazonia. *Journal of Ethnopharmacology*. 337(3): ePub.

Shepard Jr, G.H. and Daly, L. (2023). Sensory Ecology, Bioeconomy, and the Age of COVID: A Parallax View of Indigenous and Scientific Knowledge. *Top Cogn Sci*. 15 (3): 584–607.

2 Anghelescu, I.G., Kohnen, R., Szegedi, A., Klement, S. and Kieser, M. (2006). Comparison of Hypericum extract WS 5570 and paroxetine in ongoing treatment after recovery from an episode of moderate to severe depression: results from a randomized multicenter study. *Pharmacopsychiatry*. 39(6): 213–19.

Brenner, R., Azbel, V., Madhusoodanan, S. and Pawlowska, M. (2000). Comparison of an extract of hypericum (LI 160) and sertraline in the treatment of depression: a double-blind, randomized pilot study. *Comp Clin Ther*. 22(4): 411–19.

Gastpar, M., Singer, A. and Zeller, K. (2006). Comparative efficacy and safety of a once-daily dosage of Hypericum extract STW3-VI and citalopram in patients with moderate depression: a double-blind, randomised, multicentre, placebo-controlled study. *Pharmacopsychiatry*. 39(2): 66–75.

Schrader, E. (2000). Equivalence of St John's wort extract (Ze 117) and fluoxetine: a randomized, controlled study in mild-moderate depression. *Int Clin Psychopharmacol*. 15(2): 61–68.

3 Omale, S., Amagon, K.I., Johnson, T.O., Bremner, S.K., Gould, G.W. (2023 Jan); A systematic analysis of anti-diabetic medicinal plants from cells to clinical trials. *PeerJ eCollection 2023*.

Alhazmi, H.A., Najmi, A., Javed, S.A., Sultana, S., Al Bratty, M., Makeen, H.A., Meraya, A.M., Ahsan, W., Mohan, S., Taha, M.M.E., Khalid, A. (2021 May). Medicinal Plants and Isolated Molecules Demonstrating Immunomodulation Activity as Potential Alternative Therapies for Viral Diseases Including COVID-19. *Front Immunol eCollection 2021*.

Choe, J., Har Yong, P., Xiang Ng, Z. (2022 Nov); The Efficacy of Traditional Medicinal Plants in Modulating the Main Protease of SARS-CoV-2 and Cytokine Storm. *Chem Biodivers*.

Holubarsch, C.J., Colucci, W.S., Meinertz, T., Gaus, W., Tendera, M.

(2000 Dec); Survival and prognosis: investigation of Crataegus extract WS 1442 in congestive heart failure (SPICE) – rationale, study design and study protocol. *Eur J Heart Fail.*

Ng, Q.X., Venkatanarayanan, N., Ho, C.Y.J. (2017 Mar) Clinical use of Hypericum perforatum (St John's wort) in depression: A meta-analysis. *Affect Disor.*

Beer, A.M. and Wegener, T. (2008). Randomised, double-blind, placebo-controlled clinical study of the effectiveness of willow extract. *Phytomedicine* 15(11): 907–13.

Cui, Y., Shu, X.O., Gao, Y.T. *et al.* (2006). Korean ginseng and breast cancer survival. *Am J Epidemiol* 163(7): 645–53.

Daniele, C., Mazzanti, G., Pittler, M.H. *et al.* (2006). Adverse event profile of *Crataegus* spp.: a systematic review. *Drug Safety* 29(6): 523–35.

El-Kamary, S., Shardell, M., Metwally, M. *et al.* (2007). Randomised, double-blind, placebo-controlled clinical study on the efficacy of milk thistle in recovery from acute hepatitis. *Am J Trop Med Hyg* 77(5): 210.

Holubarsch, C.J., Colucci, W.S., Meinertz, T. *et al.* (2008). Randomised, double-blind, placebo-controlled study of the effectiveness of hawthorn in heart failure patients. *Eur J Heart Fail* 10(12): 1255–63.

Koo, H., Gomes, B.P., Rosalen, P.L., Ambrosano, G.M., Park, Y.K. and Cury, J.A. (2000). In vitro antimicrobial activity of propolis and Arnica Montana against oral pathogens. *Arch Oral Biol* 45(2): 141–48.

Muller, S.F. and Klement, S. (2006). Uncontrolled study of valerian/lemon balm for the treatment of restlessness and dyssomnia in children. *Phytomedicine* 13(6): 383–87.

Ozan, F., Sümer, Z., Polat, Z.A., Er, K., Ozan, U. and Değer, O. (2007). Effects of mouth rinse containing propolis on oral microorganisms and human gingival fibroblasts. *Eur J Dent* 1(4): 195–201.

Paulsen, E. (2002). Contact sensitization from Compositae-containing herbal remedies and cosmetics. *Contact Dermatitis* 47(4): 189–98.

Rouhi, H. and Ganji, F. (2007). Randomised, double-blind, placebo-controlled clinical study on the effectiveness of marshmallow extract and ACE inhibitor cough. *Pakistan J Nutr* 6(3): 256–58.

Sobenin, I.A., Andrianova, I.V., Demidova, O.N. *et al.* (2008). Randomised, double-blind, placebo-controlled clinical study of the lipid-lowering effects of garlic powder tablets. *J Atheroscler Thromb* 15(6): 334–38.

Suh, S.O, Kroh, M., Kim, N.R. *et al.* (2002). Korean ginseng and survival of patients with gastric carcinoma. *Am J Chin Med* 30(4): 483–94.

Teschke, R. and Schwarzenboek, A. (2009). Critical analysis of suspected adverse reactions to Cimicifuga racemosa. *Phytomedicine* 16(1): 72–84.

4 Zhang, Z.X., Wu, L.L. and Chen, M. (2009 Jun). Effect of lixu jieyu recipe in treating 75 patients with chronic fatigue syndrome. Randomized clinical trial 29(6): 501–05.

Chen, Y., Zhang, C., Feng, Y.J. (2024 May 23); Medicinal plants for the management of post-COVID-19 fatigue: A literature review on the role and mechanisms. *J Tradit Complement Med.* 15(1): 15-23.

Melrose, J., Smith, M.M. (Elite Ed). 2022 Oct 9). Natural and Semi-Synthetic Flavonoid Anti-SARS-CoV-2 Agents for the Treatment of Long COVID-19 Disease and Neurodegenerative Disorders of Cognitive Decline. *Front Biosci.* 14(4): 27.

Tokumasu, K., Ueda, K., Honda, H., Sunada, N., Sakurada, Y., Matsuda, Y., Nakano, Y., Hasegawa, T., Otsuka, Y., Obika, M., Hagiya, H., Kataoka, H., Otsuka, F. (2022 May) Application of Kampo Medicines for Treatment of General Fatigue Due to Long COVID. *Medicina (Kaunas).* 58(6): 730.

See, D.M., Broumand, N., Sahl, L. Tilles, J.C. (1997 Jan); In vitro effects of echinacea and ginseng on natural killer and antibody-dependent cell cytotoxicity in healthy subjects and chronic fatigue syndrome or acquired immunodeficiency syndrome patients. *Immunopharmacology.* 35(3): 229–35.

Redman, D.A. (2000 Dec); Ruscus aculeatus (butcher's broom) as a potential treatment for orthostatic hypotension, with a case report. *J Altern Complement Med.* 6(6): 539–49.

5 Zakay-Rones, Z., Thom, E., Wollan, T. and Wadstein, J. (2004). Randomized study of the efficacy and safety of oral elderberry extract in the treatment of influenza A and B virus infections. *J Int Med Res.* 32(2): 132–40.

Zakay-Rones, Z., Varsano, N., Zlotnik, M., Manor, O., Regev, L., Schlesinger, M. and Mumcuoglu, M. (1995). Inhibition of several strains of influenza virus in vitro and reduction of symptoms by an elderberry extract (Sambucus nigra L.) during an outbreak of influenza B Panama. *J Altern Complement Med.* 1(4): 361–69.

Młynarczyk, K., Walkowiak-Tomczak, D. and Łysiak, G.P. (2018). Bioactive properties of Sambucus nigra L. as a functional ingredient for food and pharmaceutical industry. *Journl of Functional Foods.* 40: 377–90.

Ho, G.T.T., Wangensteen, H. and Barsett, H. (2017). Elderberry and Elderflower Extracts, Phenolic Compounds, and Metabolites and Their Effect on Complement, RAW 264.7 Macrophages and Dendritic Cells. *Int J Mol Sci.* 18(3): 584.

Boroduske, A, Jekabsons, K, Riekstina, U, Muceniece, R, Rostoks, N. and Nakurte, I. (2021). Wild Sambucus nigra L. from north-east edge of the species range: A valuable germplasm with inhibitory capacity against SARS-CoV2 S-protein RBD and hACE2 binding in vitro. *Ind Crops Prod.* 165: ePub.

6 Mills, S. and Bone, K. (2005). *The Essential Guide to Herbal Safety.* Elsevier Churchill Livingstone.

7 Priest, A.W. and Priest, L.R. (2000). *Herbal Medication, A clinical and dispensary book.* The C.W. Daniel Company.

8 Bone, K. (2007). *The Ultimate Herbal Compendium: a desktop guide for herbal prescribers.* Phytotherapy Press.

9 Tsai, T.Y., Wang, S.H., Lee, Y.K. and Su, Y.C. (2018). Ginkgo biloba extract for prevention of acute mountain sickness: a systematic review and meta-analysis of randomised controlled trials. *BMJ Open.* 8(8): ePub.

Moraga, F.A., Flores, A., Serra, J., Esnaola, C. and Barriento, C. (2007). Ginkgo biloba decreases acute mountain sickness in people ascending to high altitude at Ollagüe (3696 m) in northern Chile. *Wilderness Environ Med.* 18(4): 251–57.

Leadbetter, G., Keyes, L.E., Maakestad, K.M., Olson, S., Tissot van Patot, M.C. and Hackett, P.H. (2009). Ginkgo biloba does – and does not – prevent acute mountain sickness. *Wilderness Environ Med*. 20(1): 66–71.

10 Bosch-Morell, F., Villagrasa, V., Ortega, T., Acero, N., Muñoz-Mingarro, D., González-Rosende, M.E., Castillo, E., Sanahuja, M.A., Soriano, P. and Martínez-Solís, I. (2020). Medicinal plants and natural products as neuroprotective agents in age-related macular degeneration. *I.Neural Regen Res*. 15(12): 2207–16.

Li, R., Ye, Z., Yang, W., Xu, Y.J., Tan, C.P. and Liu, Y. (2022). Blueberry Anthocyanins from Commercial Products: Structure Identification and Potential for Diabetic Retinopathy Amelioration. *Molecules*. 27(21): 7475.

Liu, Y., Liu, M., Chen, Q., Liu, G.M., Cao, M.J., Sun, L., Lu, Z. and Guo, C. (2018). Blueberry Polyphenols Ameliorate Visible Light and Lipid-Induced Injury of Retinal Pigment Epithelial Cells. *J Agric Food Chem*. 66(48): 12730–40.

11 Fearnley-Whittingstall, H. (2024). *How to Eat 30 Plants a Week*. Bloomsbury Publishing.

12 Li, Z,. Li, X., Cai, Z., Jin, G., Ahn, D.U. and Huang, X. (2022). Immunomodulatory effects of chicken soups prepared with the native cage-free chickens and the commercial caged broilers. *Poult Sci*. 101(10): ePub.

Brown, L. K., Miller, A. and Miller, E. (2020). Chicken soup for the treatment of respiratory infections. *E.Chest*. 158(5): 2231–32.

Hopkins, A.B. (2003). Chicken soup cure may not be a myth. *Nurse Pract*. 28(6): 16.

Jackson, P.M. (1994). Chicken soup. *Wis Med J*. 93(1): 3.

Jefferson, T. (2002). Advances in the diagnosis and management of influenza. *Curr Infect Dis Rep*. 4(3): 206–10.

Ohry, A. and Tsafrir, J. (1999). Is chicken soup an essential drug? *CMAJ*. 161(12): 1532–33.

Rennard, B.O., Ertl, R.F., Gossman, G.L., Robbins, R.A. and Rennard, S.I. (2000). Chicken soup inhibits neutrophil chemotaxis in vitro. *Chest*. 118(4): 1150–57.

Saketkhoo, K., Januszkiewicz, A. and Sackner, M.A. (1978). Effect of drinking hot water, cold water, and chicken soup on nasal mucus velocity and nasal airflow resistance. *Chest*. 74(4): 408–10.

13 Ross, S.M. (2016). Echinacea purpurea: a proprietary extract of Echinacea purpurea is shown to be safe and effective in the prevention of the common cold. *Holistic Nursing Practice*. 30(1): 54–57.

Ogal, M., Johnston, S.L., Klein, P. and Schoop, R. (2021). Echinacea reduces antibiotic usage in children through respiratory tract infection prevention: a randomized, blinded, controlled clinical trial. *Eur J Med Res*. 26(1): 33.

Mathias, A., Penman, K.G., Matovic, N.J., Bone, K.M., De Voss, J.J. and Lehmann, R.P. (2005). Bioavailability of Echinacea constituents: Caco-2 monolayers and pharmacokinetics of the alkylamides and caffeic acid conjugates. *Molecules*. 10 (10): 1242–51.

Miller, S.C. (2005). Echinacea: a miracle herb against aging and cancer? Evidence in vivo in mice. *Evid Based Complement Alternat Med.* 2 (3): 309–14.

Raduner, S., Majewska, A., Chen, J.Z., Xie, X.Q., Hamon, J., Faller, B., Altmann, K.H. and Gertsch, J. (2006). Alkylamides from Echinacea are a new class of cannabinomimetics. *J Biol Chem.* 281(20): 14192–206.

Shah, S.A., Sander, S., White, C.M., Rinaldi, M. and Coleman, C.I. (2007). Evaluation of echinacea for the prevention and treatment of the common cold: a meta-analysis. *Lancet Infect Dis.* 7(7): 473–80.

Stevenson, L.M., Matthias, A., Banbury, L., Penman, K.G., Bone, K.M., Leach, D. and Lehmann, R.P. (2005). Modulation of the immune responses of macrophages by echinacea alkyl amides. *Molecules.* 10(10): 1279–85.

14 Beasley, R., Clayton, T., Crane, J., Von Mutius, E., Lai, C.K.W., Montefort, S., Stewart, A. and the ISAAC Phase Three Study Group (2008). Association between paracetamol use in infancy and childhood, and risk of asthma, rhinoconjunctivitis, and eczema in children aged 6–7 years: analysis from Phase Three of the ISAAC programme. *The Lancet.* 372(9643): 1039–48.

15 Barak, V., Birkenfeld, S., Halperin, T. and Kalickman, I. (2002). The effect of herbal remedies on the production of human inflammatory and anti-inflammatory cytokines. *Isr Med Assoc J.* 4(11 suppl): 919–22.

Sun, J., Madan, R., Karp, C.L. and Braciale, T.J. (2009). Effector T cells control lung inflammation during acute influenza virus infection by producing IL-10. *Nat Med.* 15(3): 277–84.

Zambon, M.C. (2001). The pathogenesis of influenza in humans. *Rev Med Virol.* 11(4): 227–41.

Zhai, Z., Liu, Y., Wu, L., Senchina, D.S., Wurtele, E.S., Murphy, P.A., Kohut, M.L. and Cunnick, J.E. (2007). Enhancement of innate and adaptive immune functions by multiple Echinacea species. *J Med Food.* 10(3): 423–34.

16 Leeuwendaal, N.K, Stanton C., O'Toole P.W., Beresford T.P. (2022). Fermented Foods, Health and the Gut Microbiome. *Nutrients.* 14(7):1527.

Park, K.Y., Jeong, J.K, Lee, Y.E. (2014). Health benefits of kimchi (Korean fermented vegetables) as a probiotic food. *J Med Food.* 17(1): 6–20.

Useful resources

Recommended reading

Barker, J. (2001). *The Medicinal Flora of Britain and Northwest Europe.* Winter Press.

Bartram, T. (2002). *Bartram's Encyclopedia of Herbal Medicine.* Da Capo Press.

Bone, K. (2007). *The Ultimate Herbal Compendium.* Phytotherapy Press.

Bone, K. (2021) *Functional Herbal Therapy: A Modern Paradigm for Clinicians.* Aeon Books Ltd.

Bradley, P. (2006). *British Herbal Compendium. Vol 2: A Handbook of Scientific Information on Widely Used Plant Drugs.* British Herbal Medical Association.

British Herbal Medical Association (1983) *British Herbal Pharmacopeia.* British Herbal Medical Association.

Mills, S. and Bone, K. (2005). *The Essential Guide to Herbal Safety.* Churchill Livingstone.

Mills, S. and Bone, K. (2013). *Principles and Practice of Phytotherapy*, 2nd edition. Elsevier Churchill Livingstone.

Ody, P. (1995). *Home Herbal.* Macmillan Canada.

Pole, S. *Ayurvedic Medicine: The Principles of Traditional Practice.* Singing Dragon (15 Sept. 2012)

Thomsen, M. (2022). *Phytotherapy Desk Reference*, 6th edition. Aeon Books

Trickey, R. and Cooke, K. (2001). *Women's Trouble.* Allen & Unwin.

Trickey, R. and Cooke, K. (2002). *Menopause.* Allen & Unwin.

Websites

bmj.com – shares medical research

nature.com – scientific and medical papers

ncbi.nlm.nih.gov – a free digital archive of biomedical and life sciences journal literature

thelancet.com – scientific and medical papers

newvitalitytuition.com – free online course on using medicinal plants for self-treatment

herbalreality.com – a free educational website that aims to share traditional, scientific and practical insights into herbal medicine

Suppliers

The following are UK-based retailers, mail-order suppliers of herbs, and trade and practitioner suppliers.

Avicenna Herbs
avicennaherbs.co.uk
Supplies high-quality herbal tinctures and a large selection of aromatic waters. Sales to practitioners only.

BeeVital
beevitalpropolis.com
Sells high-quality propolis products online.

G. Baldwin & Co.
baldwins.co.uk
Stocks a large selection of good-quality herbal products. Sales online.

Granary Herbs Ltd
granaryherbs.co.uk
Specialist in high-quality tinctures made from fresh native herbs. Sales mainly to practitioners, but a small selection of products are available online.

Herbs in a Bottle
herbsinabottle.com
Sells a wide range of herbal products. Sales to practitioners and retail only.

Lamberts Healthcare Ltd
lambertshealth care.co.uk
Supplies good-quality herbal tablets and capsules. Sales to health professionals and general public.

Mediherb
mediherb.co.uk
Sells the highest-quality herbal tinctures and tablets. Sales to practitioners only.

Napiers
napiers.net
A long-established herbal clinic in Edinburgh, with many other clinics and shops in Scotland, and online sales of high-quality herbal preparations.

Neal's Yard Remedies
nealsyardremedies.com
A chain of retailers selling herbal products and natural cosmetics. Branches in most UK cities and an online shop.

Organic Herb Trading Company
organicherbtrading.com
Supplies a wide range of organically sourced herbs to practitioners and retail only.

Panacea
panaceahealthonline.com
Supplies a wide range of herbal supplements to practitioners only.

Phyto Products Ltd
phyto.uk
Supplies a wide range of herbal preparations. Sales to practitioner only.

Pukka Herbs
pukkaherbs.com
High-quality organic herbal teas often based on ayurvedic herbs, available directly online and in many supermarkets.

Rutland Biodynamics Ltd
rutlandbio.com
Biodynamic growers and manufacturers of a wide range of high-quality herbal products. Sales to practitioners, clinics and retail only.

Weleda (UK) Ltd
weleda.co.uk
Stocks a good selection of herbal creams and ointments.

Herb nurseries

Jekka's Herb Farm
jekkas.com
The UK's leading organic herb grower, with a very wide selection of medicinal herbs and seeds.

The National Herb Centre
herbcentre.co.uk
Supplies a good selection of medicinal and culinary plants.

Poyntzfield Herb Nursery
poyntzfieldherbs.co.uk
Stocks a good variety of native medicinal herbs, as well as unusual Asian species.

Organisations

The following are organisations and registers of professional herbalists in the UK:

College of Practitioners of Phytotherapy (CPP)
thecpp.uk
An organisation with a strong scientific and evidence base bias; runs a register of practitioners in the UK and abroad.

National Institute of Medical Herbalists (NIMH)
nimh.org.uk
The oldest herbalist organisation in the UK; runs a register of practitioners.

British Herbal Medical Association (BHMA)
bhma.info
An organisation that fosters research into herbal medicine. Members include growers, manufacturers and academics.

The Herb Society
herbsociety.org.uk
An educational charity that encourages the use of herbs, and organises many talks and events for the general public on herbs.

European Herbal and Traditional Medicine Practitioners Association (EHTPA)
ehtpa.org
An umbrella body that represents professional associations of herbal/traditional medicine practitioners.

Below A beautiful herb garden.

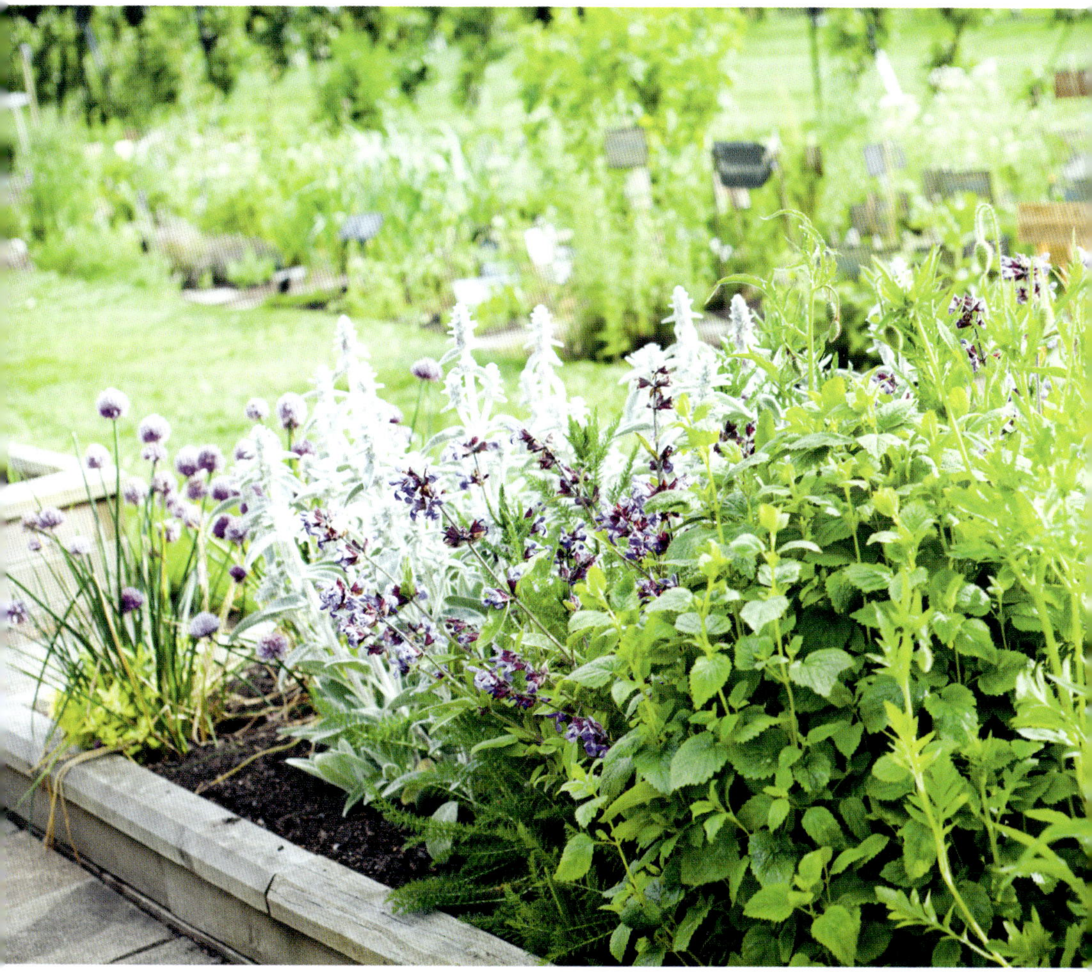

Acknowledgements

Author's acknowledgements

I would like to thank the following people: all of my patients who appreciated the value of herbal medicine and put trust in my treatment; Katie, my best young patient, who took herbal medicine although it was 'yuck'; Diana, my oldest patient who said she would sulk for the rest of her life if I retired; all my teachers of herbal medicine, who inspired me for life; my herbalist colleagues, who shared their experience; my family, for being willing to try my unusual cures; my mother, for introducing herbs into my life; my father, for instilling a dose of healthy scepticism in me towards science and non-science alike; my husband Richard, for his encouragement and advice at every stage of the production of this new edition; Monica French, for her stylistic advice; Heather Bradbury and Jenny Campbell, my editors, for the meticulous improvements to the book; Austin Taylor, for his brilliant design; Ewa Trojanowska, for the design of icons; Jo Hargreaves, my copy editor, for her amazing attention to detail; Amanda Keyte for the cover; Jacky Ferneyhough for the proofread and index, and the whole team at Green Books, Bloomsbury Publishing for their contributions to the final product.

Photo credits

Bloomsbury Publishing would like to thank the following for providing photographs and for permission to reproduce copyright material. While every effort has been made to trace and acknowledge all copyright holders, we would like to apologise for any errors or omissions and invite readers to inform us so that corrections can be made in any future editions of the book.

With the exceptions of the photographs listed on the page numbers below, all photographs in this book (including the cover) remain © Anna Newton.

Key:
SS = Shutterstock, G = Getty, A = Alamy, iS = iStock, T = Top, M = Middle, B = Bottom, L = Left, R = Right.

Front cover: G/Ivan Bajic.
Back cover: Top: SS/Madeleine Steinbach; Middle: G/Madeleine_Steinbach; Bottom: G/Madeleine Steinbach.

2: iS/MelanieMaya; 3–4: A/Connect Images; 8: SS/marcin jucha; 10: SS/Susann Guenther; 11: G/ivstiv; 12–13: SS/pixfix; 15: SS/Daisy Daisy; 18: SS/Luis Raul Torres; 19: SS/Plateresca; 21: SS/Madeleine Steinbach; 22: SS/Chuta

Kooanantkul; 23: SS/cherryyblossom; 24: SS/pixfix; 25: SS/Wirestock Creators; 28T: SS/dajingjing; 28B: SS/Luis Echeverri Urrea; 29: SS/Marie Luce; 30: SS/Heike Rau; 32: G/Alex Potemkin; 33: iS/AscentXmedia; 34: iS/RyanJLane; 35: SS/rsooll; 36: SS/Tatevosian Yana; 39: SS/White bear studio; 40–41: A/ Natallia Khlapushyna; 45R: SS/grafvison; 46L: SS/Aleksei Voronov; 48: SS/Brent Hofacker; 49: SS/OKcamera; 51: SS/ images72; 52: G/EMS-FORSTER-PRODUCTIONS; 53: SS/Madeleine Steinbach; 55: SS/iMarzi; 58L: SS/ NicoletteWollentin; 60L: SS/1989studio; 60R: SS/spline_x; 61L: SS/weha; 61R: SS/Madeleine Steinbach; 62: SS/ MaRee22; 63L: SS/Photoongraphy; 63R: SS/milart; 64: SS/Halil Ibrahim mescioglu; 65: SS/Iker Zabaleta; 66R: SS/ LianeM; 67: SS/DZiegler; 69: G/13-Smile; 70: SS/itor; 71: G/Anna Blazhuk; 73: SS/Tolikoff Photography; 74: SS/ Feyyaz Alacam; 75: iS/istockexstock; 76: SS/KieferPix; 78: SS/Nitr; 81: SS/ hadot 760; 84: SS/Fabrizio Guarisco; 86R: SS/Ihor Hvozdetskyi; 87: SS/ Nahhana; 88: SS/grafvision; 89: SS/ Madeleine Steinbach; 90: G/elenaleonova; 92: G/Anastasiia Krivenok; 94: SS/ DimaBerlin; 95: SS/Taras Grebinets; 98: SS/Melica; 100: SS/decoplus; 102: SS/JPC-PROD; 104: SS/Mykolal Mykolal; 105: SS/Pedal to the Stock; 107: SS/New Africa; 108: SS/Madeleine Steinbach; 110: SS/RBagusdiani; 113: SS/Esin Deniz; 114: SS/Peter Turner Photography; 117: SS/Karnwela; 119: SS/Kabar; 112: SS/antoniodiaz; 123: SS/Nenadmil; 124: SS/oneinchpunch; 127: SS/Cultura Creative; 128: SS/ Madeleine Steinbach; 130: SS/ monshtadoid; 131: SS/amberto4ka; 132: SS/Prostock-studio; 140: SS/Henk Vrieselaar; 141: SS/maxbelchenko; 143: SS/Maria Evseyeva; 145B: SS/ FeriDhaniHasri; 146: SS/Natalia Bostan; 147: SS/Travel Photography 2024; 150: SS/Gamzova Olga; 151: SS/phM2019; 152: SS/AndreaMonica; 153: SS/Volodymyr Plysiuk; 155T: SS/SrideeStudio; 155B: SS/Nick Alias; 156: SS/LiuSol; 159: SS/Kabar; 160L: SS/Orest lyzhechka; 161: SS/ Opulent Photos; 162L: SS/Michelle Lee Photography; 162R: SS/Nicolas Dorsaz; 164L: SS/Tibesty; 164R: A/ imagebroker.com; 165: G/Milan_Jovic; 167: SS/Olenaduygu; 168: SS/Madeleine Steinbach; 169: SS/teatian; 170: G/Justin Paget; 171: G/Helin Loik Tomson; 173: SS/Madeleine Steinbach; 176–177: A/ imagebroker.com; 178: G/miljko; 179: SS/AS CREATIVE STUDIO; 180: SS/ Azay photography; 181: SS/IgorCheri; 182: SS/New Africa; 183: SS/fizkes; 185L: SS/freedomnaruk; 186: SS/New Africa; 187B: SS/Kiran Nagare; 188: SS/ Madeleine Steinbach; 189: SS/Stock-Asso; 190: SS/OneWithNaturePhotos; 191: SS/mineoztan; 192: SS/Yuliia Kononenko; 193: SS/Diana Hlachova; 195B: SS/ AnnaNel; 196: SS/Sunart Media; 197: SS/Natalia Hanin; 199: Eugene_R (Photodeposit); 201: SS/Tavarius; 202T: SS/VisuthCreators; 203: SS/New Africa; 204–205: SS/Shyntartanya; 206: G/ Hill Street Studios; 208: SS/bubutu; 209: G/Trudie Davidson; 210T: SS/ diwali; 210B: SS/New Africa; 213TL: SS/Melica; 213TR: SS/Luca love photo; 214MT: SS/marineke thissen; 214TL: SS/asli_ti_tasik; 214BL: SS/Soleina; 215TM: SS/Chamomile_Olya; 215BR: SS/LianeM; 216BL: A/imagebroker. com; 217T: SS/Stepanych; 218B: SS/ OMfotovideocontent; 219: SS/Marketa Laschke; 221: SS/Elena Elisseeva; 224: SS/Elena_Gr; 225: G/Madeleine_ Steinbach; 226: SS/Madeleine Steinbach; 228–229: SS/JoannaTkaczuk; 247: SS/ JoannaTkaczuk.

Index

Bold text indicates the main page for that herb or ailment.